D1766825

# Dairy Herd Health

———————————

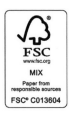

FSC
www.fsc.org
MIX
Paper from
responsible sources
FSC® C013604

# Dairy Herd Health

---

*Edited by*

## Martin Green

*University of Nottingham, UK*

*Co-edited by*

## Andrew Bradley, James Breen, Helen Higgins, Chris Hudson, Jon Huxley

*University of Nottingham, UK*

## Jonathan Statham

*Bishopton Veterinary Group, North Yorkshire, UK*

## Laura Green

*University of Warwick, UK*

*and*

## Alastair Hayton

*Synergy Farm Health, Dorset, UK*

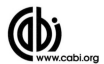

www.cabi.org

**CABI is a trading name of CAB International**

| | |
|---|---|
| CABI Head Office | CABI North American Office |
| Nosworthy Way | 38 Chauncy St |
| Wallingford | Suite 1002 |
| Oxfordshire OX10 8DE | Boston, MA 02111 |
| UK | USA |
| | |
| Tel: +44 (0)1491 832111 | Tel: +1 800 552 3083 (toll free) |
| Fax: +44 (0)1491 833508 | Tel: +1 617 395 4051 |
| Email: info@cabi.org | Email: cabi-nao@cabi.org |
| Web site: www.cabi.org | |

A catalogue record for this book is available from the British Library, London, UK.

**Library of Congress Cataloging-in-Publication Data**

Dairy herd health /edited by Martin Green, University of Nottingham, UK; co-edited by Andrew Bradley, James Breen, Helen Higgins, Chris Hudson, Jon Huxley, University of Nottingham, UK, Jonathan Statham, Bishopton Veterinary Group, North Yorkshire, UK, Laura Green, University of Warwick, UK, Alastair Hayton, Synergy Farm Health, Dorset, UK.
    p.  cm.
Includes bibliographical references and index.
    ISBN 978-1-84593-997-7 (hb : alk. paper)
    1. Dairy cattle—Health. I. Green, Martin (Martin J.)

    SF208.D37 2012
    636.2'142—dc23

                                        2012036472


ISBN-13:  978-1-84593-997-7


First printed 2012
Reprinted 2014


Commissioning editor: Sarah Hulbert
Editorial assistant: Chris Shire
Production editor: Simon Hill


Typeset by SPi, Pondicherry, India.
Printed and bound in the UK by CPI Group (UK) Ltd, Croydon, CR0 4YY.

# Contents

# Contributors

---

**Simon Archer** – svxsa@nottingham.ac.uk
**Herman Barkema** – barkema@ucalgary.ca
**Nick Bell** – njbell@rvc.ac.uk
**Andrew Biggs** – andrew.biggs@btinternet.com
**Andrew Bradley** – andrew.bradley@qmms.co.uk
**James Breen** – james.breen@qmms.co.uk
**Mark Burnell** – mark.bvet@btinternet.com
**Peter Down** – svxpd1@nottingham.ac.uk
**Laura Green** – laura.Green@warwick.ac.uk
**Martin Green** – martin.Green@nottingham.ac.uk
**Alastair Hayton** – alastair.hayton@tiscali.co.uk
**Helen Higgins** – Helen.Higgins@nottingham.ac.uk
**Chris Hudson** – chris.hudson@nottingham.ac.uk
**James Husband** – james@ebvc.eu
**Jon Huxley** – Jon.Huxley@nottingham.ac.uk
**Mike Kerby** – MKerby@delawarevets.co.uk
**Theo Lam** – T.Lam@gddeventer.com
**Aurélien Madouasse** – Aurelien.Madouasse@oniris-nantes.fr
**Sarah Potterton** – svzslp@exmail.nottingham.ac.uk
**Jon Reader** – jon.reader@synergyfarmhealth.com
**Jonathan Statham** – Jonandsianstatham@gmail.com
**Sian Statham** – Jonandsianstatham@gmail.com
**Gerdien van Schaik** – g.v.schaik@gddeventer.com
**Richard Vecqueray** – richard@ebvc.eu
**Wendela Wapenaar** – Wendela.Wapenaar@nottingham.ac.uk

# Preface

---

Currently we are in the second decade of the 21st century and there is considerable interest and concern over how we will feed the world's population in the next 40 years. Difficult choices will be made about which food products we consume and how we produce them. It appears that the demand for meat and dairy products will increase, especially as relatively underdeveloped countries become more affluent.

It is in this context that we consider how we should manage the health of farmed animals, in this case dairy cows. Philosophically we believe that if we want to consume animal products, it is ethically and morally right to care for them properly and also to respect and care for the environment in which they are kept. This means maintaining farm animals in good health; healthy dairy cows will thrive, be cost effective, are good for the environment and potentially will have 'a life worth living' – it should be a win – win situation.

Thus maintaining a healthy dairy herd is important. While care for the individual animal should never be overlooked, in this book we focus on disease prevention at the herd level. In doing this we do not wish to play down the importance of the individual animal, but we believe that in modern farming systems, preventing disease at the population level will ultimately be more rewarding. If we get this right, we can improve the lives of many animals and reduce the need for individual interventions.

Dairy cow herd health is a vast subject, and each chapter in this book could extend to a large volume in itself. The aim of the book is to cover the most important areas in sufficient detail to allow the inexperienced reader to initiate herd health programmes and to help the more experienced herd health practitioner to re-evaluate and hopefully improve their approach. We apologize if some areas receive less attention than others – inevitably we had to make difficult choices, and we based these choices on our own experiences as well as on the literature relating to herd health. On that note, we have tried, as far as the literature allows, to adopt an 'evidence-based' approach – we advocate approaches that are supported by the research literature. This inevitably means that in some areas and for some approaches uncertainty remains, and we have highlighted many of these areas. While frustrating, we would rather the reader is aware of this uncertainty rather than believe that received clinical wisdom is correct. This is particularly important in herd medicine, because interventions can be complex and expensive and implementing unproven changes can be disastrous.

Following an introductory chapter that describes the concepts of herd health (including what we mean by 'herd health'), the second chapter details how to facilitate changes on dairy farms. It is increasingly recognized that technical knowledge of dairy cow health is only one element of a successful herd health programme. The interactions between advisor and farm staff, the ability to communicate and modify day-to-day habits and the art of working as a team are all crucial when conducting herd health, and this area is discussed in detail in Chapter 2. The subsequent chapters on youngstock, reproduction, mastitis, lameness, infectious disease and nutrition provide details of how to run a herd health programme in these areas. We finish by discussing the important area of how dairy farming influences the environment in which we live.

We would like to emphasize that the book is not aimed at addressing the diagnosis and treatment of individual cows or describing the pathology of individual diseases. This has been undertaken in many texts and is simply not what we intend to cover. Instead our focus is on methods and indices for monitoring cow health, evaluating and interpreting herd patterns of disease and implementing herd-level control strategies. We feel these skills will be essential for the dairy cow specialist during the 21st century.

We hope you enjoy the book.
The Authors

# 1 Concepts in Dairy Herd Health

**Martin Green,**[1] **Laura Green,**[2] **Jon Huxley**[1] **Jonathan Statham**[3] **and Sian Statham**[3]
[1]*School of Veterinary Medicine and Science, University of Nottingham, Sutton Bonington, LE12 5RD, UK;* [2]*School of Life Sciences, The University of Warwick, Coventry, CV4 7AL, UK;* [3]*Bishopton Veterinary Group, Mill Farm, Studley Road, Ripon, HG4 2QR, UK*

---

## Context of Dairy Herd Health: Why Improve the Health of Farmed Livestock?

We believe that the veterinary surgeon and farm advisor should play a central role in preventing disease and maintaining the health of dairy cows within a framework of economic, environmentally sustainable farming. Maintaining excellent cow health and welfare are the primary and overarching aims of a herd health programme. Our aim in this book is to provide a route for a committed health professional to monitor and improve the health and welfare of dairy cows in their care, and we concentrate on the areas that we believe are most important in terms of enhancing health. In this chapter we consider the current context of livestock farming and then general concepts that underpin herd health programmes.

As long as humans continue to consume animal products, livestock will be farmed. While animal products are not essential to man's diet and survival, the taste, availability and nutritional value mean that livestock farming is likely to continue. Although many make a credible case for reducing the amount of meat and milk that we consume as a society (e.g. Tudge, 2004), there is little evidence, at a global level, that we intend to do so. The projections for animal produce required to meet the predicted increase in world population suggest that, globally, livestock farming will have to increase (Thornton, 2010). The ability of ruminants to utilize forages that are of little nutritional value to humans and to incorporate these into high-quality protein is a further reason for farming these species.

The next few decades hold many challenges for those working in the food animal sector and it is in this context that we describe the management of dairy cow herd health. The world population is forecast to grow by over two billion by the middle of the century (The Foresight Report, 2011), and increasing affluence in the huge population centres of China, India and Brazil is leading to increased global consumption of dairy and other animal products. Governments around the world are starting to prepare for the competition for food and water that may result. Agriculture will have to adapt rapidly to meet these demands and at the same time reduce its contribution to greenhouse gas emissions and climate change.

As the world continues to consume livestock products, as a global society we believe we are duty bound to look after the animals that we farm. Dairy cows are sentient beings and it is ethically right that we should care for them throughout their lives, to look after their health and welfare. It is clear that good health plays a pivotal role in good welfare, and indeed poor health is possibly the most common reason for compromise in the welfare of dairy cattle. Most of the diseases and conditions described throughout this book have an important impact on cow welfare, but we draw particular attention to lameness, mastitis, periparturient disease, dystocia and delayed treatment as being potentially large welfare issues. Whilst poor health cannot be completely avoided, it is the responsibility of the owner, herdsperson and herd health professional to work together to ensure that management policies are in place to prevent disease and maintain health at the highest possible levels: excellent management of herd health is strongly linked to (but not the only reason for) good cow welfare.

There are many other reasons to ensure the good health of our dairy cows. Healthy animals are more productive and cost effective for the keeper than unhealthy; this will be considered further in later chapters. Healthy animals are better for the environment and we discuss this in Chapter 9. Healthy animals are probably less likely to harbour zoonotic organisms and will require fewer treatments with antimicrobial agents; this has potential benefits for public health. Consequently, as well as a moral argument which dictates that farmed animals deserve good health, there are other clear benefits for us collectively, as a global society, to ensure that dairy cows are healthy.

Perhaps a more pertinent question is not whether but how much do we care about livestock health as a global community. How much, for example, is society willing or able to pay in order to consume livestock products from animals with guaranteed 'excellent' health and welfare? It is one thing to declare that we want our farmed animals to enjoy good health, another to pay for it. And this is not trivial – the infrastructure used in livestock farming needs regular renewal and significant investment to prevent difficulties arising with animal disease. Are consumers prepared to pay a sufficient sum for the products we consume to finance such investments?

In a market economy, farmers respond to circumstances that prevail; they have to be profitable to remain in business, and dairy farming is an excellent example of how farming has changed to meet the demand for a reasonably priced product. Over the last century we have witnessed a prolonged period of consolidation, intensification, mechanization and specialization in much of the global dairy industry. In highly developed dairy economies, the dairy cow lives in a herd with over 100 herd mates and often gives over 7000 l of milk per year. An average cow, giving 28 l of milk per day is working at over three times her maintenance requirement for energy; in a high-yielding cow giving 50 l, this figure is closer to five times maintenance. The consequences of breeding and managing for high yield are numerous and diverse, but as animal health professionals it is up to us to identify and mitigate the consequences for cow health.

We believe that the veterinary surgeon (veterinarian) and farm advisor should play a central role in preventing disease and maintaining the health of dairy cows within a context of economic, environmentally sustainable farming. Maintaining excellent cow health and welfare are the primary and overarching aims of a herd health programme. Our aim in this book is to provide a route for a committed health professional to monitor and improve the health and welfare of dairy cows in their care, and we concentrate on the areas that we believe are most important in terms of enhancing health. In the rest of this chapter we consider general concepts that underpin herd health programmes.

## What is Herd Health?

It is important to distinguish clearly the approach that we define here as 'herd health management' from that of solving a specific herd problem (a one-off herd investigation) or the production of a 'health plan' (essentially an annual review). Whilst both of these approaches have merit, and both can contribute to a full herd health programme, we would like to differentiate them from our definition.

We define 'herd health management' as a method to optimize health, welfare and production in a population of dairy cows through the systematic analysis of relevant data and through regular objective observations of the cows and their environment, such that informed, timely decisions are made to adjust and improve herd management over time. A critical aspect is the regularity of contact between the herd health advisor and the dairy farm personnel, with consistent, methodical evaluation of data to ensure that health and welfare are under continual scrutiny. Herd health management is therefore a continuous process, not just a short-term response to a herd problem. Regular interactions require a good working relationship between the herd health advisor and the farm staff, and this critical component is discussed further in Chapter 2.

Successful herd health management requires that the attending veterinary practitioner and farm advisor have sufficient knowledge of technical issues that relate to cow health and production and have a detailed knowledge of the participating dairy unit. Some of the skills required are beyond graduate level and continuing professional development, and specialization are essential. It should be recognized, however, that an attending veterinary surgeon may not be sufficiently expert in all necessary areas but instead may coordinate a team of experts to produce the best results. Examples of areas where additional expert advice may be sought include housing, nutrition, agronomy and genetics. Thus, understanding and coordinating the views of experts for the benefit of an individual unit is an important element of herd health management and success relies on a mutual trust between all parties involved in the decision-making process.

It is also important to recognize that herd health is not an exact science: there will always be some uncertainty in outcome when decisions are taken. Whilst this uncertainty can be hard to accept in practice, it is real and has to be dealt with. In fact, it is only by implementing the continuous approach of herd health, accepting that there may be need for iteration, and making further changes if initial ideas do not work as expected that uncertainty can be overcome. This is why the monitoring and re-evaluation phases associated with herd health are so crucial, because these allow a repeated evaluation of management

practices to occur, which facilitates a gradual improvement in cow health and welfare over time. Therefore, the implementation of a dairy herd health programme involves a continuous cycle of events aimed at the gradual improvement of cow health on a dairy unit, and this is illustrated in Fig. 1.1.

## Practical Implementation of Herd Health: Getting Started and Structuring the Health Visits

An outline of the approach to herd health management is shown in Fig. 1.1, and we describe below the most important aspects of implementing a herd health programme.

### Appreciating client aspirations

Starting a herd health programme on a dairy unit can be difficult. An understanding of what the client wants and needs is crucial, and several studies have illustrated that, unsurprisingly, farmers vary in values and motivations. When embarking on a herd health programme, an understanding of what drives the farmer and the context within which he/she sees their own farm is essential. Such an understanding often develops from a close working relationship between veterinary surgeon and client and will form the basis of how goals are set and what decisions are taken. The role of 'understanding, cajoling and convincing' in the provision of dairy herd health is probably as important as having the technical expertise in the specifics of bovine health, and this is discussed further in Chapter 2. Gaining an appreciation of the primary motivator – for example, money, family or professional pride – will help when it comes to making management choices relating to herd health. Whilst it is essential to establish farmer motivations in terms of their business, the importance of the relationship between farmer and herd health professional cannot be overstated and this is pivotal to what can be achieved in herd health. The trust and closeness of this relationship will develop over time, and it is this relationship that forms the foundation of a herd health programme.

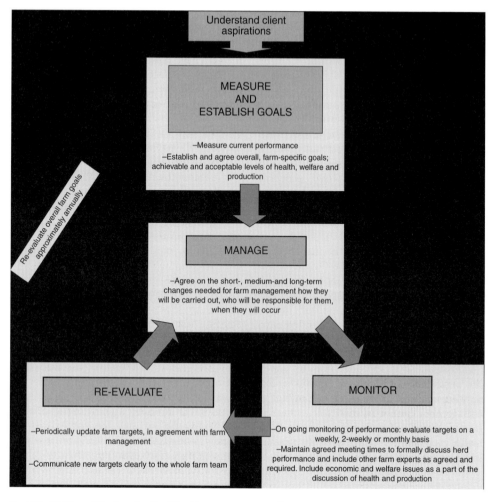

**Fig. 1.1.** Outline of the iterative herd health management cycle.

### Establishing farm-specific goals

Once a farmer's motivations and aspirations are established, a clear discussion about the type of herd health programme that is suitable and how this will meet the farm's needs should follow. General objectives when undertaking dairy herd health are to:

- meet the farmer's specific aims and ambitions. These should be discussed and transparent from the start;
- maximize the health and welfare of the cows within an ethical and environmentally sustainable framework;

- meet targets for production and profitability as well as quality and safety; and
- meet the expectations of the local and global marketplace and dairy consumers.

Therefore, a veterinary surgeon's approach to dairy herd health should not only meet the specific requirements of an individual but should also be placed in the context of the farmer's life beyond the farm gate. Before starting a herd health programme, it is necessary to make some initial calculations and decisions:

- Evaluate initial herd performance: in particular, measures of fertility, lameness, mastitis, culling rate (and reasons) and production.

- Estimate the costs and benefits (to farm finances, cow welfare and staff working conditions) that are possible if improvements can be made.
- Agree on an initial course of action for herd health by identifying and concentrating on specific areas that will produce the greatest improvements.
- Agree a structure for the health visits (which will depend on herd size, see below).
- Agree on the farm staff and any external experts that are to be involved in the health programme.
- Agree a time to review the initial phase of herd health, often after the first six or twelve months.

### Measuring performance and setting targets: the importance of data recording and analysis

The importance of high-quality data recording and analysis in successful herd health management cannot be overstated: it forms the cornerstone of a modern, accurate herd health programme. Using data to measure and monitor performance allows assessment of management strategies and highlights whether improvements can be made. Indeed, the monitoring of a parameter or performance index has to go further than just measure an overall level of performance; it should be recorded, analysed and fed back in such a way as to inform *where* improvements can be made. For example, it is not sufficiently useful to know simply that a herd's clinical mastitis incidence rate has increased if the increase is in one specific area (e.g. detail required is a high rate of clinical mastitis in first-parity cows, immediately after calving, in the summer months). This extra detail in analysis guides us to the specific area of management that requires attention; this is a principle of monitoring we emphasize in subsequent chapters.

For data monitoring to be effective as an early warning system in terms of cow health, it is important that the indicators measured are meaningful in the short term. Monthly or three-monthly rolling average incidence rates and prevalence estimates are often useful. A balance has to be struck between examining too many parameters and involving unnecessary complication or choosing too few and omitting those that are important. With computer systems in place, however, regular examination of a variety of indicators becomes trivial, and suggestions for health and production parameters to be used as regular indicators are provided throughout the book.

Thus routine data evaluations are central to herd health management, and the herd health professional has the opportunity to take responsibility for this and to direct the herd health process. The herd health advisor is in an excellent position to offer perspective on a unit's performance and to suggest interference levels for health and production indicators. One reason that there has been a general lack of monitoring of dairy cow health is because we have often not analysed and fed back information in a way that is sufficiently useful, and thus the motivation to maintain excellent records can deteriorate. In recent years improvements have been made to the on-farm monitoring of disease and there are a variety of computer software packages available to help this process. We do not intend to recommend the use of any one software package over another, but when considering computerized recording for herd health, the following features are important:

- easy data entry, including some inbuilt data quality checks;
- clear definitions of the events being recorded (with staff training to ensure consistency);
- easy access to individual cow records and also herd health and production indices;
- transparency and accuracy of methods used to calculate herd indices; and
- outputs that facilitate good reporting.

### Structure of the herd health visit

The frequency and duration of the visits required, and also the time allotted for data evaluation, depend to some extent on herd size. Smaller herds accumulate information more slowly and therefore patterns become apparent more gradually. However, in practice, all herds need a minimum monthly evaluation. Large herds (>500 cows) will generally require weekly attention and have the huge advantage that data patterns become clear relatively quickly, which enables more rapid decision making. The duration of a herd health visit will be dependent not only on herd size, but also on what is being included in the specific health programme. However, in general, a weekly or fortnightly visit will require 2–4 h to allow time for cow and environmental observations and discussion around the data. Periodically, extra time may be needed to attend milking or observe cow time budgets, for example. Therefore it is useful to budget for more time at longer intervals (~3-monthly) to carry out such assessments.

Whilst the exact nature of the herd visit will be based on the aims of the overall programme and will depend on the major areas to be tackled, the framework should include:

- time on farm for the regular assessment of cows and the environment, to include reproductive examinations if required;
- time for data analysis;
- time for less frequent but more time-consuming assessments (e.g. milking routine, mobility scoring);
- time for discussion sessions; and
- time for collaboration with other external advisors.

As an example, a 200-cow dairy herd with a fortnightly routine visit might require approximately:

- a two-weekly farm visit of 2–4 h;
- 1–2 h per month for data analysis; and
- an extra visit every 3 months, of approximately 4 h, to focus on a specific area.

### Charging for herd health

Before initiating a dairy herd health programme, it is essential that both provider and recipient have a clear view of the aims and structure of the programme. This includes agreement on the exact nature of services to be provided, time to be allocated and the fee structure for the services provided. Charging for herd health services can be approached in a number of ways, but for the service to be sustainable, a regular (generally monthly) fee for a pre-agreed amount of time is recommended. For the veterinary practice, linking herd health provision to a reduced price for medicines is a popular option with clients, and one that can be built into a practice business model to ensure minimal dependence on profit from medicine sales. Options for different herd health fee structures are shown in Box 1.1.

### Other Factors to Consider for Successful Implementation of a Herd Health Programme

#### Training of farm staff

For herd health programmes to be successful, the quality of stockmanship and animal husbandry is critical, and without adequate training this can be a limiting factor. The herd health professional can play a useful role in improving the working skills of farm staff through the provision of relevant training. Training courses should be designed to deliver more than improved technical proficiency; training should also foster team bonding within the staff, encourage ownership of particular areas of management/ husbandry and provide clarity over the importance of each person's role and why it is important in the context of the overall farm business. Examples of areas in which training can have a beneficial impact on herd health are milking procedures, foot trimming, mobility scoring, oestrus detection and body condition scoring. Communication and motivation are key issues when training farm staff, and we discuss this further in Chapter 2. It is also worth noting that the stockperson has an important influence on the interaction between cows and their environment, and this relationship certainly affects cow health. In general the calm,

**Box 1.1.** Charging options for providing a herd health programme.

| Method of charging | Comments |
| --- | --- |
| Fixed monthly fee | A fee is charged based on the pre-arranged time required for the herd per month and charged as a fixed monthly fee. The advantage of this method is that the time and fees are agreed and transparent. It is essential that the agreed time is adhered to, otherwise one of the parties involved can become disgruntled. A monthly fee could also include non-herd health activities – for example, a specified amount of time for emergency visits or surgical procedures. Once again, the main issue is transparency and agreement, such that all parties know and are happy with what is included in the health agreement. To this end, it is usually worth specifying the agreement in a written document. |
| A fee per litre of milk production | A monthly fee is charged according to the annual number of litres produced by the herd and split into 12 equal monthly payments. An advantage of this method is that payment is linked to production and thus both parties benefit from increased output. Also, for higher-yielding cows, herd health can become more time consuming and this is accounted for by linking payment to production. |
| A per-cow fee | A monthly fee is charged according to the number of cows in the herd. If herd size increases, the time needed for herd health will generally increase and therefore this is accounted for. However, the fee per cow may have to vary according to cow yield since herds with higher-yielding cows may need more time per cow than those with lower-yielding cows. |
| Charge for the time required for each visit | A fee is charged according to the time spent during each health visit. The advantage of this method is that all time is charged appropriately, but a major disadvantage is that there can be an inclination on the part of the farmer to minimize time at each visit in an attempt to reduce costs. This can lead to insufficient time being available to conduct an adequate programme. Additionally, the fee per month will vary depending on the level of input required over the month, making farm budgeting more difficult. |
| Other options | Other fee structure options are possible, including linking the fee to farm profit or specific health/production performance. This type of approach is often problematic because the actual implementation of health management is not under the direct control of the herd health advisor. As herd sizes increase and veterinary surgeons become an ever more integral part of the farm management team, such methods of remuneration may become more popular and may extend to a veterinary advisor being completely employed by a single large farm enterprise. |

quiet, authoritative handling of cows is important to minimize health problems and enhance cow well-being.

### The cow's environment

Whether at pasture or when housed, the environment of the dairy cow has a fundamental impact on health and welfare. The environment is a potential source and reservoir for a variety of pathogens, and monitoring the environment within which a dairy herd is kept is an important element of herd health. Rather than deal with this in separate sections on housing and pasture, we have chosen to describe important features of the cow's environment throughout the book, when discussing relevant health issues. However, many aspects of environmental management for dairy herds are not clear-cut and the herd health advisor will require thought and imagination to find solutions for individual herds. This again demonstrates the importance of the cyclical nature of herd health (Fig. 1.1) because it is vital to evaluate the impact of changes made to the environment and to iterate management decisions if necessary. As a general rule, it is often true that housed cows benefit from more space than has conventionally been considered appropriate: wide passageways, large loafing areas and substantial feed areas seem to allow cows to express normal behaviours (including oestrus) and in general improve well-being.

We recommend that cows are assessed and monitored within their environment rather than solely when separated for clinical examination. Environmental conditions will change over time as climatic conditions, management practices and cow numbers change. Regular assessment of environmental conditions during the health visit allows the practitioner to understand areas that could pose a risk to cow health and we describe details of important elements of environmental management in the following chapters.

### Relevance of genetics in herd health

The manifestation of ill health or poor performance depends on a balance between a cow's genetic makeup and the environment (including for infectious disease, the virulence of a pathogen), and therefore genetics has an important influence on herd health. Heritability is the term used to describe the variation between animals caused by genetic as opposed to environmental effects. In general, traits related to fertility, disease and survival have a relatively low heritability in dairy cows (generally <0.15) whereas production traits are higher (often 0.30–0.40). The heritability of specific dairy cow diseases is generally low, indicating that the environmental component is relatively important for these conditions and, whilst genetic selection has a role to play, altering environmental management to control these conditions is likely to be

more rewarding. Heritability estimates for major health and production characteristics are provided in Appendix 2.

It is also clear that animals of different genotypes are more or less suited to different management or production systems. For example, cows bred to produce large milk yields (such as the Holstein) are not well suited to systems based mainly on pasture grazing. The full implications of selecting specific genotypes for specific systems are not yet fully understood, but this is an area that should progress in the next few years.

In the last decade genetic research has accelerated and, with studies of the bovine genome, has provided greater insights into specific genetic regions, or combinations of regions, that are associated with different susceptibilities to disease. Whilst these have not yet come fully to fruition, it is likely that groups of genetic markers will be identified for specific dairy cow diseases, such as mastitis, lameness and displaced abomasum. However, genomic investigations are complex and progress may be slow if a vast number of genes (or gene combinations) have to be identified to determine an animal's susceptibility to a specific disease. There may be some genetic elements (e.g. those associated with general immune function (Heriazon *et al.*, 2011)) that are associated with overall disease resistance, and this is an area of current research. To further add to the complexity, it is also clear that the presence of genes may be insufficient for complete prediction of their effects, since gene function can be altered after birth environmental influences. Further research in this area (epigenetics) will be needed to clarify the hugely complex interactions between gene function and the environment.

Therefore, although genetics will not provide all or even most of the answers to poor health in dairy cows, it has a role to play in the medium- to long-term strategies in a herd health programme. A detailed description of bovine genetics is outside the scope of this book, and it is an area for which the herd health practitioner may wish to enrol external advice. Indeed, this is an excellent example of the need for a co-coordinating role in herd health for the herd health advisor – the need to balance the influences of genetics and management system/environment is critical. An outline of the terms and methods used in genetic evaluations of dairy cows are provided in Appendix 2.

## Conclusion

An efficacious herd health programme on a dairy unit delivers improved cow health and welfare, and also improved environmental sustainability. The herd health advisor has the opportunity to take a pivotal role in the application of dairy herd health management, and it is essential to have a full understanding of both the farmer and dairy unit for the best herd health service to be provided. Transparency, agreement and a close working relationship between herd health advisor and farmer forms the foundation of herd health provision.

In the following chapters we describe specific routes for delivering optimal herd health and, for convenience, we have separated herd health management into discrete topics. However, we emphasize that, in practice, these different areas are addressed simultaneously and a herd health programme represents a holistic approach that incorporates all elements. We have structured our descriptions of herd health management as follows.

Chapter 2: facilitating change; encouraging farmers to take action; barriers to herd improvement; Chapter 3: rearing youngstock and replacing cows; Chapter 4: Control of herd reproduction; Chapter 5: control of mastitis; Chapter 6: control of lameness; Chapter 7: control of infectious disease; Chapter 8: nutritional management in herd health; Chapter 9: dairy farming, food security and environmental issues; Appendices: sample sizes and disease prevalence estimates; genetic indices.

## References and Further Reading

Heriazon, A., Hamilton, K., Huffman, J., Wilkie, B.N., Sears, W. *et al.* (2011) Immunoglobulin isotypes of lactating Holstein cows classified as high, average, and low type-1 or -2 immune responders. *Veterinary Immunology and Immunopathology* 144, 259–269.

The Foresight Report (2011) *Foresight. The Future of Food and Farming.* Government Office for Science, London.

Thornton, P.K. (2010) Livestock production: recent trends, future prospects. *Philosophical Transactions of the Royal Society: B* 365, 2853–2867.

Tudge, C. (2004) *So Shall We Reap: What's Gone Wrong with the World's Food - and How to Fix it.* Penguin Books Ltd, London.

Zwald, N.R., Weigel, K.A., Chang, Y.M., Welper, R.D. and Clay, J.S. (2004) Genetic selection for health traits using producer-recorded data. II. Genetic correlations, disease probabilities, and relationships with existing traits. *Journal of Dairy Science* 87, 4295–4302.

# 2 Facilitating Change in Herd Health

**Helen Higgins, Martin Green and Aurélien Madouasse**

*School of Veterinary Medicine and Science, University of Nottingham, Sutton Bonington Campus, Leicestershire LE12 5RD, UK*

## Introduction

Real improvements in dairy herd health will occur only if farmers successfully implement management changes on their farms that prevent and control disease. This chapter focuses on ways in which veterinary surgeons can facilitate the necessary changes on the farm by encouraging and assisting farmers to take action, when required. We discuss many of the challenges involved and apply concepts sourced from human behavioural science and related disciplines, in order to promote understanding and provide solutions.

We close the chapter by noting that an essential (but by no means sufficient) requirement for facilitating improvements in dairy herd health is technical knowledge. Since up-to-date veterinary advice is provided in the following chapters of this book, we finish by providing a short overview of the principles of evidence-based veterinary medicine; developing these skills will enable practitioners to rapidly incorporate new research findings into their clinical decision-making processes in the future.

## Encouraging farmers to take action: context and challenges

Over time, humans have genetically selected for an extraordinary dairy cow – a creature that is capable of phenomenal production performances. However, when compared with her predecessors, today's dairy cow requires the application of substantial expertise and significantly higher levels of management, not only to ensure the attainment of full production potential but also in order that cow health and welfare are maintained. It is evident in the subsequent chapters of this book that the veterinary profession has tried to keep pace with this genetic change by expanding its understanding and knowledge of the modern cow, and is continuing to do so. Privileged to many years of university teaching, veterinary surgeons qualify today as highly knowledgeable professionals and as a result have bestowed upon them a considerable responsibility for the health and welfare of livestock.

However, it is farmers who must take care of the dairy cow; they must provide for a cow's daily needs and this gives farmers final control over every aspect of the dairy cow's life. As a result, it is farmers who are the keepers of dairy cow health and welfare and this confers a considerable responsibility to the farmer. Ultimately, the successful delivery of herd health hinges entirely on whether herd health advisors can encourage farmers to take action and execute decisions. Thus while veterinary surgeons need to acquire technical knowledge and then transfer that knowledge to farmers, this alone is far from sufficient. Crucial to all herd health programmes is the practitioner's ability to facilitate changes to human behaviour relating to stockmanship, management and investment. Unquestionably some of the most frustrating aspects of herd health can involve attempts to initiate and then sustain the necessary changes on the farm. Moreover, for practitioners to shoulder responsibility for the dairy cow in the absence of any real control can be an important source of stress, yet is seldom articulated as such; we know that if we fail to implement change then all is lost and we are accountable for the professional role that we have played.

Nevertheless, modifying the behaviour of our human colleagues is perhaps the most challenging task of all facing a herd health advisor. Generally speaking, we want farmers (who work long hours) to do more work every day, which may compromise their own physical health, with any positive health benefit going to a third party, the cow. Given this, perhaps it is not surprising that simple economic arguments regarding financial cost–benefit are rarely enough to alter human behaviour in the way that is required for effective herd health. Any estimated financial or other benefits to the farmer, however large, may swiftly dwindle to nothing when weighed against the two greatest factors of all, the farmer's own health and time. Moreover, the simple fact that *Homo sapiens* are highly evolved creatures should lead us to expect that altering behaviour is inevitably going to be significantly more complicated than that. Thus while further research to demonstrate the cost-effectiveness of different disease control strategies is certainly necessary and important, this alone will never be enough.

Given this context, a better understanding of what drives human behaviour will enable practitioners to help farmers initiate and sustain the necessary changes in management on the farm. We divide this subject into two areas. The next section provides an overview of what determines human behaviour and the subsequent section builds on this by describing, for each step along the path to implementing change, the most important points to consider and approaches to take in order to facilitate further action on the farm. Several theories from health behaviour science are relevant and are discussed.

## To Change Human Behaviour, We Need First to Understand It

The aim of behaviour research is to (i) understand why people perform a variety of behaviours and (ii) design interventions to alter behaviour. Over the last two decades there has been an explosion of research in the specific area of human health behaviour – and with good justification. In wealthy societies, human morbidity and mortality from the most common diseases are strongly associated with particular behaviour patterns (e.g. obesity and smoking) that are modifiable; people living in these societies can significantly improve their own health by consciously choosing to alter their own behaviour (e.g. by exercising or not smoking). There has also been a recent rapid surge in research aimed at designing intervention studies to modify people's behaviour in favour of a sustainable environment (e.g. recycling and reducing carbon emissions). Altering human behaviour for the benefit of our own health or for the long-term survival of the planet (and hence the survival of our own species) will subsequently be referred to as 'selfish' health behaviour.

In the context of herd health, practitioners require humans to alter their behaviour in circumstances where the health benefit is for another non-human species (the cow), with the possibility in many instances of a negative effect on their own health, referred to hereafter as 'self-less' health behaviour. Given this, some readers may already feel discouraged; the rocketing levels of obesity in some wealthy societies is just one example that illustrates the difficulties involved in changing selfish human behaviour, and some may feel that self-less health behaviour is likely to be even more difficult to influence. However, there is no evidence for this and it is likely to be a simplistic assumption. It should be kept in mind that farmers spend the entirety of their very long working days in the company of their animals, possibly spending substantially more time with the cows than with their own family and friends. As a result they often form exceptionally close bonds with their cows and may be prepared to make sacrifices for the good of their own animals that they wouldn't make in any other context. Indeed, the very fact that many farmers have work-induced health problems is testimony to this; the truth is they are already putting their own health second. That said, it is of course very important to appreciate that implementing management changes on the farm may have negative health implications for the farmer, a point we will return to later.

As has been alluded to, when trying to modify people's behaviour the exact type and context of the behaviour is important. It is unfortunate that, in stark contrast to selfish health behaviour, there has been virtually no research into self-less health behaviour per se. Yet nevertheless much of the research into selfish behaviour (which includes the fields of social science and psychology) is useful and is starting to be applied in a herd health context (Edwards-Jones, 2006; Rehman *et al.*, 2007; Heffernan *et al.*, 2008; Jansen *et al.*, 2009; Ellis-Iversen *et al.*, 2010). We describe below research that has originated from the field of selfish health behaviour which is relevant to herd health.

### Selfish human behaviour research applied to herd health

Many factors can affect whether an individual will carry out a given behaviour. These can be broadly categorized into those which are 'extrinsic' or 'intrinsic' to the person themself. Extrinsic factors include inconvenience or

unpleasantness of the task, finance (e.g. market price, milk contracts, penalties, incentives, taxes) and legislation. Intrinsic factors include demographic variables (e.g. age, gender, ethnicity), personality, social background (e.g. parental influences, culture) and cognitive factors (e.g. beliefs, attitudes, knowledge).

Whilst numerous theories and frameworks aimed at explaining human behaviour exist, with respect to the intrinsic factors, research into understanding how cognitive factors influence health behaviour has received by far the most attention, possibly because these factors are regarded as the most amenable to change. Several so-called 'social cognition models' have been devised that attempt to identify important cognitions and how they combine to influence behaviour. These theoretical models form the framework upon which formal interventions to alter behaviour are often based. For an in-depth review of the six main social cognition models we recommend Conner and Norman (2005), who describe their theoretical background and many behavioural intervention studies that have been designed based upon them, along with a critical appraisal and comparison of the models.

However, since there is considerable overlap in these models and none are perfect, we present and critique a conceptual framework, placed within a herd health context, that involves the integration of two commonly applied social cognition models along with extrinsic factors. For our purposes this provides a useful overview of the main determinants of human behaviour by illustrating in one diagram the main concepts involved (Fig. 2.1). A similar framework has also recently been applied in the context of implementing zoonotic control measures on cattle farms (Ellis-Iversen *et al.*, 2010). The coloured circles in Fig. 2.1 together comprise what is termed a 'stage model', which simply means that certain 'stages' of behavioural change are identified through which a farmer must progress in order to implement changes on the farm; success involves moving from left to right, failure from right to left. Different numbers and types of stages are discussed in a variety of models described in the literature, but in Fig. 2.1 just four simple stages are recognized (circles, from left to right): (i) no intention to perform the behaviour; (ii) intention to perform the behaviour (i.e. willingness to begin); (iii) implementation of control measures (i.e. taking action); and (iv) sustaining the control measures over time. Different factors (boxes) are shown as being capable of influencing whether an individual progresses through different stages. Which factors are most important at any point is largely unknown, but are likely to depend on both the specific behaviour change itself and the individual farmer.

In Fig. 2.1 the theory of planned behaviour (Ajzen, 1985) is summarized within the box at top left. This is one of the most popular and widely applied of the social cognition models, stating that a person's intention (willingness) to perform a given behaviour is influenced by three factors: (i) attitude (do I believe this is a good or bad thing to do?); (ii) social norms (do people important to me in this context, think it is a good or bad thing for me to do, and how much do I want to please these people?); and (iii) perceived behavioural control (do I believe I can do it?). The latter, also referred to as 'belief in self-efficacy', is closely related to self-confidence. For a given behaviour, establishing which of these factors is the most important can help to target interventions to change behaviour. For example, Ellis-Iversen *et al.* (2010) found that with respect to the farmers who currently had no intention to implement zoonosis control measures on their farms (half of the 43 farmers surveyed), attitudes were generally positive but a lack of belief in self-efficacy and/or unsupportive social norms was hindering their willingness to start; in other words,

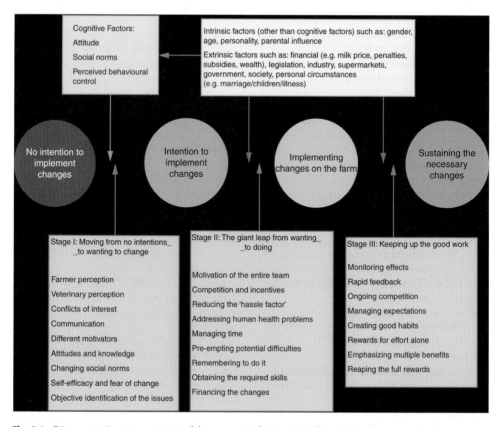

**Fig. 2.1.** Diagrammatic representation of the conceptual steps to implementing changes on the farm.

in general they believed it was a good thing to do, but they had no intention of doing anything about it, either because they believed that they themselves couldn't do anything about it or because they believed that they personally shouldn't have to do anything about it.

As illustrated in Fig. 2.1, the theory of planned behaviour is of primary importance in influencing a farmer's intention to implement changes. However, it is possible that in some instances the initial intention to change may pervade, to some degree at least throughout the stages, such that the greater the intention to implement change is, the more likely it is that action will, in fact, be taken and subsequently sustained. It is also worth noting that the theory of planned behaviour is particularly important because it is the first step on the pathway to implementing change and it contains intrinsic cognitive factors (beliefs, attitudes, social norms) that are amenable to change. The other intrinsic factors (e.g. gender, personality) and the extrinsic factors (e.g. finance, legislation, government) are shown in the box at top right (Fig. 2.1). While these other factors are known to affect behaviour, with the exception of finance, their influence is discussed here only with respect to their effects on the cognitive factors, since otherwise they are largely beyond the direct influence of practitioners.

While Fig. 2.1 gives a useful overview, it merely describes planned behaviour – in other words, actions that we consciously deliberate over, also called 'cold cognition'. To deliberate consciously over an issue is to take the time to weigh in our minds the advantages and disadvantages in order to reach a decision over how we want to behave in the future. However, the vast majority of our behaviour comprises spontaneous actions that simply happen in response to the daily events around us without any real time for deliberation, so-called 'hot cognition'. We do not consciously deliberate getting up, having breakfast, getting to work, working, having lunch and so forth, not least because we

simply do not have the time to deliberate consciously about it all – rather, it just happens. This distinction is very important. We may have the very highest of intentions (have made a conscious decision at some point in the past) to change our behaviour but it is a giant leap from intention to action Fig, 2.1). We need to find a way to force our new intentions into our daily routines (which, by necessity, will always be dominated by spontaneous actions) in order to reach the stage of implemented control; and then to continue our efforts through time in order to achieve the stage of sustained control, even when adverse events might hinder us and our initial enthusiasm and good intentions have waned. A major criticism of all social cognition models has been that they do not explicitly consider hot cognition or describe the optimal ways to implement change in a practical way (Rutter and Quine, 2002). The three lower boxes (Fig. 2.1) summarize the most important issues to consider and ways to help a farmer to progress along the conceptual steps and to implement changes successfully on the farm. These are discussed in full in the following section.

## How to Assist Farmers in Implementing Changes on the Farm

While many of the ideas in this section have arisen from reflections upon experiences in practice in combination with general research, some have also been sourced from techniques used in social marketing that aim to promote sustainable behaviour amongst communities. For further reading on this approach, we recommend McKenzie-Mohr and Smith (2000), which includes examples of its highly successful application in a variety of selfish health behaviour contexts. These methods are also now starting to be applied to good effect by animal welfare scientists in self-less health behaviour contexts – for example, Whay and Main (2009) describe practical ways to promote changes on the farm, including the use of extrinsic factors and a specific project that involved the application of social marketing techniques to improve lameness in dairy cattle.

We have structured this section by first describing the importance of correctly identifying where a farmer has reached on the pathway to change, and then for the transition between each stage, what we consider are the most important issues to be aware of and ways to facilitate action. The latter are summarized in the lower boxes in Fig. 2.1. However, Fig. 2.1 is presented for conceptual purposes only and overlap clearly exists – for example, 'communication' is obviously applicable at all stages of this process.

It is important to emphasize at this point that greatest success will ensue when (i) we can gain a true perspective and understand all the issues involved and (ii) we use several different methods in combination to facilitate change sensibly. It is also useful to distinguish between two different types of change, because the issues faced in trying to implement their action can be different: 'one-time' behaviours (such as laying a new cow track) and 'repetitive' behaviours (such as the regular sweeping of stones off the cow track). Typically in a herd health context, one-time behaviours can involve moderate to large capital investment.

### First identify which stage the farmer has reached

To avoid considerable frustration from the outset, it is *very* important to appreciate that different motivators may be more or less relevant depending on which stage the farmer has currently reached (in Fig. 2.1). The work of Ellis-Iversen *et al.* (2010) suggests that with respect to implementing zoonotic control measures on cattle farms, financial incentives are not important motivators for farmers who currently have no intention to implement control measures (far left circle, Fig. 2.1). Instead they identified their private veterinary surgeon as their preferred motivator; extrinsic factors such as money did not appear relevant as long as intrinsic cognitive factors such as belief in self-efficacy and social responsibility were lacking. This

makes perfect sense. If we have reached the point where we want to make changes (Fig. 2.1), then how much they will cost to implement may be important in our conscious deliberations over whether we will actually go ahead and do it. However, if we are in fact still at the 'no intention to implement control measures' stage, such that we don't want to (or see a need to) change, then money could well be largely irrelevant as a means of motivation for us. The true importance of this is illustrated by a very common mistake that practitioners make when trying to implement changes on farm, which we describe in the following paragraph.

A common approach to alerting a farmer that he has a disease problem is to tell him about it. For example, we might mobility score the milking cows and report the percentage that are lame. We often then contextualize this for the farmer, by telling him how this compares to other farms and may point out some of the disadvantages of lameness, especially in terms of reduced milk yield, cost of treatment, culling and so forth. Thereafter we often make two (rather large) assumptions. First, because we have told the farmer that there is a problem and have discussed it on numerous occasions, we assume that he must now know that there is a problem; and in particular we assume that he must now perceive the entire problem in exactly the same way that we do. Secondly, we assume that the farmer must want to do something about it, probably because we ourselves really want to do something about it. In other words, we automatically assume that he has now reached the second from left circle in Fig. 2.1. As a result of our two previous assumptions, we now make a third assumption. That is, we assume that because the farmer knows there is a problem and wants to do something about it, we assume that money will play a part in his decision over whether he decides to do anything about it. This third assumption would be sensible, but only if the other two assumptions are correct. As a result of all these assumptions, we proceed carefully to calculate the economic cost–benefits of making the necessary changes and report these to the farmer. When this fails to motivate them to take any action we feel dismayed and conclude that he is acting irrationally. Indeed, why this doesn't motivate the farmer can seem incomprehensible to us. And then it is tempting to make a fourth (final and fatal) assumption. Since the economic arguments are so overwhelming in favour of change we assume that if this will not motivate him, then nothing will.

Probably the single biggest mistake we could make when trying to implement changes on the farm is to believe at the outset that the farmer has reached the stage of wanting to change (second from left circle, Fig. 2.1). Quite often, and for a variety of reasons that will become clear, the farmer may have no genuine desire of his own to change at all and is still waiting, oblivious to our angst, at the far left circle in Fig. 2.1. Identifying what stage a farmer is currently at is the first thing to establish because, as we will see, the most important issues to consider, obstacles to overcome and motivating factors differ depending on where you are on the pathway to change. Economic motivation is a good example of this, because financing the change can be utterly irrelevant if you have no intentions to change to start with, and this is not irrational behaviour at all. If in any doubt, the safest thing to assume is that the farmer currently has no intention to change (Fig, 2.1) and work from there.

### Stage I: moving from no intentions ... to wanting to change

An important point raised in the previous section was that we often make two assumptions: (i) just because we have discussed a disease problem with a farmer, he must know that there is a problem and (ii) if he knows that he has a problem he must want to do something about it. Understanding why the first assumption may not be true and what can be done about it requires us to truly appreciate the importance of *perception* and *communication*. With respect to the second assumption, the theory of planned behaviour can help our understanding and

ways to facilitate intention to change. We will tackle each in turn.

#### *Perceiving a problem*

FARMER PERCEPTION: SEEING A PROBLEM THROUGH DIFFERENT EYES. Given (just for now) that the herd health advisor has an accurate perception of the disease situation, as mentioned, we often assume that by merely telling a farmer about the disease, and what can be done about it, that he must perceive the entire problem exactly as we do. This may not be true. Farmers may never have had the time, or been encouraged, to really think through, step by step in their own minds, what having this scale of disease really means for them. We should also be conscious of the fact that it is not good news that we are bringing to their attention and unsurprisingly, therefore, some farmers may not want to hear it. If this is the case and all we ever do is 'tell' farmers about a problem, this approach may have no impact at all, irrespective of how often we repeat the message.

In many cases we may need to help the farmer to explore the disease situation fully in his own mind and think about all the implications. To achieve this requires us to ask the farmer a series of open questions and listen to his answers, in order to stimulate thought around the subject, rather than just 'telling' him what the answers are. For example in the case of lameness, it might involve asking him to describe what effect he thinks lameness has on the cows themselves, to estimate what the time costs of treating the lame cows are for the herdsman, in what ways does he think that lame cows cost money, what costs are involved, and so forth. This is a different approach. In essence it is forcing the farmer to think in depth about what having a disease really means to him personally, and for his animals and the business. Clearly it is much quicker just to tell the farmer all the negative outcomes, and for some farmers this may enable them to perceive the problem in its entirety. But for others, doing this will never give them the opportunity to appreciate the disease problem properly at all, let alone consider what they might want to do about it. This approach is also useful for farmers who don't want to hear they have a problem, because if we ask them questions such that they have to describe the disease situation and its consequences to us, it is much more difficult for them to withhold the issue from their mind.

There is inevitable overlap here with the next section, because creating intentions to change (far left circle, Fig. 2.1) and considering some of the issues involved in actually making a start (second from left circle) in reality may often be thought about simultaneously and hence discussed in one conversation. An important barrier to change at this point concerns the fact that, in the context of the life of a farmer (with its long and antisocial hours), the apparent impossibility of doing anything different can be very real. It can be a fundamental step forward to help farmers to start to think through for themselves some possible ways to implement changes and, in particular, to help them realize that there may be scope to make existing tasks more efficient and/or to make some jobs more convenient than they might immediately perceive them to be. This can involve walking round the farm with the farmer and asking him open questions about parts of the infrastructure/management that are likely to be a risk factor for the disease, then to encourage him to think through what action might be taken, and especially to help him to consider fully all the advantages as well as the disadvantages of making changes. Overall therefore, it can be a much more supportive approach to invite farmers to describe a disease using open questions, listen to their answers and then constructively start to help them to consider possible solutions and the pros and cons of making changes. Whay and Main (2009) describe this concept as 'ownership of change', which is 'about creating opportunities for farmers to explore and realise their problem and allowing them to be a partner in generating ideas for possible solutions'. They also note that for some farmers, true perception and acceptance of the problem may only occur when they have been able to discuss the problem with other farmers.

Ultimately, it is vitally important that, as a starting point to implementing change, the farmer does perceive and understand the true extent of a problem for himself. For some diseases, part of the difficulty with obtaining an accurate perception of the disease problem relates to difficulties with measurement per se. For example with respect to lameness, the subjectivity involved in scoring cows for lameness and ensuing disagreements over what constitutes a lame cow can hamper efforts to establish an accurate perception of the disease situation. Clearly a giant leap forward in tackling a disease is a cheap, quick, objective and indisputable way to measure it; disease measuring and monitoring is discussed in depth in subsequent chapters.

There is certainly evidence that perception of a problem by farmers is an important issue and dairy cow lameness provides a good example of this. A recent UK research study by Leach *et al.* (2010b) found that out of 222 dairy farms, 90% of farmers did not perceive lameness to be a major problem on their farm, although the mean lameness prevalence scored by the researchers was 36% (range 0–79%).

VETERINARY PRACTITIONERS' PERCEPTIONS CAN FADE.     It is also important for the implementation of change that veterinary practitioners perceive the true extent of a problem. However, the high prevalence of some diseases on of commercial dairy farms can make it much more difficult to maintain an objective perspective over the course of a professional career; if unacceptable levels of disease exist on many farms, disease can become tolerated as time progresses just because it is encountered everywhere and consequently our perception of the problem fades. This happens, not through any fault of our own per se, but just because we are human. Eventually only farms with extreme levels of disease may be noticed at all. We should be aware of this and consciously strive to maintain our perspective over time. Moreover, if the same practitioner is the sole provider of veterinary services to a dairy farm for prolonged periods of time, perception can be lost altogether; some diseases can insidiously increase and reach very high levels without recognition by either the practitioner or farmer, both of whom can become habituated to the problem. Needless to say, if diseases are properly recorded and regularly reviewed (the cornerstone of implementing herd health programmes effectively) this should not happen. One way to address this is for different practitioners to visit the same farm on a regular basis. Besides reducing the chance of diseases creeping up on us unnoticed, it allows the injection of new ideas and variety and challenge for practitioners themselves.

PERCEPTION, FRIENDSHIP AND CONFLICTS OF INTEREST. From a practitioner's point of view, for some diseases, helping farmers' to truly perceive their own problem can be particularly challenging for those farmers who are unwilling or unable to perceive it at all. The reason resides within one of the most enjoyable aspects of being a bovine practitioner, namely the relationship that we frequently forge with dairy farmers; regular farm visits over many years often result in strong, sometimes lifelong, friendships being formed. It is for this reason that practitioners are repeatedly identified as 'farmers' most trusted advisors', and the implicit assumption that usually follows is that our friendship with farmers can only be of benefit to the cow (DEFRA, 2004). Yet this is not necessarily true: it depends on both the disease and the situation. It is useful here to draw a distinction (albeit simplistic) between two types of endemic disease: 'emotive diseases' (e.g. lameness) and 'non-emotive' diseases (e.g. bovine viral diarrhoea, BVD); while the latter can undoubtedly cause devastation, it is often considered of lesser welfare importance for the adult cow. Emotive diseases carry with them the capacity to quickly upset, offend and even anger people. Discussing emotive diseases with farmers can put us in a difficult position; no one wishes to upset or anger their friends, especially not when their own business depends on that friendship. In an idealistic, purely disease-tackling world, we would be completely free of any potential concern of causing angst to a close friend (or losing a client) and be able instead to concentrate on the disease in question – to talk absolutely frankly and objectively with farmers about the problem. Instead, in reality, conflicts of interest inevitably exist for practitioners and this can cloud our objectivity, place us in difficult situations and hamper our abilities to implement changes on farm. Often we may have to tread a very fine line: to balance our need to improve herd health and make changes on farm, with a real risk of causing grievance, potentially to the point where a long-standing relationship is broken. Clearly the latter could be counterproductive since any subsequent veterinary involvement may not be trusted. It is worth noting that this can be an important source of stress for veterinary surgeons that is infrequently acknowledged.

### Communication

Effective communication between farmers and practitioners is essential in order to initiate and sustain behavioural change. 'Communication' as a subject can be divided into two quite distinct but equally important areas: 'verbal' and 'non-verbal'. We specifically discuss 'non-verbal' communication later, under the section heading 'perceived behaviour control'.

As previously discussed, removing important obstacles to change requires practitioners to employ verbal communication skills that encompass facilitation, active listening, asking open questions and so forth. It is accepted that the communication style has to be appropriate for the personality of the farmer involved. However, communicating effectively to a very diverse range of people such as farmers is difficult and it is perhaps not surprising that recent research has suggested that practitioners would benefit from improving their communication skills (Jansen, 2010). In particular, this research reported that of the 17 tape-recorded veterinarian–farmer conversations held during regular herd health visits in the Netherlands, none of them included active listening; furthermore, 'less than 1% of all spoken sentences were devoted to eliciting farmers' opinions and values'. Another study involved interviews with 24 Dutch dairy farmers who were nominated by their own veterinary surgeons as difficult to approach with regard to advice on udder health management (Jansen *et al.*, 2010). The researchers concluded that 'there are ample opportunities to reach hard-to-reach farmers provided the communication strategies are tailored to their specific needs'. They divided these farmers into four categories based on 'their trust in external information sources and their orientation towards the outside world', namely: proactivists, do-it-yourselfers, wait-and-see-ers and reclusive traditionalists. They commented that 'there is especially much to be gained in communication with do-it-yourselfers and wait-and-see-ers, but this demands a more proactive role on the part of veterinarians'.

In addition, since a key element of herd health management is the regular monitoring and analysis of farm data, decisions over how best to communicate the results of our analyses are crucial ones; the content, format and presentation of this information will vary enormously between farmers depending on their individual requirements and preferences. Such decisions need careful thought and should be reviewed over time, including asking for feedback from farmers as to the usefulness of the methods employed. It is also sensible to identify and report on the disease and performance outcome measures to which the farmer attaches greatest importance, regardless of whether they happen to be routinely encountered in veterinary textbooks.

There are many different ways that practitioners can improve their communication and presentation skills: numerous books, training courses and on-line resources exist. In addition, two recent articles reviewing the role and importance of communication skills in a herd health context have been published (Atkinson, 2010a; Lam *et al.*, 2011), the former highlighting the importance of agenda setting. It is vital at the outset to ascertain fully (in detail) the goals and ambitions of the farmer, which may often be very different to our own; it will avoid the considerable frustration that arises from attempting to motivate a farmer to make changes that are targeted in the context of achieving an end result about which he is simply not primarily concerned. However, whilst it is crucial to respect and understand the wishes of the farmer, practitioners may feel that diseases that carry the greatest welfare implications should be given the highest priority. If there appears to be a disparity between the current goals of the farmer and our own ambitions, then we should link our goals to that of the farmers, and often this is not difficult. For example, if the farmer's primary objective is to improve his fertility but our greatest aim is to improve nutrition or lameness, then since these diseases are inexorably linked, if we place the changes that will improve nutrition and lameness *very firmly* in the context of the poor fertility, then more action is likely to be taken. Establishing the farmer's agenda is closely related to understanding farmer motivations, and these are considered further in the section below.

### Different things motivate different people

Many different 'types' of dairy farmer exist; examples include family-owned farms passed down through generations, tenant farmers, business entrepreneurs and hobby farmers. It goes almost without saying that because farmers can have *very* different reasons for farming they can also have very different goals and ambitions. As a result, how factors that can motivate behavioural change are perceived and valued by farmers can be markedly different, and this will influence their agenda setting and also their decisions over whether to implement changes on the farm (Edwards-Jones, 2006; Kristensen and Jakobsen, 2011). This adds a layer of complexity because not only do different motivating factors (e.g. money, time, reputation, lifestyle choice, environmental concerns, social pressure, empathy) become more or less relevant depending on where on the pathway to change you are (Fig. 2.1), they can also vary enormously depending on the individual person, their reasons for farming and the benefits they are seeking from it. This latter issue is so important that several research studies have sought formally to develop behavioural typologies for farmers that broadly reflect differences in motivating factors, and two such examples are provided in Table 2.1. There are two points to note with regard to these classifications. First, the labels and key features merely reflect the most dominant themes for this broad type of farmer and there is overlap between categories: for example, it is clearly not only the 'custodians' who care about the environment (Pike, 2008). Second, they are predominantly derived from questions concerning long-term values and aspirations (Garforth and Rehman, 2006).

In view of the differences between farmers, it is important for herd health advisors to clarify the short-, medium- and long-term goals of an individual farmer, along with what will currently motivate them to take action. It is dangerous to make simplistic assumptions based on first impressions, particularly as these can easily become fixated in our minds. If we don't take the trouble to identify what factors motivate a farmer, we have a tendency to assume that they will be motivated by the same factors that would motivate ourselves, and this can easily be wrong.

**Table 2.1.** Summary of two research projects into farmer behavioural typologies.

| Farmer behavioural types ascribed by the University of Reading, following a postal survey of 3000 farmers in England[a] | Farmer behavioural types ascribed by DEFRA, following a review of current literature[b] |
| --- | --- |
| *Family orientation* <br> • stewardship; <br> • sensitive to environmental issues; <br> • working alongside family members; <br> • handing over viable business to next generation; and <br> • content with prevailing institutional and communal outlook on farming. | *Custodians* <br> • protecting the countryside; <br> • guardians of farming heritage; <br> • feeling proud to look after and enhance the farm; and <br> • less of a business focus. |
| *Business/entrepreneur* <br> • farming is a business; <br> • expansion/investment; <br> • debt avoidance; <br> • staff management; and <br> • dissatisfaction with public view of farming. | *Lifestyle choice* <br> • farming unlikely to be main source of income; <br> • preference for traditional farming methods; <br> • less focused on making money; and <br> • aspiring to farm well. |
| *Enthusiast/hobbyist* <br> • alternative / additional source of income; <br> • diversification; <br> • quality of life away from farm; <br> • leisure; and <br> • job satisfaction. | *Pragmatists* <br> • love of farming; <br> • making enough money to break even; <br> • enjoying life; and <br> • prepared to diversify to keep farm running. |
| *Lifestyler* <br> • quality of life; <br> • quality of leisure; <br> • investment for the future; <br> • concern about uncertainty in farming; and <br> • feeling let down by government and society. | *Modern family business* <br> • future focused: farming is passed down through generations; <br> • growth; <br> • profit/business orientated; and <br> • efficiency. |
| *Independent small farmer* <br> • family standard of life; <br> • job satisfaction; <br> • independence; and <br> • indifference to profit. | *Challenged enterprises* <br> • struggling: perhaps inherited through obligation; <br> • falling out of love with farming; <br> • feeling isolated & unsupported; and <br> • anxious about survival of the farm. |

[a] Garforth and Rehman (2006); [b] Pike (2008).

It is also worth appreciating that, in general, pride can be a very strong motivator for farmers; in the context of lameness, a recent study reported that 'pride in a healthy herd' was the motivator most commonly given high importance in a survey of 222 UK dairy farmers (Leach *et al.*, 2010a). Hence fostering a sense of pride is likely to be useful. As an example, in the right situations, it may be appropriate to highlight just how important the role of the farmer is – that it is farmers who are the guardians of the dairy cow's health and welfare. Our encouragement and praise also count for a great deal – everyone likes to hear when they are doing well.

### Perceiving a problem does not necessarily equate to wanting to change

Assuming that both the farmer and the practitioner accurately perceive the true scale and extent of the disease problem, it is still entirely possible that the farmer may have no intention of doing anything about it. As described in the previous section, the theory of planned behaviour is a social cognition model that defines three main constructs (attitudes, social norms and perceived behavioural control) that combine to determine a person's intentions to take action. Identifying which of these factors are the biggest obstacles to initiating change, and taking measures to address them, can help to generate a genuine desire to change and facilitate transition to the next stage – intention to implement changes. We consider each in turn.

### Changing attitudes: knowledge is vital, but is never enough

Attitudes are formed from a person's beliefs about the chance of a behaviour resulting in a possible outcome and how much value they attach to that outcome. Practitioners can influence a farmer's attitude by providing information (based on scientific evidence when available) about the outcomes of disease control measures and the probability of success. However, while it is essential to provide such information, there is substantial

evidence to suggest that providing knowledge alone is usually not sufficient to initiate changes in behaviour (McKenzie-Mohr and Smith, 2000). To maximize the likelihood that knowledge will be influential in facilitating change we must take great care to ensure we provide information to farmers in a format that best matches their current information needs (and this should be discussed and clarified with each client), and that it is presented in a manner that appeals to them in order to initiate change (see earlier sections 'Communication' and 'Different things motivate different people').

### Changing social norms: follow the leader?

Our behaviour is heavily influenced by the behaviour of others; in particular, people are considerably more likely to want to change their behaviour if they know that everyone else already has, or that they are different to what is 'socially acceptable'. Some farmers may simply not be aware that implementing certain types of disease control measures is 'normal expected' activity, especially since farmers may work exclusively on their own farms. 'Social norms' is a term that embraces this concept but also refers more generally to the social pressure a farmer feels under to perform the behaviour in question. Practitioners can change social norms by, for example, organizing facilitated farmers' meetings or through pre-existing farmers' groups. However, not all farmers will attend such meetings (or join such groups), and these are the very farmers for whom social norms may be lacking. Actively identifying these farmers and raising their awareness of the actions of other farmers is important.

Moreover, within a farming community there may be a 'ringleader' farmer, often an entrepreneurial character, someone who is usually the first to try out new ideas on their farm – and hence the other farmers keenly observe the behaviour of this individual, in a 'wait and see what he does' philosophy. Clearly the 'ringleader', if he exists, is a key farmer to persuade to implement changes since others may well follow. Obtaining permission from such a key player to write up the changes they have made and the benefits generated (for example in a practice newsletter) is a good way to disseminate information about their behaviour to others.

Formal 'benchmarking' can also have a role to play in influencing social norms; gathering data from similar farms and reporting this information to farmers allows them to identify how their farm compares to others. However, care should be exercised because this has the potential to hinder change in some instances. For example, it may demotivate the 'best' farmers out of the group, who may become complacent, even though the 'best' farms may still have unacceptable levels of disease. Furthermore, for the 'worst' farms in the group, it may evoke a sense of futility, with farmers demoralized by the gulf between themselves and others, and this may exacerbate their perceptions of the difficulties of making changes. Of course benchmarking a farm against itself over time, with realistically achievable (but movable) goalposts avoids these potential issues, and indeed is essential to implementing herd health programmes effectively.

*Perceived behaviour control: trying and failing can perpetuate the inertia to change*

Failed attempts to implement change on farms in the past can make it much more difficult for farmers and advisors to even begin to want to change anything in the future. Mostly this occurs through the cognitive variable, perceived behaviour control ('Do I believe I can do it?'). As mentioned in an earlier section, perceived behaviour control is related to self-confidence and is of fundamental importance; if we don't believe we can actually change something then we won't have any intention to try.

The more practitioners have failed in the past to initiate changes on the farm, the more we believe the farmer will never change, especially if we have put a considerable amount of effort into the process of trying to help him, albeit perhaps not always in the most optimal way. As a result of this we have a natural tendency to start prejudging what we think farmers will and won't want to do, or the money we think they will

be prepared to invest, and then tailor our advice to them accordingly; from our point of view, not only does this save wasting time but we also feel that it will save any embarrassment by making suggestions that we believe are outwith the capabilities, ambitions or finances of this farmer. This is often done semi-consciously, but is obviously unhelpful. To do so is to presume not only that we know precisely a farmer's values, along with their financial situation and personal circumstances, but also how they will then balance everything to reach a final decision. It also assumes that, in the past, the reason they didn't initiate change was entirely due to their own failings, not ours to help them, and therefore they are immune to making certain changes in the future. It is essential to make farmers fully aware of all the options, no matter how unlikely we believe they may be to follow some of the potential routes we offer. Whilst some of the time our initial presumptions about the options chosen may prove correct (and this may very quickly become apparent in our discussions), if we take this approach we will also be surprised on other occasions by their decisions. Most importantly, to explain all the options to a farmer is to convey a very positive attitude regarding their abilities because to do so is to send a clear message that we believe that they are capable of achieving any of the options – a major boost to self-confidence. Moreover, it may also inspire farmers to work towards new goals that hitherto had simply not existed for them. If we label a farm as recalcitrant to change then it certainly will be, even though (i) a farmer's circumstances, financial situation, values and goals can change considerably over time and (ii) despite considerable effort, it may still be us who have failed to recognize how best to help them change.

In a similar vein, we should make conscious efforts not to bias overtly the opinions of newly employed practitioners when they first join the veterinary practice, but allow them, at the very least, to take their first step onto every farm with an open mind; this is particularly true for new graduates who may be more impressionable, but who also, by virtue of their lack of experience, often possess an abundance of enthusiasm and new ideas and hence can often be in a good position to initiate change. It is also worth noting that it is often our most junior colleagues who deal predominantly with farms that have, so far, progressed least along the pathway to change and hence are at greatest risk of going out of business. In contrast, there is a natural tendency for our most experienced practitioners to gravitate towards the farmers who are quickest to implement change, and who are also in many respects, and for a variety of reasons, more appealing to work with. However such an allocation of veterinary expertise is not optimal for two reasons. First, if our most experienced and highly qualified practitioners concentrate their efforts on the most proactive farms, this could serve to increase the variation in the health of dairy herds. Secondly, a report into veterinary career choices describes the 'spiral of disillusionment' encountered by veterinary surgeons within their first five years of working with farm animals (Robinson *et al.*, 2004). If, early in their careers, veterinary surgeons have active and tangible involvement in the herd health management being conducted on the most progressive farms, it may help to curb the migration of some promising young practitioners towards other disciplines within just a few years of qualification.

Another way that a farmer's perceived behavioural control may be inadvertently negatively affected is via our non-verbal messages which are as, if not more, important than merely the words we say. The spoken word evolved long after *Homo sapiens* had cohabited in social groups and spoken language developed over and above non-linguistic communication. Research in this field began in earnest in the 1960s, but improved technology has recently brought new advances, with wearable electronic devices capable of recording subtle body movements and other non-verbal messages (Pentland, 2010). A research experiment in 2005 fitted telesales operators with electronic devices that measured variations in the tone and pitch of their spoken words but not the specific words uttered (Buchanan, 2009). The researchers devised an algorithm capable of predicting whether a call would result in a sale from just the first few seconds of data; successful operators it transpired, spoke little and listened more. When they did speak, their voices varied markedly in amplitude and pitch, implying interest and responsiveness to the caller. This understanding is now used commercially by call centres to recruit and train operators, and such measures alone have been estimated to improve sales success by 20%. With respect to herd health, how often do we (subconsciously) convey our own lack of faith in the farmer's ability to successfully implement change via our non-verbal communications? To do so is to reinforce the farmer's own negative belief of self-efficacy and make the situation worse. In order to convince the farmer it is crucial that we truly believe ourselves that he can and will do it. Thus, to implement change on farms, practitioners must be in the correct frame of mind themselves before they attempt to communicate anything at all.

We can of course take active steps to increase a farmer's belief in self-efficacy, and many practitioners do. Examples of this include arranging open visits to demonstration farms; by observing other farmers carrying out the behaviour successfully, farmers are more likely to believe they can actually do it themselves. In this respect, probably most useful is for a farmer to visit another farm with infrastructure similar to his own, so that it is easier to believe that carrying out the changes would be feasible at home. Building up a practice catalogue that can be taken on to farms is useful; this could contain photographs of farmers at various stages of implementing changes (such as laying a new cow track) along with contact details (obtained with permission) of farmers who are willing to discuss the changes they have made with others (Whay and Main, 2009). This catalogue could also contain details of local suppliers of materials and equipment that would need to be ordered to complete the task, or other advisors whose advice may need to be sought (such as building experts or nutritionists).

It is also essential to recognize that many people are simply afraid of change itself. An important element of herd health can be, when possible, to 'trial' the new task for a period of time, which may be a less daunting initial step. This allows time for a farmer to hone and get used to a new management procedure. For some disease control measures it also provides an opportunity to measure its immediate efficacy in terms of cow health; however, for some diseases a rapidly observable benefit will not be seen and this is discussed further in Stage III. It is obviously vital that this pilot step is successful if the management change is to become permanent. As described by Atkinson (2010b), it is the veterinary practitioner's role to support the farmer through this 'experimentation phase' and to actively help him to overcome any teething problems, but it is also, as he comments, 'very often a weak area in the farmer–vet relationship'. In short, we must follow changes through.

In summary, the more frustrated we get when farmers don't make changes, the more we believe they never will. Not only may we loudly voice this message non-verbally but we may also prejudge what farmers will or won't do and hence fail to give them all the options. Beyond that we may bias other colleagues with our negativity, thereby quashing any chance of change in the future. It is important to understand objectively the issues involved because if we don't, over time, we ourselves may become a major part of the inertia to change. An admittedly difficult, but nevertheless key clinical skill for all practitioners to acquire is the ability to maintain an open mind over the course of their career. It is unfortunate, but unlike most other clinical skills, our abilities to facilitate changes on the farm do not necessarily improve with clinical experience.

### Summary: intention to change

We have described what we consider to be the main issues involved (and approaches to take) in order to help a farmer move from having 'no intention to change' to having a genuine desire to initiate changes on the farm. Our natural tendency is often to assume that because farmers are humans like us, they must see the world through our eyes – to think, value, understand, decide, perceive and be driven as we are; yet it is more likely that another person will perceive the situation in a completely different way to us. An important point is that simply telling farmers about their disease situation and what they can do about it will often have no impact at all. Asking farmers to describe their disease problem to us, listening to their answers and helping them to overcome their natural fear of change by assisting them to consider the pros and cons of making changes is a considerably more supportive approach to take and should prove to be more helpful in many cases.

If having tried various activities, good intentions are still lacking, it is worth considering whether any of the extrinsic factors (upper right box, Fig. 2.1) are currently playing a major role in a farmer's ability to move forward; for example, changes in personal circumstances or fortunes can have a major impact on whether a farmer intends to make changes.

### Stage II: the giant leap from wanting … to doing

For farmers who have good intentions to change (i.e. they have now reached the second from left circle, Fig. 2.1), as mentioned previously it is still a giant leap from wanting to change to taking action. However, there are several ways to facilitate this, as summarized in the lower boxes, Fig. 2.1. These are discussed below.

### It's a team effort

Almost invariably, implementing a proactive approach to herd health involves a concerted effort and often requires new actions to be taken by all members of the farm 'team', which includes: relief milkers, tractor drivers, part-time staff, tanker drivers and other regular visitors to the farm. Vital to a successful outcome is that everyone involved understands what needs to change and why; the entire team must feel included and 'buy into' the new ethos. Not only can one person's negative actions undo the hard work of many, but a genuine team effort brings multiple benefits such as encouraging and reminding one another to make changes. Practitioners need to work hard to foster a working relationship with all team members. This involves regularly seeking out those people who are not routinely encountered to ensure that they are being kept informed and that their contributions are acknowledged and appreciated. Such an approach also demonstrates a close interest in (and hence great care for) the farm's success. Always relying on messages to be passed on will often prove ineffective. It is also wise to apply our previous comments about uncovering what motivates individual farmers to the entire farm team. It is highly likely that different team members will be motivated by very different things. The shrewd practitioner will take the trouble to identify what motivates each person and use this knowledge to good effect.

*Putting our competitive nature to good use: everyone likes to win*

Many people have a competitive streak and can be motivated by the desire to outperform a rival. Turning routine farm tasks into an ongoing competition amongst farm workers, with a weekly or monthly prize to be won, has several advantages. Drawing on this natural human trait can go some way to making the job more fun. It also means that people are more likely to remember to do it and to carry it out to the best of their abilities. The 'prize' does not need to be expensive; the fact is that people just like winning a prize, whatever it is. One of the reasons for this is that the prize is (and must be) awarded in front of as many other people as possible; hence it is a reward from our peers for what may be perceived to be a mundane job, done well. For many people this type of public recognition of their work can be just as, if not more, important to them than their salary. It makes people feel valued and helps them to truly appreciate the importance of the work they do; a task may be considered unimportant and therefore not worth doing

well, simply because it is perceived as being mundane. This perception is reinforced over time if nobody ever says 'well done'. For example, the person milking the cows should be regularly acknowledged for protecting cow health and welfare and for the work they do being extremely important and far from ordinary.

*The all-important 'hassle factor'*

For repetitive behaviours, making the task as easy to perform as possible is absolutely vital to success. It may sound obvious, but jobs that are easy to do, get done. Anything that can make the task more convenient to complete is worthwhile and the effects can be very dramatic. The provision of recycling bins by councils to individual households is a good example where making a task more convenient has had a substantial impact on human behaviour (Perrin and Barton, 2001). The importance of identifying specific measures that need to be put in place to facilitate the specific behaviour required cannot be overemphasized. It is useful to put yourself in the farmer's shoes and imagine that it is you who has to perform the task you want doing on the farm every day: What would make it easier for you to do? For example, lame cows are not going to get treated promptly if the crush does not have a proper winch or blocks for the front feet, if hoof knives cannot be kept sharp, if there is no light to see by in winter or if the crush is positioned with the exit against a brick wall so that cows do not readily want to enter into it. Indeed, any of these factors, by themselves, are easily enough to stop the task getting done at all. The hassle factor *must* be addressed (McKenzie-Mohr and Smith, 2000). A useful tool to help here is the practice catalogue (discussed in Stage I, under 'Perceived behaviour control'), which contains useful information the farmer will need in order to get started.

*Human health problems: a weighty yet silent obstacle to change*

Many farmers suffer from bad backs or other chronic injuries that they have sustained whilst working on the farm, and some of the changes required may aggravate these conditions. This may be a major factor that is given a great deal of weight in the farmer's decision over whether a management change will be implemented. However, farmers may find it difficult to admit that they are not physically capable of performing a task or they may be unwilling to concede that it will cause themselves pain and suffering. This may be an important obstacle to change that is unlikely ever to be voiced by farmers themselves, and there is also a need to handle the issue with sensitivity. Persuading farmers to seek medical attention to alleviate their own health problems or diplomatically helping to delegate more physically demanding tasks to others may be an important step towards implementing change.

### Make time, because there isn't any

Many of the changes we would like to see implemented will take more of the farmer's time, their most precious resource. Whilst it is obviously important to make the new changes as quick as possible to implement, it will often also be necessary to seriously consider ways to create more time if we really want the new changes to get done. Making time may often involve being inventive and helping the farmer to find ways to save time on other tasks by making these quicker and more efficient. Hence implementing changes can involve an in-depth appraisal of each person's working day and how people work together, in order to identify where and how time savings can be made, along with identifying any measures that could be taken to speed up existing tasks. Clearly it is important that the new changes do not result in existing tasks being carried out suboptimally (such as rushing cows in for milking), but honing time management skills can be rewarding and greatly increase the chances of action being taken.

There is also no escaping the fact that buying time may be necessary in some instances, but of course this doesn't have to involve a full-time member of staff: creatively sourcing a few hours of extra help per week can be enough to greatly facilitate change.

### Make 'tried but not feasible' work

A seemingly powerful argument presented by a farmer when faced with the proposition of implementing a change is to say he has already tried it, but it wasn't feasible. It can be, and often is, the end of any action because many practitioners simply accept this as an insurmountable obstacle to change and at this point abandon all their efforts to help the farmer. In this respect there are two points worth considering. First, we should be very encouraged because the farmer has reached the point of having high enough intentions that he has been prepared to try something. Secondly, we can now ask the farmer to describe in full how he found carrying out the task and what exactly the problems are, and as a result we have more precise information about the inconvenience of the task. The latter point means that, far from forsaking the cause, we can work creatively to find ways to make the task more feasible.

In general however, wherever possible, foreseeing, honestly discussing and pre-empting potential obstacles that may be encountered by the farmer when he actually begins to take action are advisable. For example, if we know that an important management change to control mastitis is obviously going to prolong milking time, it is shrewd to acknowledge and discuss ways to overcome this right at the very start.

### Remembering

Perhaps an obvious yet easily overlooked fact is that, being only human, spontaneous unplanned behaviour dominates our days and we often simply forget to do what we said we would do. This is more likely to happen if the task is to be carried out by one person, or at unsociable hours when there is nobody around to remind us. In this case triggers to help us remember are important; they need to portray a very clear and simple message and be placed as close in space and time to the point where the behaviour occurs (McKenzie-Mohr and Smith, 2000): for example, a waterproof/laminated card attached with baler twine to the crush to remind farmers to record every case of lameness they treat. Such a trigger could also be informative, with pictures of the most common causes of lameness to aid recognition of lesions. Other examples include: a notice by the switch to the milking machine to remind the herdsman to start filling up the footbath, or a notice hanging down in the middle of the parlour reminding milkers to post-dip the cows. It may sound too simple to work, but triggers have been proved in many intervention studies to increase the behaviour of interest and they are of trivial cost (Austin *et al.*, 1993). In short, it would be foolish not to use them. However, we should issue a word of warning. Triggers should not be used as just another way of telling people what to do; this will not work very effectively because people will simply ignore them. Triggers are for reminding people who want to do something to do it. Hence they must only be used when all the people who must carry out the task actually want (or at the very least have agreed) to do it. If a notice suddenly appears in the parlour and the relief milker knows nothing about it, it will often be counterproductive!

### *Obtaining the required skills: do no harm*

However much farmers may want to implement changes on the farm, they cannot achieve anything unless they have the necessary skills to perform the task properly. Fortunately many practitioners already provide training for farmers in a variety of formats, including on-farm practical workshops. However, some farmers may believe they have the necessary skills to implement a change, when in fact they don't. We need to make absolutely sure when we make recommendations that the people who will be carrying out the tasks have the skills to do them; and in particular that they do not suddenly start doing more harm than good. An example of this is the farmer who begins using an internal teat sealant at drying off following the good advice of his veterinary surgeon, but iatrogenic infections then occur due to unhygienic administration. Several dead cows later it is fair to assume that this

excellent management practice is never again going to be used on this farm. If there is even the slightest doubt and/or the consequences of getting it wrong are severe, it is vital that we ensure that farmers have the skills they need. However, we should also be conscious of the fact that some farmers may be reluctant to admit that they do not have the necessary skills; they may be embarrassed to ask how it should be done, or simply feel uncomfortable being taught by someone younger than themselves. In this respect, veterinary students can be useful; to explain and demonstrate a skill to a student in the presence of a farmer overcomes these possible issues.

### *Financing the changes*

In the medium to long term, practitioners can and must influence how much a farm is able to reinvest, but at any given moment in time, being unable to make a capital investment can obviously be a fundamental obstacle to change on farm. However, as mentioned, it is important that we do not prejudge what a farmer can or cannot afford to do and we should not make recommendations simply based on what we perceive is affordable to the farmer. If a capital investment is required and agreed to but currently cannot be made, it should be worked towards as a medium- to long-term goal, and alternative interim measures of disease control implemented.

### Stage III: keeping up the good work

Clearly, one of the most important factors to influence a farmer's decision to continue implementing a control measure is whether any benefits are (i) rapidly observable and (ii) directly attributable to the action taken. Wherever possible, measuring outcomes and providing as rapid feedback as possible is vital to sustaining action, and the subsequent chapters of this book provide detailed advice on monitoring the outcomes of herd health programmes. As an example, monthly zinc sulphate turbidity (ZST) tests are a cheap easy way to feed back changes in colostrum management, helping farmers to quantify the results of their efforts. Indeed some farmers incorporate such monthly outcome measures into their ongoing competitions to motivate staff. Similarly, if farmers can be persuaded to start recording disease incidences, they are much more likely to continue to do so if they see immediately that the information they record is being used to good effect.

Diseases for which benefits are not quickly demonstrable are usually more challenging to control. In this respect it is important to manage farmer expectations, such that a realistic appreciation about the observable effects of their endeavours is known from the outset; avoiding disappointment is crucial. For these diseases, creating good habits becomes more important. Eventually, if a particular action is repeated often enough, it slips out of our conscious thoughts and becomes embedded into our subconscious, automatic actions. Clearly, the major advantage of forming a good habit is that not only does the chance of forgetting to do the task virtually vanish, but since all conscious perception of it disappears, so too does the inconvenience that was once associated with it; no longer do we have to 'internally battle' with ourselves over whether to carry out the task. It is difficult to know how long a particular behaviour has to be performed in order for it to become a habit, but for diseases such as Johne's, striving to create good habits on farms is clearly a must. It is worth remembering that it is just as easy to reward people for their efforts as it is for an actual disease reduction.

Wherever possible it also makes good sense to stress the multiple benefits that may originate from a single management change and, in particular, to link controlling diseases that may have less obvious or immediate benefits to other areas where benefits are clear. Farmers are often more likely to take action if the rewards are greater. For example, raising the standard of hygiene in the dry cow accommodation not only reduces the risk of spread of Johne's disease, but also the risk of intra-mammary infections and digital dermatitis; the latter may also mean that cows are more likely to have a reference heat observed post-calving. We are often guilty of thinking in terms of either 'mastitis' or 'lameness' or 'fertility' or 'Johne's', when instead we need to be thinking holistically, an essential element of herd health. Eventually, over time, farmers will reap the full rewards of preventing and controlling disease in numerous ways and hence ultimately, successfully implemented herd health programmes will perpetuate themselves.

## A final reflection

To gain an overall perspective it is useful to take a final look back at Fig. 2.1. There are many steps that need to be taken, and many potential hurdles to overcome, in order to sustain the necessary changes on the farm. Needless to say, veterinary surgeons will not always be successful at encouraging farmers to take action. If our own previous attempts to implement change have failed, it is natural to become disheartened, conclude that change is impossible and simply resort to delivering reactive/emergency healthcare. Hopefully, however, the preceding pages have provided some alternative insight that may spark ideas and inspiration for facilitating change in the future. Perhaps it is not that farms will not change, but rather that we have not yet managed to identify correctly where on the pathway to change they currently are, what will motivate them and what barriers prevent actions from being taken. It may be that the first person who needs to change is ourselves; to set aside our previously formed opinions and start completely afresh, equipped with a better understanding of human behaviour and how to initiate and sustain changes on the farm.

## Facilitating Change: Evidence-based Veterinary Medicine

While understanding ways to facilitate change on the farm is essential to making improvements in dairy herd health, a prerequisite to success is the quality of the technical advice provided and this is discussed in detail in subsequent chapters. However, not only is it impossible for a single textbook to answer all clinical questions, but research is continually being published. The ongoing identification and incorporation of best available evidence in the context of the individual requirements of a particular farmer can be achieved under a framework generally termed 'evidence-based medicine'. We briefly outline below the key principles of evidence-based veterinary medicine.

## What is evidence-based medicine?

It is widely accepted that it is important to base clinical decisions, including those on herd health, on valid evidence and this is the endeavour of evidence-based veterinary medicine. Its most cited definition was given by Sackett *et al.* (1996), which was made in the context of human health: 'Evidence-based medicine is the conscientious, explicit, and judicious use of current best evidence in making decisions about the care of individual patients'. The practice of evidence-based medicine means integrating individual clinical expertise with the best available external clinical evidence from systematic research. Evidence-based medicine now forms an integral part of human medicine and it has even entered popular culture through the excellent book *Bad Science* (Goldacre, 2009). Although its importance is growing in veterinary medicine (Cockcroft and Holmes, 2003), further progress in large-scale implementation is still needed.

The application of evidence-based medicine can be divided into five steps (Sackett, 1997):

1. Ask an answerable question.
2. Find the best evidence to answer it.
3. Critically appraise the evidence.
4. Integrate the appraised evidence with our clinical expertise and apply it to the situation at hand.
5. Evaluate performance.

A clear and concise description of these five steps can be found in Heneghan and Badenoch (2006). We now consider each of these areas in terms of herd health.

*Ask answerable questions*

The aim is to lay out clearly the question we need to answer in order to find the evidence that is relevant to the problem at hand. A well-formed question should contain four distinct parts summarized by the acronym PICO, which stands for:

P = patient/population and problem: What are the characteristics of the herd and problem we wish to address?

I = intervention: What is the main intervention(s) available to address the problem?

C = comparison: What are the alternative (comparator) interventions?

O = outcome: What outcome are we interested in? Mortality, morbidity, production, finances, welfare …?

An example of such a question could be:

In a high-yielding Holstein dairy herd, housed all year around, with an elevated incidence of clinical mastitis (P), does the use of an iodine-based pre-dip solution during milking preparation (I) result in a cost-effective reduction in clinical mastitis (O) compared with the milking routine without the pre-dip being used (C)?

*Find the evidence*

Having formulated a question, what are the sources of evidence available to answer it and how do we use them? Some general principles have been laid out regarding the validity of different types of evidence and have led to the concept of 'hierarchy of evidence', often represented as a pyramid (see Fig. 2.2 below). At the base of this pyramid is relatively weak evidence that should carry little weight and at the top are meta-analyses and systematic reviews that pool the evidence from similar and well-designed studies and are thus considered strong evidence. Large studies are deemed superior to small studies. Systematic reviews are starting to appear in cattle veterinary medicine, and it is likely that their number will increase in future.

Identifying relevant scientific articles is important, and this can be done by querying

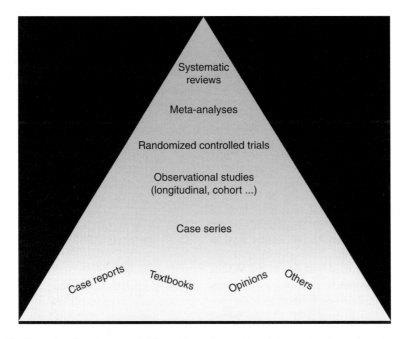

**Fig. 2.2.** The hierarchy of evidence available: evidence is considered strongest at the peak and weakest at the base.

one of the databases available on the Internet such as:

- Pubmed (http://www.ncbi.nlm.nih.gov/pubmed/);
- Scopus (http://www.scopus.com/);
- Scirus (http://www.scirus.com/); or
- Google Scholar (http://scholar.google.co.uk/).

Although there is a large overlap between these, the databases do not always contain the same information.

### Appraise the evidence

Much has been written about how to appraise evidence. Since we cannot begin to cover this vast subject within the space available, we direct the reader to two easy-to-read references, Crombie (2008) and Greenhalgh (2010). Crombie provides six areas that form a structure to assess the quality of a study:

- Is it of interest?
- Why was it done?
- How was it done?
- What has it found?
- What are the implications?
- What else is of interest?

Evaluating a study under these headings helps to determine whether the study is relevant to our own question, whether the research design was suitable, whether the conclusions drawn were appropriate and what the implications are to the clinical question of interest.

A useful way to learn how to appraise the evidence is by doing it! A regular journal club, where a paper is chosen and discussed around a table, provides an excellent means of developing these skills while obtaining detailed knowledge in specific areas of research.

### Facilitating change: integrating evidence into practice

A component of evidence-based medicine is that best evidence does get translated into clinical practice. However, as discussed in detail throughout the earlier sections of this chapter, identifying evidence for the best way to prevent or treat a condition does not necessarily lead to its use in practice. Thus, understanding the elements of human behaviour and barriers to change described previously is vital to the successful performance of evidence-based medicine.

*Evaluate performance*

The final component of evidence-based medicine lies in the evaluation of our decisions, once they are made. This should occur automatically as a part of true herd health management (Fig. 1.1, and further described in subsequent chapters). Indeed dairy herd health, carried out in this way, is essentially based on, and is an extension of, the principles of evidence-based medicine; we try to incorporate the best evidence when making a decision and then continually evaluate the outcome to judge its success.

## Conclusion: Facilitating Changes in Dairy Herd Health

In this chapter we have emphasized that facilitating the necessary changes on dairy farms is essential for successful herd health management in practice. Making changes is challenging and the speed with which farmers adopt change is very variable. Not unsurprisingly, farmers may not take action for a host of complex reasons that depend on both the individual farmer and where they are on the pathway to implementing change. Veterinary surgeons must address these issues if they are to make a real difference in practice. However, this requires consideration of subjects and challenges that go beyond the conventional technical advice associated with dairy herd health. We believe that much can be gained by understanding and applying concepts developed in the human behavioural sciences and related disciplines, but this may require practitioners to equip themselves with new skills. It is unquestionably a major challenge when undertaking dairy herd health to identify both the best clinical evidence and the best methods to facilitate changes for a particular farm situation. However, this is a challenge we must meet if we are successfully to play our part in making sustained improvements to the health and welfare of dairy cows, and lay claim to the countless rewards that follow. If farmers are not making the necessary changes then it is important to identify objectively why this is, for if we fail to do so then we ourselves can become part of the inertia to change. Farmers who are slowest to embrace change are the most likely to go out of business, and it is these farmers who are in greatest need of herd health advisors who have a good understanding of human behavioural science and the skills to apply it successfully in practice.

## References and Further Reading

Ajzen, I. (1985) From intentions to actions: A theory of planned behaviour. In: Kuhl, J. and Beckman, J. (eds) *Action-control: From Cognition to Behaviour*. Springer, Heidelberg, Germany, pp. 11–39.

Atkinson, O. (2010a) Communication in farm animal practice 1. Farmer–vet relationships. *In Practice* 32, 114–117.

Atkinson, O. (2010b) Communication in farm animal practice 2. Effecting change. *In Practice* 32, 163–165.

Austin, J., Hatfield, D.B., Grindle, A.C. and Bailey, J.S. (1993) Increasing recycling in office environments – the effects of specific, informative cues. *Journal of Applied Behaviour Analysis* 26, 247–253.

Buchanan, M. (2009) Behavioural Science: Secret signals. *Nature* 457, 528–530.

Cockcroft, P.D. and Holmes, M.A. (2003) *Handbook of Evidence-based Veterinary Medicine*. Wiley-Blackwell Publishing, Ltd, Oxford, UK.

Conner, M. and Norman, P. (eds) (2005) *Predicting Health Behaviour: Research and Practice with Social Cognition Models*. Open University Press, Milton Keynes, UK.

Crombie, I.K. (2008) *Pocket Guide to Critical Appraisal*. BMJ Publishing Group, London.

DEFRA (2004) *Animal Health and Welfare Strategy for Great Britain*. DEFRA, http://archive.defra.gov.uk/foodfarm/policy/animalhealth/index.htm (last accessed 16 September 2011).

Edwards-Jones, G. (2006) Modelling farmers decision-making: concepts, progress and challenges. *Animal Science* 82, 783–790.

Ellis-Iversen, J., Cook, A.J.C., Watson, E., Nielen, M., Larkin, L., Wooldridge, M. *et al.* (2010) Perceptions, circumstances and motivators that influence implementation of zoonotic control programs on cattle farms. *Preventive Veterinary Medicine* 93, 276–285.

Garforth, C. and Rehman, T. (2006) Final Report, DEFRA Project EPES 0405/17: Research to understand and model the behaviour and motivations of farmers in responding to policy changes (England). University of Reading, http://archive.defra.gov.uk/ evidence/economics/foodfarm/reports/documents/Behaviour.pdf (last accessed 17 September 2011).

Goldacre, B. (2009) *Bad Science*. Harper Perennial, London.

Greenhalgh, T. (2010) *How to Read a Paper: The Basics of Evidence-based Medicine*. John Wiley Publications, Ltd, Oxford, UK.

Heffernan, C., Nielsen, L. and Thomson, K.G. (2008) An exploration of the drivers to bio-security collective action among a sample of UK cattle and sheep farmers. *Preventive Veterinary Medicine* 87, 358–372.

Heneghan, C. and Badenoch, D. (2006) *Evidence-based Medicine Toolkit*. Wiley-Blackwell Publishing, Ltd, Oxford, UK.

Jansen, J. (2010) Mastitis and the farmer mindset: Towards effective communication strategies to improve udder health management on Dutch dairy farms. PhD thesis, Wageningen University, The Netherlands.

Jansen, J., van den Borne, B.H.P., Renes, R.J., van Schaik, G., Lam, T.J.G.M. and Leeuwis, C. (2009) Explaining mastitis incidence in Dutch dairy farming: The influence of farmers' attitudes and behaviour. *Preventive Veterinary Medicine* 92, 210–223.

Jansen, J., Steuten, C.D.M., Renes, R.J., Aarts, N. and Lam, T.J.G.M. (2010) Debunking the myth of the hard-to-reach farmer: Effective communication on udder health. *Journal of Dairy Science* 93, 1296–1306.

Kristensen, E. and Jakobsen, E.B. (2011) Challenging the myth of the irrational dairy farmer; understanding decision-making related to herd health. *New Zealand Veterinary Journal* 59, 1–7.

Lam, T.J.G.M., Jansen, J., van den Borne, B.H.P., Renes, R.J. and Hogeveen, H. (2011) What veterinarians need to know about communication to optimise their role as advisors on udder health in dairy herds. *New Zealand Veterinary Journal* 59, 8–15.

Leach, K.A., Whay, H.R., Maggs, C.M., Barker, Z.E., Paul, E.S., Bell, A.K. *et al.* (2010a) Working towards a reduction in cattle lameness: 2. Understanding dairy farmers' motivations. *Research in Veterinary Science* 89, 318–323.

Leach, K.A., Whay, H.R., Maggs, C.M., Barker, Z.E., Paul, E.S., Bell, A.K. *et al.* (2010b) Working towards a reduction in cattle lameness: 1. Understanding barriers to lameness control on dairy farms. *Research in Veterinary Science* 89, 311–317.

McKenzie-Mohr, D. and Smith, W. (2000) *Fostering Sustainable Behaviour: An Introduction to Community-based Social Marketing*. New Society Publishers, Gabriola Island, Canada.

Pentland, A. (2010) *Honest Signals: How They Shape Our World*. Bradford Books, MIT Press, Cambridge, Mass.

Perrin, D. and Barton, J. (2001) Issues associated with transforming household attitudes and opinions into materials recovery: a review of two kerbside recycling schemes. *Resources, Conservation and Recycling* 33, 61–74.

Pike, T. (2008) Understanding behaviours in a farming context: Bringing theoretical and applied evidence together from across Defra and highlighting policy relevance and implications for future research. DEFRA Discussion Paper, http://archive.defra.gov.uk/evidence/statistics/foodfarm/enviro/observatory/research/documents/ACEO%20Behaviours%20Discussion%20Paper%20(new%20links).pdf (last accessed 15 September 2011).

Rehman, T., McKemey, K., Yates, C.M., Cooke, R.J., Garforth, C.J., Tranter, R.B. *et al.* (2007) Identifying and understanding factors influencing the uptake of new technologies on dairy farms in SW England using the theory of reasoned action. *Agricultural Systems* 94, 281–293.

Robinson, D., Hooker, H. and Barber, L. (2004) Institute for Employment Studies Report, Vet Career Choices, http://www.scotland.gov.uk/Publications/2005/01/20499/49568 (last accessed 15 September 2011).

Rutter, D. and Quine, L. (eds) (2002) *Changing Health Behaviour: Intervention and Research with Social Cognition Models*. Open University Press, Milton Keynes, UK.

Sackett, D.L. (1997) Evidence-based medicine. *Seminars in Perinatology* 21, 3–5.

Sackett, D.L., Rosenberg, W.M.C., Gray, J.A.M., Haynes, R.B. and Richardson, W.S. (1996) Evidence-based medicine: what it is and what it isn't. *British Medical Journal* 312, 71–72.

Whay, H.R. and Main, D.C.J. (2009) Improving animal welfare: Practical approaches for achieving change. In: Grandin, T. (ed.), *Improving Animal Welfare: A Practical Approach*. CABI Publishing, Wallingford, UK.

# 3 Restoring the Dairy Herd: Rearing Youngstock and Replacing Cows

James Breen,[1,2,3] Peter Down,[1,] Mike Kerby[4] and Andrew Bradley[1,2]
[1]School of Veterinary Medicine and Science, University of Nottingham, Sutton Bonington Campus, Leicestershire LE12 5RD, UK; [2]QMMS Ltd, Cedar Barn, Easton Hill, Easton, Wells, BA5 IDU, UK; [3]Orchard Veterinary Group, Glastonbury, Somerset, UK; [4]Delaware Veterinary Group, Fulford House, Torbay Road, Castle Cary, Somerset, BA7 7DT, UK

## Introduction

Maintaining a healthy, productive group of cows is an overarching aim of a herd health programme, and thus replacing unhealthy or unproductive cows and rearing replacements are important elements of herd health management. In this chapter we describe how rearing youngstock and replacing cows can be incorporated into a herd health programme.

In many dairy herds today, the health of adult milking and dry cows is often prioritized over the health and management of youngstock. Youngstock are often observed less frequently than adult cows by both veterinary advisors and farm staff, resulting in delayed disease detection and treatment; veterinary attention becomes focused on diseased individuals as they arise rather than working towards producing groups of healthy calves.

The rearing period should be productive but the measurable outputs are different to the adult herd; productivity in this period means weight gain and appropriate body size as well as optimizing overall health. This chapter aims to provide the herd health advisor with a logical approach to managing and monitoring youngstock health and performance.

## Dynamics of the dairy herd structure: culling and replacements

The importance of monitoring health and losses during the rearing period becomes clear when we consider the balance between availability of replacement heifers and the rate of culling of adult cows. Restrictions on the availability of replacement heifers will have an impact on management strategies to control disease in the adult herd, as well as affecting calving pattern and production. Examples include poor contagious mastitis control because of an inability to cull chronically infected cows and ineffective infectious disease control because latently infected animals are not removed in a timely fashion. Furthermore, an excess of healthy, well-grown replacement heifers can result in a source of income for the farmer through their sale.

The herd health advisor needs to be aware of the number of replacement heifers required given the herd's culling and death rate. For example, for a herd with a culling rate of ~25% and loss in youngstock before first calving of ~20%, this will typically be around 30 heifers per year for a 100-cow herd. This means around two-thirds of the adult herd need to be inseminated with dairy semen each year.

Many dairy herds use natural service in nulliparous heifers, but this requires careful management of the stock bull and restricts genetic progress. Artificial insemination (AI) of nulliparous heifers is recommended because this generally provides greater control over genetic improvements, calving pattern and potential disease risks. However, the use of AI requires planning, the ability to detect oestrus and/or use synchronization programmes and good handling facilities. Breeding decisions for nulliparous heifers therefore require careful thought and the herd health advisor is well positioned to offer advice on heat detection, synchronization programmes and expected pregnancy rates; this area is discussed later in this chapter and in Chapter 4.

It is also important to organize when heifers will enter the herd, and this is dependent on the management system. If the dairy herd has a seasonal calving pattern, then typically heifers will calve into the herd before the cows, to allow for extra attention and additional growth in the 1st lactation, as well as a longer interval between first calving and first service. If the herd has cows that calve all year round, then entry of new heifers is more flexible, and multiple 'batch' systems are often easier to manage than entry of individuals over prolonged periods.

The source of the replacement heifers is an important consideration. They may be 'home-bred' (i.e. the herd is completely closed), 'bought-in' (i.e. the herd is open) or a mixture of the two. Advantages and disadvantages of these approaches are presented in Table 3.1. Breeding heifer replacements from current heifers does have advantages: (i) heifer calves are born at the right time of year (this will depend on the age at first calving, but ideally ~2 years) and (ii) an increased rate of genetic progress. However, the disadvantages include an inability to know which heifers are phenotypically best (because they haven't yet begun milk production) and the fact that passive transfer of antibodies will be from heifer to heifer (the most immunologically naive animals in the herd) means there is increased risk of calfhood disease.

### Mortality and disease in youngstock

Mortality rates and disease incidence in youngstock are extremely variable between farms, and this is an area in which the herd health advisor can have a major influence on cow welfare and herd profitability. Although data are relatively sparse, we illustrate this below by summarizing relevant research findings.

**Table 3.1.** Advantages and disadvantages of home-bred versus bought-in replacement heifers.

| | Home-bred replacements | Bought-in replacements |
|---|---|---|
| Advantages | Control of genetic selection | Potential for step change in genetic progress |
| | Direct responsibility for nutritional management of replacements means good control of body condition at calving | Outsourcing replacements allows for increased focus and input of labour into the milking herd |
| | Allows for control of infectious disease through increased biosecurity | |
| Disadvantages | Capital costs required including buildings, bedding, feed, labour | Potential for poor disease status of heifers depending on previous management and routine |
| | The space required to rear animals may be incompatible with adult herd requirements | Biosecurity: a continual potential source of infectious disease |
| | Restricted genetic progress if not using AI and over-reliance on own bull | Lack of control of the future of the herd; wholly reliant on consistent quality of replacements |

A US study 30 years ago reported calf mortality rates of between 3.5 and 30.6% over a 2-year period in 16 dairy herds in California (Martin *et al.*, 1975) and a study in the UK more than 10 years ago suggested that a significant proportion of calves are born dead or die during the rearing period (8 and 13%, respectively (Esslemont and Kossaibati, 1996)). The latter authors identified that calf mortality within 24 h of birth, in 43 herds over 10 seasons, was between 7 and 8% (Esslemont and Kossaibati, 2002) and therefore understanding and monitoring wastage of replacement heifers must begin with an assessment of current perinatal calf mortality (PCM): those that are stillborn or die within the first 24 h of life. A more recent UK study reported an average perinatal calf mortality rate of 8% from 19 herds (Brickell *et al.*, 2008); other research has reported a 9.3% perinatal calf mortality rate over one year from 46 herds in Thuringia (Hoedemaker *et al.*, 2010). In a post-mortem survey, 46% of perinatal calf mortalities had non-inflated lungs and a further 23% had severe trauma to the thoracic region (for example, spinal fractures; McCoy *et al.*, 1997). The main risk factors for perinatal calf mortality are summarized in Box 3.1. Dystocia has a role in perinatal calf mortality and incidence rates of dystocia vary enormously between herds.

The pre-weaning period also represents a time of significant losses in the dairy industry. Data from a recent USDA survey (USDA, 2010) indicate an overall pre-weaned calf mortality rate of 7.8%. This is broadly in line with a 5% calf mortality rate between 1996 and 2004 from more than 4000 herds in Minnesota (Silva del Río *et al.*, 2007), although a recent Danish study that conducted a genetic analysis of calf and heifer losses on more than 840,000 calves and heifers born between 1998 and 2007 found lower mortality rates of 3.2% (first month of life) and 2.7% (months 1–6) (Fuerst-Waltl and Sørensen, 2010).

The two main disease processes implicated with morbidity and mortality in youngstock are diarrhoea and pneumonia. The USDA survey (USDA, 2010) reported that around 12.4% of pre-weaned heifers were affected with pneumonia and 23.9% with digestive problems, and the mortality rates were 56.5% for diarrhoea and 22.5% for pneumonia. A recent 3-year study of 135 dairy herds in Norway reported lower incidence rates for diarrhoea and respiratory disease in the first 180 days of life (3.8 and 2.9%, respectively; Gulliksen *et al.*, 2009), although when calf health records were examined and underestimation taken into account the 'true' incidence of these diseases was estimated at 5.5 and 4.1%, respectively. A Swedish study on calf morbidity in 3081 calves in the first 90 days of life in 122 dairy herds found the incidence rate of disease recorded by farmers and veterinarians to be 0.08 cases per calf-month at risk (Svensson *et al.*, 2003). Disease (in cases per calf-months at risk) included arthritis (0.002), diarrhoea (0.035), omphalophlebitis (navel ill; 0.005), respiratory disease (0.025) and ringworm (0.009). A separate study by

---

**Box 3.1.** Risk factors for perinatal calf mortality (after Mee, 2007).

- Gender: PCM is greater in male compared with female calves.
- Calving assistance: PCM increases with greater assistance.
- PCM increases with twin compared with single calves.
- Season: PCM is lower in summer.
- A previous PCM event means that PCM is four times more likely in that cow.
- The sire predicted transmitting ability (PTA) for PCM (see Appendix 2).
- Parity interactions: PCM is higher in primiparous than multiparous cows; PCM is greater in twins born to heifers than twins born to older cows; PCM is increased with low age at calving in primiparous cows.
- Duration of second-stage labour: PCM is significantly greater if the duration of second stage labour exceeds 120 min (Gundelach *et al.*, 2009).

the same authors that followed 2947 heifer calves in the same herds and monitored morbidity from three to seven months of age reported that the percentage of calves to succumb to diarrhoea, ringworm and clinical respiratory tract disease was 2.7, 5.6 and 5.7%, respectively (Svensson et al., 2006).

The costs of youngstock disease are difficult to quantify but are linked to a reduced growth rate and increased mortality rate (Andrews et al., 2000). There is evidence that a diagnosis of pneumonia in the first 6 months of life results in reduced growth rates, decreased future milk production, decreased fertility and increased probability of mortality (Waltner-Toews et al., 1986; Virtala et al., 1996; Warnick et al., 1997; Donovan et al., 1998). For this reason, prevention and control of diarrhoea and pneumonia needs to be a primary focus during the pre-weaned period, as well as the provision of adequate nutrition.

Losses associated with youngstock continue through the growth period and into the first lactation. A recent UK study investigating mortality, growth and fertility of Holstein-Friesian calves in 19 herds reported that on average, in approximately 15% of a cohort of 506 heifers, calves born alive did not reach their first calving (Table 3.2; Brickell et al., 2008), resulting in the authors suggesting that the situation remained unchanged compared with previous UK data. This situation is mirrored in Europe: a study in Sweden reported that 22% of heifers did not reach the first calving, of which 5% died, 10% were culled and 7% were sold live (Hultgren et al., 2008). A recent Spanish study on a large cohort of more than 7000 heifers born between 2004 and 2006 found that more than 8% did not complete their first lactation and, of these, >30% had left the herd in the first 50 days after calving (Bach 2011).

## Culling of adult cows

Monitoring culling and deaths from the dairy herd is crucial to understanding the pressures on maintaining herd structure, production and fertility as well as understanding any restrictions that may impact on advice to reduce and control endemic disease. Culling cows refers to a decision taken to remove an

**Table 3.2.** Summary of reasons for dairy heifers in 19 herds failing to reach first calving (after Brickell et al., 2008).

| Stage | Description | Heifers born alive but failing to calve for the first time (%) | |
|---|---|---|---|
| | | Mean | Range among herds |
| Perinatal | Stillbirth and mortality <24 h (all calves; n = 1097) | 7.9 | 2.7–14.3 |
| Neonatal | Died 24 h to 28 days (heifers only; n = 494) | 3.4 | 0–12.1 |
| Calves | Died or culled between 1 and 6 months (heifers only; n = 506) | 3.4 | 0–28.6 |
| Heifers | Died or culled between 6 months and start of breeding (heifers only; n = 489) | 3.5 | 0–18.5 |
| Heifers | Died or culled between breeding and calving (heifers only; n = 450) | 4.2 | 0–21.1 |
| Overall | Total heifers born live that failed to calve for first time | 14.5 | 0–28.6 |

otherwise healthy cow from the herd and replace her with another cow (referred to as 'voluntary culling'), or to remove an unhealthy/diseased cow and replace her with another cow (referred to as 'involuntary culling'). We include on-farm deaths as involuntary culls. A high culling rate will result in increased replacement costs and will have an impact on other areas (for example, herds with high culling due to *Mycobacterium avium paratuberculosis* may be forced to keep cows that have problems with chronic mastitis or lameness that would normally be eligible to be culled). In contrast, herds that cull too few cows may struggle to increase milk production and overall genetic merit. In reality, culling rates usually exceed an optimum level of around 15–20% (depending on the economic situation) and thus can often be improved. A crucial area for monitoring herd health is the herd culling rate and pattern (which should include reasons for voluntary and involuntary culling). A range of culling rates including on-farm deaths has been reported, and examples are summarized in Table 3.3.

The ratio of voluntary to involuntary culls will vary between herds and farms; for example. a recent study in a single herd in Scotland using 3498 lactations over 18 years showed that 68% of all culls were *involuntary* and that the main risk factors identified for these involuntary culls were abortion, assisted calving and mastitis (Bell *et al.*, 2010). The ratio of voluntary to involuntary culls was more extreme in a UK study of 50 herds 20 years ago, where voluntary culling

(for example, age and low milk yield) accounted for only 11.3% of all disposals from the adult herd (Esslemont and Kossaibati, 1997). A study of 45,220 cows in 340 dairy herds in the UK reported an average total culling rate of 22%, comprising infertility (5.6% of all cows), mastitis (3.6% of all cows) and poor milk yield (2.0% of all cows) (Whitaker *et al.*, 2000) – not a dissimilar pattern to that from a UK study of 80 herds in East Anglia nearly 30 years ago (Young *et al.*, 1983). Mortality and culling patterns were investigated in Pennsylvanian dairy herds, for 'high' and 'low' culling rate herds, and it was reported that high culling rate herds (>8% mortality in one year and >12% culling in the first 60 days in milk) produced more milk in lactations 1 and 2 but less in later lactations, resulting in a loss of production and increased replacement costs (Dechow and Goodling, 2008). Another recent, large US study that evaluated >3.5 million lactation records between 2001 and 2006, in more than 2000 dairy herds, reported reasons for culling (Pinedo *et al.*, 2010). The most common reason was 'died' (20.6% of all culls), followed by 'reproduction' (17.7%), 'injury/other' (14.3%) and 'low production' and 'mastitis' (both 12.1%). A large French study between 2005 and 2006, on >3.5 million cow-years, identified an annual average cow mortality rate of 3.8% (Raboisson *et al.*, 2011).

Stage of lactation influences the risk of culling. A large-scale US study (2.3 million lactation records from 727 herds between

**Table 3.3.** Published mean annual culling rates in dairy herds.

| Reference | Mean annual culling rate (% including death) | Number of herds |
|---|---|---|
| Caraviello *et al.*, 2006 | 34.0 | 103 |
| De Vries *et al.*, 2010 | 32.0 | 727 |
| Dechow and Goodling, 2008 | 27.7 | 2574 |
| Esslemont, 1992 | 23.1 | 91 |
| Esslemont and Kossaibati, 1997 | 23.8 | 50 |
| Hadley *et al.*, 2006 | 31.6[a] | 6264[b] |
| Pinedo *et al.*, 2010 | 25.1 | 2054 |
| Whitaker *et al.*, 2000 | 22.1 | 340 |

[a] Average culling rate for 10 states, 1993–1999. [b] Number of herds available for analysis in 1995 – a greater number of herds were used in subsequent years of the analysis.

2001 and 2006) reported that the risk of culling peaked approximately 30 days after calving (but was much earlier for 1st-lactation heifers at around 10 days after calving) and increased with more difficult calvings, the birth of male or twin calves, being in a herd with shorter days to first insemination or being in a herd with longer days to conception (De Vries et al., 2010). A survival analysis conducted on >3500 cows in 47 French herds concluded that mastitis before peak lactation, teat injuries, non-traumatic udder disorders, metritis or early abortion were all associated with a premature exit (Beaudeau et al., 1995).

Culling of cows in early lactation is generally avoided because of the potential for yield and profit during the remainder of lactation. As a consequence of this, increased culling rates in early lactation (for example, in the first 60 days) can be used as a possible indicator of poor cow health. In a large-scale review of 1.5 million whole lactation records from herds in the US, 42% of all cattle that died did so in the first 60 days of lactation (Hadley et al.. 2006); in a separate study, 26.2% of all culls occurred between 21 days prior to and 60 days post-calving, with 52% of all cow mortality occurring in this time period (Dechow and Goodling, 2008). Monitoring of mortality and culling rates in the first 60 days should be viewed with caution, because under-reporting is not uncommon and we consider the monitoring of culling rates in later sections of this chapter.

## Financial costs associated with culling of cows

The cost associated with the culling of a cow can be calculated from the income for the culled animal minus the cost of the replacement. The losses associated with a cull will generally be increased if culling is the result of a disease that reduces live weight (e.g. Johne's disease) or is a result of disease/injury such that the animal does not enter the food chain. The overall cost of culling is therefore highly dependent on the reasons for culling and varies greatly between herds. In this section, we outline the losses associated with culling.

### Value of a cull cow

The value of a cull cow is dependent on carcass quality and current market value. The value may be quoted per kilogramme of live weight or deadweight. For example, a 700 kg Holstein-Friesian cow, at a market price of 108 pence/kg live weight will be worth approximately £750. The value of culled cows can be obtained directly from farm financial records.

### Cost of a replacement heifer

The cost of a replacement heifer is more difficult to calculate and will vary depending on whether replacements are home-reared, contract-reared or bought-in. Replacement costs should be evaluated for the individual herd rather than assigning an average value. The costs associated with rearing replacement heifers are affected by the cost of keeping and feeding to first calving, the cost of disease and differences in the age at first calving. A US study reported that the average rearing costs for a 100-cow dairy herd were more than US$30,000 and that a reduction in the herd culling rate from 25 to 20% caused these rearing costs to fall by nearly 25% (Tozer and Heinrichs, 2001). A sample breakdown of costs for a heifer calving at 25 months of age on a medium input system in the UK is shown in Table 3.4.

### Cost of a cull cow

Using the example values in the sections above, the cost of a cull would be estimated as £750 (cull cow price) − £1165.60 (replacement heifer cost) = £415.60.

## Welfare considerations of youngstock rearing

The health and well-being of young animals is of the utmost importance, and for dairy calves the most common health issues arise from enteric and respiratory disease. These can lead to a severe compromise of welfare and their prevention is discussed in detail later in the chapter. We also emphasize the

**Table 3.4.** Example of a heifer rearing cost calculation (with additional detail provided for the first 12 weeks: source, DairyCo heifer rearing cost calculator, http://www.dairyco.net). Such a calculation would be conducted for individual farms to estimate the costs associated with culling and replacing an adult cow.

| | Notes | Unit cost (£) |
|---|---|---|
| Initial value of the calf | | 250.00 |
| Birth to 12 weeks old | | |
| Milk powder (@ £1500/t) | Calf requires ~5 l/day fed at ~10% concentration (colostrum for first 3 days); total fed 23 kg (weaned @ 7 weeks) | 34.50 |
| Calf starter mix (@ £230/t) | Fed from 3 days of age; average 0.75 kg/day until weaning; 2.5 kg/day until 12 weeks; total amount fed 120 kg | 27.60 |
| Barley straw (£80/t) | Feeding and bedding; assume 100 kg/calf until 12 weeks | 8.00 |
| Vet. and medical spend (e.g. vaccination) | May be increased with other treatments | 8.00 |
| Other (e.g. water heating for milk) | — | 10.00 |
| Mortality rate | Most calf deaths neonatal/first week of life: 4% mortality rate and £250 calf value | 10.00 |
| Labour (@ £10/h) | Includes feeding, bedding and cleaning out: 3.5 h/calf until weaning for twice-daily bucket feeding; 1.5 h/calf until 12 weeks | 50.00 |
| Total cost (birth to 12 weeks of age) | | 398.10 |
| 12 weeks to 7 months | Includes grass silage, concentrate, bedding straw, vet./medical (e.g. lungworm vaccine) and labour | |
| Total cost (to 7 months) | | 531.60 |
| 7–14 months | Includes grazing (land opportunity cost), fertilizer applications, vet./medical (e.g. anthelmintics) and labour | |
| Total cost (to 14 months) | | 676.22 |
| 14–19 months | Includes grass silage *ad lib.*, wheat straw bedding, vet./medical (e.g. anthelmintics at housing), artificial insemination (@ £18 per straw; assume 55% pregnancy rate) and labour | |
| Total cost (to 19 months) | | 977.44 |
| 19–25 months | Includes grazing (land opportunity cost), fertilizer applications, vet./medical (e.g. anthelmintics) and labour | |
| Total cost (to 25 months) | | 1165.60 |

following areas that are common causes of concern in relation to calf welfare.

- inadequate provision of colostrum;
- inadequate housing or management to allow expression of normal behaviours, such as suckling, grooming and exercise;
- inadequate provision of shelter, for example exposure to draughts;
- inadequate routines that prevent sufficient rest and sleep;
- lack of dietary iron or fibre;
- lack of fresh and clean water; and
- infestation with parasites, for example lice (*Linognathus vituli*; *Bovicola bovis*) and mites (*Chorioptes* spp. and *Sarcoptes* spp.).

It is now common for national organizations to produce laws, codes or recommendations for cattle welfare that include youngstock. Examples in the UK include The Welfare of Farmed Animals (England) Regulations 2000 (SI 2000 No. 1870), the

DEFRA code of recommendations for the welfare of livestock (cattle) 2003, and the Assured Dairy Scheme. It is essential that codes relevant to an individual farm situation are adhered to.

## Monitoring Youngstock Health

The variability in herd performance described in the earlier sections of this chapter demonstrates why the monitoring of youngstock health and performance is an important component of a herd health programme. In this section, we present methods for measuring and monitoring the performance of heifer calves from birth until first lactation. We have split monitoring into four sections: the neonatal period, pre-weaning, post-weaning and first lactation. Targets for the monitored indices are presented in the next section.

### Monitoring the neonatal period (including calving)

The indices recommended to monitor neonatal calf health are focused primarily on colostrum management and survival rates in the first 24 h of life.

#### Perinatal calf mortality and disease

Accurate health records are required for all heifer calves, including those that do not survive beyond the first 24 h. For the assessment of PCM, the denominator population is all calves that are born to cows calved >260 days gestation. Perinatal calf mortality is usefully expressed as a monthly incidence rate (number of cases per cow calving per month). Monthly incidence rates for dystocia and calf disease within the first 24 h of life should also be evaluated.

#### Colostrum

COLOSTRUM QUALITY. Colostrum quality should be measured at the first or second milking from all cows by using a hydrometer (colostrometer). A hydrometer can be used to assess the level of IgG in colostrum through measurement of specific gravity. There is a curvilinear relationship between specific gravity and IgG that is temperature dependent, and levels of fat and non-immunoglobulin proteins may also affect the specific gravity. Approximately 750 ml of colostrum should be used to obtain a reading using a standard measuring cylinder; the colostrum should be at room temperature (20°C) and only colostrum in which the density meter floats to the marked 'green' area (i.e. a specific gravity reading of 1.035–1.075) should be used to feed calves.

PASSIVE TRANSFER OF IMMUNITY. The success of passive transfer (PT) can be defined as a calf that has attained a serum level of greater than 10 mg IgG/ml serum by 48 h of age. Serum IgG levels provide a reasonable prediction of the probability of survival when used on a group basis. Optimal measurement accuracy is obtained if a test for serum IgG is performed within the first week of life (and ideally between 24 and 48 h of age), because after 8 days of age, calves can synthesize significant amounts of IgG. Several different methods of measuring the success of PT are summarized in Box 3.2, the most common being the zinc sulfate turbidity (ZST) test. The test is carried out by taking a jugular venous blood sample from recently born calves and following the steps outlined in Box 3.3. This can be used for all heifer calves born, but a randomly selected group of 6–10 calves sampled each month is recommended as an achievable, practical compromise.

### Monitoring the pre-weaning period

The indices recommended for pre-weaning health monitoring are focused primarily on disease incidence, mortality and growth rates. Additional information regarding seasonality, type of housing, stocking densities, post-mortem results and calf management should also be collated (McGuirk, 2008; see later section on disease control).

---

**Box 3.2.** Methods of assessing passive transfer of immunity in the calf.

---

- Zinc sulfate turbidity (ZST) test: there is good correlation between total serum immunoglobulin and ZST, although both specificity and sensitivity alter with the concentration of the test solution; see Box 3.3 (the sodium sulfite precipitation method is similar to ZST).
- Refractometer: this measures total plasma protein. The test may give false-positive values if a calf is dehydrated.
- γ-glutamyl transferase (GGT): this can be used indirectly to assess PT because the level in colostrum is ~300 times that of the dam's serum and it is absorbed across the neonatal calf's small intestine in the first 24–30 h of life.
- Radial immuno-diffusion assay (RID): this is considered to be the gold standard for measurement of serum levels of immunoglobulin.

---

**Box 3.3.** Outline of the zinc sulfate turbidity test.

---

The solutions required for the test are:

**1.** Zinc sulfate solution ($ZnSO_4.7H_2O$) at a concentration of 208 mg/1000 ml distilled water.
**2.** A barium chloride standard solution ($BaCl_2.2H_2O$) at a concentration of 1.15 g/100 ml distilled water (standard $BaCl_2$ is included to check that all the reagents are working).
**3.** A solution of 0.2N $H_2SO_4$ (used in the standard solution).

The test requires a colorimeter with a blue-green filter or spectrophotometer, which is read at 550 nm. Conducting the test:

**1.** For each calf, mix 2 ml of distilled water with 50 μl of serum in one tube and 2 ml of the $ZnSO_4$ solution with another 50 μl of serum in another tube. These quantities may need to be adjusted on a pro rata basis depending on the size of the cuvettes in a particular spectrophotometer.
**2.** Leave the samples at room temperature for 30 min.
**3.** Meanwhile, make up the reference $BaCl_2$ standard by adding 200 μl of the $BaCl_2$ to 1.8 ml of the $H_2SO_4$.
**4.** To read the first calf sample:

  a. Blank the colorimeter/spectrophotometer with the distilled water and serum mixture.
  b. Read the $BaCl_2$ standard sample. This value (an opacity reading) will equate to approximately 25 ZST units; calculate the conversion factor required for the serum samples by dividing 25 by the opacity reading. For example, if the spectrophotometer reading was 2, the conversion factor required would be 25/2 = 12.5.
  c. Read the value of the $ZnSO_4$ sample and multiply by the calculated factor above to convert to ZST units.
  d. Read the next calf $ZnSO_4$ sample; multiply all readings of serum samples by the same conversion factor.

**5.** A positive and negative control can be used for each farm by using a sample of adult cow serum and neonatal (pre-colostrum) calf serum, respectively.

---

*Pre-weaning mortality*

This should include deaths from 24 h of age until weaning, and is expressed as a proportion or percentage of all calves born. We recommend reviewing these data 1–3 monthly depending on herd size.

*Disease incidence rates including omphalophlebitis, diarrhoea and pneumonia*

Calculating disease incidence is of great importance, but is difficult if disease recording is poor. A first step is often to ensure accurate and consistent reporting of all treatments and especially those for navel ill, calf diarrhoea and bovine respiratory disease. The incidence rate of each disease (the number of events per week or per month, depending on herd size, divided by the calves at risk) should be calculated, and we recommend reviewing these data 1–3 monthly depending on herd size.

### Growth rate

This is perhaps the most important parameter to monitor during the pre-weaning period as it reflects the overall outcome of management and husbandry. We recommend using heart girth measurements (measuring tapes to convert girth to kg live weight) and suggest that all calves are measured after birth, at least monthly through the pre-weaning period and at weaning. An average daily gain is calculated from serial girth measurements.

### Calf environment

Monitoring calf husbandry should include assessment of housing (space, hygiene and ventilation), slurry management, isolation facilities and the hygiene associated with feeding. We recommend these are evaluated and discussed on a monthly basis. The number of calves, the amount of space available (e.g. number of individual pens/ hutches, bedded area available), a subjective assessment of bedding quality and availability and cleanliness of the feeding and loafing area are all useful. Temperature and humidity can be assessed using digital meters and air flow checked if required using a smoke bomb.

## Monitoring the post-weaning period

The indices recommended to monitor health in the post-weaning period and prior to calving are described below.

### Post-weaning mortality

This is calculated as the proportion or percentage of calves that die between weaning and first calving, and is usually expressed as a percentage of all calves weaned. We recommend reviewing these data 1–3 monthly depending on herd size.

### Incidence rate of pneumonia

Bovine respiratory disease treatments should be carefully recorded to allow monitoring. The incidence rate of disease is calculated as the total number of treatment events per animal at risk, in a specified time period. We recommend reviewing these data 1–3 monthly depending on herd size.

### Growth rate

Measuring and monitoring growth rate post-weaning is vital to ensure heifers are performing well throughout the growth phase. Body weight change can be measured by either weighing scale or heart girth tape. Measurements should be made at least monthly on several animals in a group to provide an estimate of the overall group performance. Ideally all animals should be measured at least twice yearly and a daily live weight gain calculated. Body condition scoring should also be performed in older heifers (see Chapter 8).

### Monitoring anthelmintic efficacy

This should be undertaken following treatment in the first season by performing a faecal egg count reduction test (FECRT). This allows for early detection of reduced efficacy and potential increased selection pressure; the FECRT is outlined in Box 3.4.

### Exposure to parasitic disease

This is an important item to monitor because clinical signs of parasitic infestation may go unnoticed and infestation can have a substantial impact on health. Monitoring can consist of worm egg counts (WECs), serum pepsinogen estimation and bulk milk antibody testing (this occurs in the adult milking herd but can provide information on the likely challenge to replacement stock). Key features of these options are outlined in Box 3.5.

---

**Box 3.4.** The faecal egg count reduction test (after Coles, 2003).

---

- A group of 10 heifers is weighed and ear tag numbers recorded. Faecal samples are obtained prior to an accurate dose of anthelmintic being administered to each heifer using a calibrated dosing gun.
- Faecal samples are collected again following treatment (7 days after levamisole/morantel; 8–10 days following benzimidazole; 14–18 days after a macrocyclic lactone product).
- A modified McMaster method can be used for the faecal egg count; however, the development of a new multivalent, more precise method (FLOTAC) allows for improved monitoring and is accurate to 1 egg/g (Cringoli *et al.*, 2010).

---

**Box 3.5.** Outline of laboratory methods used to assess exposure to endoparasites during the post-weaning period.

---

- Monitoring faecal WEC is a simple and inexpensive method to quantify exposure of growing dairy heifers to nematode parasites. The McMaster technique allows estimation of the number of eggs/g of faeces and has a sensitivity of <50 eggs/g in cattle (MAFF, 1986). We recommend composite sampling from each group of heifers midway through the first (and second) season at pasture to decide whether treatment is required for the group. If a composite sample returns a WEC of <100 eggs/g and weight gains are as expected, then treatment should be delayed (Coles *et al.*. 2010).
- Serum pepsinogen levels, measured at housing, may be used to identify nulliparous cows from the current season that have experienced minimal exposure (potential immunity issues) or too high an infection level (insufficient control), and also to inform parasite control measures in the following year. A Belgian study of 41 groups of first-season grazing animals across 15 herds exposed to gastrointestinal nematodes (Dorny *et al.*, 1999) found serum pepsinogen levels gave a clearer division between treated nulliparous cows (<2.6 units of tyrosine) and untreated nulliparous cows (2.0–4.1 units of tyrosine for subclinical infections and 3.7–6.3 for clinical infections), when compared with WEC, pasture larval count and weight gain. Another recent study found more variation in serum pepsinogen levels between herds than between animals, highlighting the usefulness of the test at the herd level, and reported a sample size of seven nulliparous cows as sufficient to estimate the mean serum pepsinogen level of a group of up to 40 animals with an error of 0.5 units of tyrosine (Charlier *et al.*, 2011). The same study used herd mean serum pepsinogen results alongside length of pasture season and worming strategy to advise on chemoprophylaxis for the following season. Using this approach, in 39% of the 82 herds followed, reducing the intensity of chemoprophylaxis resulting in more targeted use of anthelmintics was advised. In summary, we would recommend sampling seven nulliparous cows at the end of the first grazing season to estimate a mean serum pepsinogen level for the nulliparous cow group and follow the strategy outlined in Fig. 3.1.
- The bulk milk *Ostertagia ostertagi* (MOO) test is used to monitor levels of parasitic infection in a dairy herd by determination of antibodies to *O. ostertagi*. Significant negative relationships have been reported between milk production and bulk milk antibody levels to *O. ostertagi* in Canada (Sanchez and Dohoo, 2002) and Belgium (Charlier *et al.*, 2005). While this has resulted in many studies that have investigated the effects of whole-herd anthelmintic treatment on milk production (see Gross *et al.*, 1999), a MOO test at the end of the grazing season in the adult herd may aid with planning worming strategies for replacement cows in the next season. For example, a test with a low antibody value at the end of the grazing season in the adult herd may indicate that exposure for first-season grazing animals in that year was not sufficiently large to ensure adequate immunity going into the second season (e.g. a dry summer). It may therefore be prudent to consider a MOO ELISA test result as a lead-in to serum pepsinogen testing as outlined above.

### Fertility performance

Fertility performance in heifer replacements should be monitored in a similar way to adult cows (see Chapter 4), but with a focus on the following indices.

- age at first service (including the distribution of ages within heifer cohorts born at different times, see Fig. 3.2);
- service rate: proportion of eligible heifers served in each available 21-day period;

- pregnancy rate: proportion of services resulting in a pregnancy (see Fig. 3.3); and
- age at first calving.

## Monitoring first calving and lactation

First-lactation heifers are an important cohort to monitor. The indices used should include (i) age at first calving (AFC); (ii) dystocia and mortality rate at first calving;

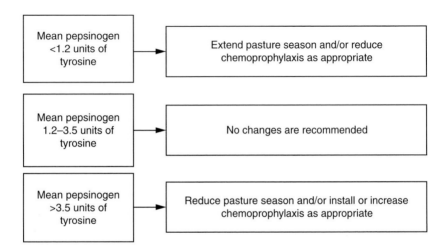

**Fig. 3.1.** Outline of a strategy to incorporate serum pepsinogen testing in a group of seven nulliparous cows (see Box 3.5) to inform a farm policy on prevention of gastrointestinal nematodes (from Charlier *et al.* 2011).

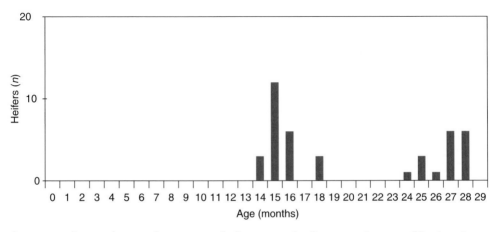

**Fig. 3.2.** Distribution of services by age in months for a group of nulliparous and a group of first-lactation cows. The number of heifer services (y-axis) is plotted by month since birth (x-axis); some heifers are still being served at 18 months in this herd example.

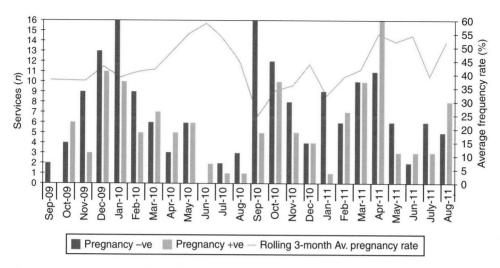

**Fig. 3.3.** A pregnancy rate plot for nulliparous heifers in a sample herd. The x-axis shows an 18-month period of service data for nulliparous animals; in each month the number of services resulting in a pregnancy and the number not resulting in a pregnancy are shown. For example, in April 2011 a total of 27 nulliparous heifers were served, 16 resulting in a pregnancy and 11 not, giving a pregnancy rate for the month of 16/27 = 59%, and the rolling 3-month average pregnancy rate reached 55%.

(iii) first milk recording test-day parameters (for example, proportion with a somatic cell count >200,000 cells/ml, see Chapter 5); (iv) mean daily yield in the first lactation; (v) the proportion that are culled involuntarily (and reason for the involuntary cull); (vi) the proportion detected with clinical mastitis within the first 30 days of lactation; and (vii) the proportion of heifers with a mobility score of 2 or 3 during the first lactation. Monitoring heifers at this stage incorporates the concepts described in later chapters on health and nutrition.

### Age at first calving

The median, mean and range for AFC should be monitored for each group of heifers that calve into the herd. An example is shown in Fig. 3.4.

### Dystocia and mortality at first calving

Dystocia and deaths at first calving should be monitored and can be expressed as either monthly or yearly incidence rates. Dystocia can be further categorized by degree of assistance, after agreeing definitions with farm staff (simple scales are recommended such as calved alone, slight assistance, great assistance). Mortality at first calving should include all deaths and involuntary culls at or within seven days of calving.

### Incidence rates of metabolic and infectious disease

These should be monitored at least every three months during the first lactation and should include the monthly incidence rate of retained fetal membranes, endometritis, lameness, mastitis and abomasal disease. Monitoring of these conditions is described in detail in subsequent chapters covering mastitis, fertility and nutrition.

### Monitoring culling in the adult herd

It is essential that cows culled from a herd are recorded, and this should include reasons

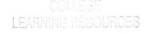

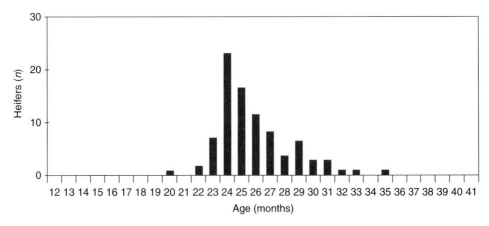

**Fig. 3.4.** Distribution of first calvings by age in months. The number of first calvings (*y*-axis) is plotted against months since birth (*x*-axis); despite a high number of calvings at 24 months, the distribution is highly right-skewed with some first calvings at >30 months in this herd example.

for culling and the stage of lactation at which culling occurs. Recommended analyses that provide useful information for a herd health programme are described below.

### Incidence rate of all culls

The incidence rate of all culls (voluntary and involuntary, including deaths) should be reviewed every 1–3 months, depending on herd size. The reasons for culling (e.g. mastitis, lameness, poor milk yield, increased somatic cell count) should be reviewed and particular note made of the rate at which cows die or are destroyed on the farm (as an indicator of severe disease and injury). Fertility culls are also of particular importance and are discussed in Chapter 4.

### Incidence of culling by stage of lactation and parity

In addition to the overall rate of culling, the stage of lactation at which culling occurs should be monitored. For example, an increased rate of culling shortly after calving suggests an increased incidence of periparturient disease. Monitoring of culling and mortality rates in the first 30 and 60 days of lactation is helpful to identify involuntary exits, again suggestive of herd

health problems. Analysis of culling rates in cows of different parity is useful to identify specific problems, particularly in parity-one cows. A cumulative survival plot of time until culling for all cows, starting either from birth or from first calving, provides an excellent picture of herd longevity and highlights periods of increased risk of culling for further investigation (Fig. 3.5).

## Targets for Youngstock Rearing and Dairy Cow Culling

Setting achievable targets for the indices discussed in the previous section is not straightforward; targets should be 'SMART' (farm-specific, measurable, attainable, realistic and time-based) and therefore these will need adjusting for individual herds over time. We outline below recommendations for targets for monitoring of replacement heifers and culled cows.

### Targets for the neonatal period (including calving)

Recommended targets for the neonatal period are summarized in Table 3.5.

### Targets for the pre-weaning period

Recommended targets for the pre-weaning period are summarized in Table 3.6.

### Targets for the post-weaning period

Recommended targets for the post-weaning period are summarized in Table 3.7.

### Targets for first calving

Recommended targets for monitoring health and performance at first calving are summarized in Table 3.8.

### Targets for monitoring culled cows

Recommended targets for monitoring the culling of adult cows are summarized in Table 3.9.

**Table 3.5.** Outline of targets for monitoring the neonatal period.

| Herd monitor | Target | Comment |
| --- | --- | --- |
| Stillbirth (%) | <2 | Born dead (lungs not inflated) |
| Perinatal calf mortality (%) | <5 | Losses in first 24 h (of calves born live) |
| *Assessment of passive transfer* | | |
| Colostrum quality (hydrometer; specific gravity) | >1.05 | Do not use for calves if <1.035 |
| ZST (ZST units) | >15 | Calves within the first week of life |
| Refractometer (g/l) | >65 | |
| Serum GGT (iu/l) | >75 | |
| Radial immunodiffusion assay (RID; mg/dl) | >1000 | IgG |
| | >80 | IgM |
| | >22 | IgA |
| | | Values are for calves at >48 h old |
| Proportion of calves with serum IgG <10g/l (%) | <15 | |

**Table 3.6.** Outline of targets for monitoring the pre-weaning period.

| Herd monitor | Target | Comments |
| --- | --- | --- |
| Mortality rate (%) | <2–5 | From 24 h old to weaning |
| Incidence rate of navel ill | <0.05 cases per calf during the rearing period | |
| Incidence rate of neonatal diarrhoea | <0.08 cases per calf during the rearing period | |
| Incidence rate of respiratory disease | <0.05 cases per calf during the rearing period | |
| Growth rate (g/day) | >750 | Holstein-Friesian |
| Age at weaning (weeks) | 6–8 | Dependent on feed and management |
| Weight at weaning (kg) | >70 | Holstein-Friesian |
| Chest circumference at weaning (cm) | 90 | Holstein-Friesian calving at 24 months |
| Approximate airspace (m³/calf) | >6 | Depends on ventilation |
| Approximate floor area (m²) | >3 | Depends on ventilation |
| Relative humidity (%) | 50–80 | Meter to assess |
| Ventilation | >4 changes per hour | See later sections |

**Table 3.7.** Outline of targets for monitoring the post-weaning period.

| Herd monitor | Target | Comment |
| --- | --- | --- |
| Mortality (%) | <2 | From weaning to calving |
| Incidence rate of respiratory disease | <0.05 cases/calf during the rearing period | |
| Growth rate (g/day)[a] | >800 | Holstein-Friesian |
| Age at 1st heat (months) | <12 | |
| Weight at 1st heat (kg)[a] | >275 | Holstein-Friesian |
| Age at service (months)[a] | 15–16 | |
| Weight at service (kg)[a] | >360 | Should be 60% of mature body size |
| Chest circumference at service (cm)[a] | >160 | Holstein-Friesian |
| Height at withers at service (cm)[a] | >125 | Holstein-Friesian |
| Pregnancy rate to first service (%) | >50 | Possible 10% reduction if sex-sorted semen is used |
| Faecal WEC[b] (eggs/g) | <100 | Dependent on stage of the season; pooled sample |
| Serum pepsinogen (units of tyrosine[c]) | 1.2– 3.5 | See text |

[a] Target body measurements for heifers calving at 24 months based on 60% adult weight at service, 80% adult weight at calving (Kertz et al., 1998; Brickell et al., 2009). [b] Worm egg counts – see text.

**Table 3.8.** Outline of targets for monitoring the first calving and first lactation.

| Herd monitor | Target | Comment |
| --- | --- | --- |
| Age at 1st calving (months) | 24–26 | |
| Weight at 1st calving (kg) | >500 | Holstein-Friesian (or 80% of mature weight) |
| Chest circumference at calving (cm)[1] | >200 | Holstein-Friesian |
| Height at withers at calving (cm)[a] | >130 | Holstein-Friesian |
| Mean BCS[b] at 1st calving | 2.5–3.0 | |
| Assistance at 1st calving (%) | <20 | |
| Cow mortality at 1st calving (%) | <2 | |
| Affected by RFM (%)[c] | <5 | |
| Affected by endometritis (%) | <10 | See Chapter 4 |
| Affected by abomasal disease (%) | <5 | See Chapter 8 |
| Affected by clinical mastitis in early lactation | <1 in 12 | First case in first 30 days of lactation – see Chapter 5 |
| Heifers with SCC[d] >200,000 cells/ml on 1st test day recording (%) | <10 | See Chapter 5 |

[a] Target body measurements for heifers calving at 24 months based on 60% adult weight at service, 80% adult weight at calving (Kertz et al., 1998; Brickell et al., 2009) [b] Body condition score. [c] Retained fetal membranes. [d] Somatic cell count.

A graphical illustration of cow longevity in two dairy herds is shown in Fig. 3.5.

## Disease Control in the Rearing Period

The general aim of disease control during the rearing period is to implement evidence-based, practical strategies, informed by the results of detailed health monitoring. A holistic approach is essential to address the multifactorial nature of the common diseases. We therefore present in this section a route for the herd health practitioner to evaluate problems and implement preventive strategies. We divide the description of different age groups into feeding, management of the environment,

**Table 3.9.** Outline of targets for monitoring culling in the adult dairy herd.

| Herd monitor | Target | Comment |
|---|---|---|
| Percentage of cows culled (after the first calving) per annum. This should be evaluated on a 1–3 monthly basis (depending on herd size) and include an assessment of reasons for culling. If any single reason exceeds 30% of all involuntary culls, further investigation is warranted. | 15–22 | Includes voluntary and involuntary culling (including deaths). The target could be higher than this if the cost of replacing adult cows is low. The target could be lower than this if a herd is undergoing expansion. |
| Deaths (after the first calving) per annum (%) | ≤2 | Includes cows destroyed on the farm as casualties |
| *Culling by parity* | | |
| Culled in 1st lactation (%) | ≤10 | |
| Culled in 2nd lactation (%) | ≤5–10 | |
| Culled in 3rd lactation (%) | ≤5–10 | |
| *Culling by stage of lactation* | | |
| Culled <60 days in milk (%) | ≤3 | |
| Mortality <60 days in milk (%) | ≤1–2 | |

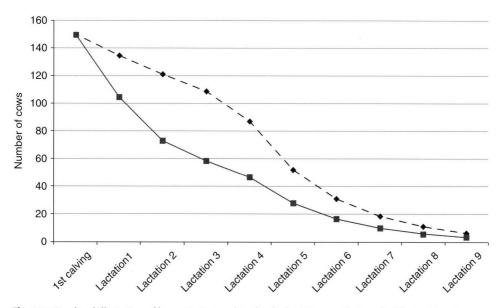

**Fig. 3.5.** Graphical illustration of longevity in two dairy herds, for 150 cows that reached first calving. In one herd (dashed line) the culling rate in parities one, two and three was 10%, in parity four was 20% and in later parities was 40%. In contrast, in the second herd (solid line), the culling rate in parities one and two was 30%, in parities three and four was 20% and in later parities was 40%. The shape of the curves allows visualization of culling rates at different life stages and could be compared with a curve that defines a herd target.

general husbandry and relevant preventive medicine. However, we stress that we do not intend to describe all possible systems of youngstock rearing, but instead to consider areas that are related to health and to describe the major principles important for all systems in terms of youngstock health.

### Disease control in the neonatal period (including calving)

#### Management at calving

A structured approach to calving cows is vital. If the rate of perinatal calf mortality is above target, calving management should be reviewed and discussed with farm staff. Training staff on good calving management (see paragraphs below on the environment) and the correct approach to a case of dystocia are important roles for the herd health advisor. Suggested approaches to providing assistance at calving, umbilical care and resuscitation of the newborn calf following dystocia are summarized in Boxes 3.6 and 3.7. Management of the cow and calf at calving time can be usefully demonstrated during staff training and summarized in a standard operating procedure if required.

#### Feeding

Ingestion of colostrum by calves in the first 24 h after birth is fundamental to neonatal health, as it allows the passive transfer of immunity from dam to calf. Immunoglobulin provides passive immunity both via absorption into the bloodstream and also locally

---

**Box 3.6.** Management of calving assistance.

- Separate the cow and move to a calving pen (calving cows should be separated from herd-mates but other animals should remain visible and audible).
- Disinfection of the perineum is recommended.
- Assistance during stage 1 of labour should be given if progress to stage 2 (cow becoming recumbent and straining) does not occur within 4–8 h. A vaginal examination should be carried out to check for torsion of the uterus.
- Assistance during stage 2 of labour should be given if regular and forceful straining is unproductive (i.e. there is no emergence of the calf's legs and muzzle through the vulva). Straining can last for between 30 min and 4 h (heifers take longer), but unproductive straining for 1 h (cow) or 2 h (heifers) should indicate that assistance is required.
- Assistance must be given if signs of reduced vigour become apparent in the calf.
- Calving ropes with manual traction are preferred to mechanical traction. If used, mechanical aids should not forcibly remove the calf, rather they act to prevent retrograde movement of the calf when the dam relaxes.
- Immediate veterinary attention should be sought if malpresentations cannot be corrected, progressive movement of the calf cannot be achieved or the operator is faced with a situation they are unfamiliar with or cannot resolve.
- The umbilical cord should be left to rupture spontaneously and a topical disinfectant applied; it is recommended that tincture of iodine is used.

---

**Box 3.7.** Resuscitation of the newborn calf by farm staff (after Grove-White, 2000).

- Establish a clear airway by positioning the calf with the neck extended. Hanging the calf upside down (for example, over a gate) may assist the removal of excess fluid from the airway but must be for a short duration of time only, as the weight of the gut contents on the diaphragm will restrict breathing.
- A mask-type ventilator can be used by appropriately trained staff.
- Stimulant drugs such as doxapram and etamiphylline act to increase tidal volume via stimulation of peripheral chemoreceptors (doxapram) or relax airway smooth muscle and increase heart rate (etamiphylline). They can be dispensed for use on farm by appropriately trained staff.
- Other stimulants should be used with caution, such as using straw placed into the nares, cold water shock, acupuncture (nasal philtrum) and thoracic massage.
- Request immediate veterinary attention if the calf fails to raise its head after 20 min or fails to stand after 60 min.

within the intestinal lumen; $IgG_1$ returns to the small intestinal lumen in high concentrations from the circulation and retains its antigen-binding capacity. Adequate passive transfer (PT) of immunity requires ingestion of 200g of immunoglobulin, mainly $IgG_1$, within 12–24 h of birth. The apparent efficiency of absorption of IgG is 20–35%, and this declines with age with no further absorption taking place after 27–30 h.

Important constituents of bovine colostrum are summarized in Box 3.8.

Where a failure of passive transfer is identified (see earlier section on monitoring), it is essential to assess and address the possible reasons for poor quality and inadequate intake of colostrum (Tables 3.10 and 3.11). Identification of the possible cause(s) will require a detailed assessment of the protocols and procedures in place on the unit and

---

**Box 3.8.** Important constituents of bovine colostrum.

- a rich source of energy (carbohydrate and fat);
- protein, mainly casein;
- trypsin inhibitor;
- fat-soluble vitamins A, D and E;
- calcium;
- immunoglobulin present in colostrum is typically ~80% $IgG_1$, with the remainder being made up of approximately 7% IgM, 5% $IgG_2$ and 5% IgA. These provide passive immunity both via absorption into the bloodstream and also locally within the intestinal lumen;
- immune cells: >$10^6$ maternal immune cells including T and B lymphocytes, polymorphonucleocytes (PMNs) and macrophages; these may be absorbed and be functional and probably have a role in the development of the calf's immune system;
- growth factors (e.g. $IGF_1^a$ and $IGF_2$, epidermal growth factor, nerve growth factor, etc.), although the role these may play in stimulation and development of the gastrointestinal tract and other organs in neonatal calves is unclear;
- hormones (e.g. insulin, cortisol, thyroxine); and
- other non-specific protective systems (e.g. lactoferrin, lactoperoxidase, thiocyanate, cytokines).

[a] Insulin-like growth factor.

---

**Table 3.10.** Factors affecting colostrum quality.

| Factor | Comments |
|---|---|
| Breed of dam | Holsteins reported to have inferior IgG content compared with other breeds (e.g. Muller and Ellinger, 1981) |
| Yield of dam | Inversely correlated with immunoglobulin content (Guy et al., 1994; Morin et al., 2010) |
| Parity of dam | First-lactation cows have both lower volume and lower concentration of immunoglobulin (Besser and Gay, 1994) |
| Length of dry period | Negative correlation with colostrum quality if dry period ≤14 days and slightly negatively correlated if dry period is excessively long (Pritchett et al., 1991) |
| Pre-partum milking/leakage | Reduces volume of colostrum and density of immunoglobulin |
| Poor body condition score at calving | Reduces volume of colostrum and also serum IgG content (Petrie, 1984) |
| Intercurrent disease in dam | Reduces IgG content (e.g. liver fluke infestation) |
| Interval between calving and first milking | Colostral IgG content declines by ~4% during each hour following calving due to post-parturient secretion by mammary tissue (Morin et al., 2010) |

**Table 3.11.** Factors affecting passive transfer of immunity to the neonatal calf.

| Factor | Comments |
| --- | --- |
| Timing and quantity of the first two feeds | A calf requires 100 g of immunoglobulin at both of the first two feeds; ideally the first feed should occur within 4 h of birth and the second within 12 h. Depending on colostrum quality (see section on monitoring), this means that ~2 l of colostrum are required at each of these feeds |
| Colostrum quality | (see Box 3.8) |
| Size of udder and teat placement | Low udders in older cows can reduce colostrum intake |
| Presence of dam | This can improve efficiency of immunoglobulin absorption by up to 80% compared with that when dam not present |
| Environment | Field-born calves have been reported to have higher serum IgG levels than calves born in confined calving boxes |
| Ambient temperature | In extremes of hot and cold, IgG content in colostrum decreases, neonates have lower volume intakes and IgG absorption is reduced |
| Dystocia or Caesarean section | These pose a higher risk of post-natal respiratory acidosis in the calf; such acidotic calves both consume significantly less colostrum and also absorb significantly less IgG than normal calves (Besser *et al.*, 1990) |
| Maternal recumbency | e.g. hypocalcaemia or musculoskeletal/nerve damage restrict and may prevent colostrum intake altogether |

an assessment of herd records to identify trends (e.g. is the problem predominantly one of calves born to heifers or at certain times of year?). While this investigation takes place, a suggested immediate action is to supplement all calves with 150–200 g IgG by feeding 4 l of good-quality colostrum (minimum 50 g IgG/l) within 6–12 h of birth (alongside strict hygiene in the calf environment). Providing colostrum by oesophageal tube can prove useful; in one study, only 10.8% of calves that were tube-fed colostrum were diagnosed with failure of passive transfer, compared with 19.3% fed via a teat on a bottle and 61.4% that suckled their dams (Besser *et al.*, 1991).

Where the problem is one of poor colostrum quality (a common issue in high-yielding Holstein herds), colostrum can be replaced with stored/frozen colostrum from donor cows of known good immunoglobulin status. Best practice is to take the first milking colostrum (milked out as soon after calving as possible) from second-parity cows of known disease status (e.g. negative for Johne's Disease, BVD, *Salmonella* spp. and enzootic bovine leukosis). Hygienic collection and storage is essential to minimize bacterial contamination. Fresh colostrum can be stored at 4°C for up to a week or frozen for prolonged storage with minimal degradation of IgG over time. If the colostrum is to be stored then it should be refrigerated/frozen in suitably sized aliquots (e.g. 2 or 4 l) and not pooled. Mixing of colostrum is only of value if it is of known high IgG concentration, but since it carries a much higher risk of spread of disease, this not recommended.

Identification of cows with good-quality colostrum can be problematic in some high-yielding herds because poor-quality colostrum may be produced by the majority of animals. In this situation options are to use beef cross cows to provide additional high-quality colostrum for storage (taking appropriate biosecurity measures when animals are introduced) or to use artificial replacers. Commercial colostrum replacers and substitutes are available, and their usefulness is determined by the quantity, specificity and apparent efficiency of absorption of the IgG. The apparent absorption of colostrum replacers based on serum is equivalent to maternally derived colostrum (20–35%), while that based on colostrum/whey is lower (5–25%). Colostrum supplements (defined as products unable to raise blood IgG concentration above 10 mg/ml and typically containing less than 100 g IgG per dose) cannot replace high-quality colostrum. Colostrum replacers (defined as products able to raise blood IgG concentration to greater than 10 mg/ml, typically containing a minimum of 100 g IgG per dose along with fat, protein, vitamins and minerals) can provide an effective and convenient method of supplying adequate passive immunity to calves, in the short term.

Finally, the specificity of IgG can be an issue in some situations (i.e. immunoglobulins do not provide protection against diseases to which the calf is exposed). This can be a problem with colostrum replacers and when nulliparous heifers are added late to a herd, having been reared in another location, or when calves are reared in a separate unit to that where they were born.

### Environment

After birth, the first time a calf is exposed to pathogens is in the calving environment; the management of cows and the calving pen will impact upon this. Cows in transition should be kept as clean as possible by housing them in well-bedded environments at a low stocking density; cleanliness can be monitored over time by routine hygiene scoring (see Chapter 5). While obviously dirty cows (especially the udder and perineum) can be cleaned by hand as a short-term measure, ensuring transition cows are kept in clean environments is the key. The use of clean individual calving pens, compared with other calving accommodation, has been shown to reduce the risk of both calf diarrhoea and pneumonia (Frank and Kaneene, 1993; Svensson et al., 2003); ideally the cow should not be moved into the pen until just before she calves, to minimize contamination. If possible, cows should be moved to the calving environment once stage 2 of labour (commencement of calving, regular and forceful straining) is under way. Calving pens should be cleaned out, disinfected (see Box 3.9) and provided with clean bedding after each calving.

### Preventive treatment

Vaccination of cows in the last trimester of pregnancy can be useful in providing immunoglobulins in colostrum specifically

---

**Box 3.9.** Spectrum of activity of various disinfectants.

Disinfection (the elimination of microorganisms that may cause disease) may be natural or artificial. Natural disinfection includes sunlight, heat, cold and desiccation from fresh air and wind. Steam-cleaning can provide an excellent means of disinfection if performed well, including removal of coccidial oocysts. The major farm chemical disinfectants are listed below. All disinfection should be preceded by cleaning of the area to remove organic matter, which may interfere with the disinfection process.

*Quaternary ammonium compounds* are cationic neutral detergents that are broad-spectrum (active against both Gram-positive and Gram-negative bacteria), but are not active against bacterial spores, fungi or viruses. They have a high residual activity but are inactivated in the presence of organic material.

*Formalin* (40% formaldehyde gas in water) is widely used as a disinfectant at 4–5% solution and is bacteriocidal, virucidal and fungicidal as well as active against anthrax spores. It requires prolonged contact time and warm temperatures to be optimally effective.

*Oxidizing disinfectants* such as peracetic acid and propionic acid are active against a wide range of bacteria, spores, viruses and fungi at low concentrations.

*Halogens* such as chlorine are often used for cleaning milking equipment as they have a rapid action, particularly when warm, and are effective against viruses. They are inactivated in the presence of organic material.

*Iodine and iodophors* have a broad bacteriocidal and fungicidal action and are also active against bacterial spores, viruses and vegetative forms of bacteria.

*Ammonia* used as a 10% solution is effective against coccidial oocysts but has no other applications as a disinfectant on the farm.

against certain diseases (e.g. *Escherichia coli* K99, rotavirus, coronavirus clostridial diseases and *Salmonella* spp.). Enhancing specific immunoglobulins in colostrum by this method is particularly useful for control of calf diarrhoea. While vaccination strategies of this type can be helpful, they are not infallible because of (i) variations in the titre and duration of the specific antibody response that are achieved; (ii) the amount and timing of the antibody ingested by the calf; and (iii) the size and pathogenicity of the challenge faced by the neonate (Crouch *et al.*, 2001). Ultimately, vaccination cannot replace excellent hygiene and husbandry in the neonatal period.

Oral solutions of concentrated bovine lactoserum containing specific immunoglobulins against *E. coli* F5 adhesin (e.g. Locatim Oral Solution; Vetoquinol UK, Ltd) can be considered in specific situations. These may reduce mortality in calves when used in conjunction with colostrum, but not as a substitute. We suggest that any requirement for supplementary treatments to aid the reduction of neonatal calf diarrhoea is a cause for reviewing and monitoring adequate passive transfer of immunity and hygienic management of the environment.

### Disease control in the pre-weaning period

#### *Feeding*

Calves can be fed colostrum, milk from the dairy herd or artificial milk replacer during the pre-weaning period, using a variety of different feeding systems. The success or failure of any feeding method in terms of calf health depends on important underlying principles, which we highlight below.

Continued feeding of colostrum during the pre-weaning period allows prolonged enhancement of the immune system, with the presence of specific antibodies within the gut lumen exerting a local protective effect. Feeding colostrum from cows in the herd has the advantage of increased levels of protective antibodies to pathogens on the farm, and may be boosted by the use of vaccination; antibodies against rotavirus,

coronavirus and *E. coli* F5 (K99) in colostrum and milk have been demonstrated for at least 28 days in one UK study (Crouch *et al.*, 2001). However, as described earlier, the feeding of mixed (pooled) colostrum is a significant risk for spread of infectious disease (see Chapter 7) and thus should be used with caution and only when the disease status of contributing cows is known.

Saleable milk from the dairy herd is not often used to feed calves because of its market value. Feeding waste milk from adult cows (i.e. milk discarded from cows currently under antibiotic treatment, for example for mastitis) is not recommended because of potential bacterial and antibiotic contamination. Feeding low levels of antibiotics to calves is a particular concern because of the potential to enhance selection of resistant bacterial strains, and we strongly recommend this is avoided.

There are many systems for feeding calves including bucket feeding (once or twice daily), use of artificial teats and automatic machines. No method is always superior, the success of each depending on the management routines involved. Important principles to minimizing disease during the pre-weaning period associated with feeding management are set out in Box 3.10.

#### *Environment*

Pathogens responsible for neonatal calf diarrhoea and calf pneumonia are generally ubiquitous and may be present in healthy as well as diseased animals. The aim of environmental management in this age group is therefore not to eliminate all pathogens but to maintain infection pressure at a sufficiently low level, while providing shelter, a suitable temperature and a comfortable lying surface. There are a variety of management systems and types of housing, including individual pens, grouped pens and hutches, all of which can be managed successfully, or otherwise. We highlight the key principles of environmental management during the pre-weaning period in Box 3.11. While a detailed account of all ventilation systems is outside the scope of this book, we outline methods to evaluate adequacy of air quality in Box 3.12.

---

**Box 3.10.** Principles of feeding management to minimize disease during the pre-weaning period.

- Continue to feed colostrum for first 3–4 days of life: in addition to the benefits of local immunity (see main text), the immaturity of the pepsin digestive enzyme system in the abomasum (due to lack of hydrochloric acid-secreting parietal cells) means that calves should continue to be fed on colostrum (or moved on to whole milk) until 4 days old.
- Concentration of milk powder: this should be checked against the manufacturer's recommendations and the accuracy of mixing monitored. Most artificial replacers are mixed at a concentration of 125–150 g/l, but can vary between products.
- Temperature: milk or milk replacer is best mixed at 45–50°C to be fed at ~42°C (although some acidified milk replacers can be fed cold; follow the manufacturer's instructions).
- pH: cold milk is acidified so it remains fresh for several days in ad lib feeding systems.
- Mixing: milk powder and water must be well mixed to avoid aggregation.
- Hygiene of equipment and utensils: equipment should be washed at least once daily and buckets after every feed; use of the same buckets for each pen limits disease transmission between calves.
- Quantity fed: this is usually 10–12% bodyweight (l/day). For twice-daily feeding this equates to around 2.0 l per feed at birth up to 3.5 l per feed by 6 weeks of age. However, on ad lib (or regular feed) systems, calves are able to consume greater quantities (up to 20% bodyweight) and achieve greater growth rates; limiting intakes prior to weaning may be required to encourage intake of concentrate feed.
- Height of feeders: teats/buckets must be positioned at a natural height (~0.6m from the floor) to mimic udder position and ensure optimal closure of the oesophageal groove.
- Calm handling and a consistent feeding routine are essential – feeding should occur at the same time every day.
- Care should be taken with feeding immediately after a stressful event (noise, travel, disbudding) – consider a feed of electrolytes at this time.
- Avoid sudden changes of feed or ingredients. Increases in the amount fed (e.g. increasing the volume of milk) should be done gradually over several days to allow the calf to adapt.
- Fresh, clean water should be available to calves at all times. This will stimulate calf starter ration intake, weight gain and ruminal development.
- Transition to post-weaning ration: the calf should be consuming ~1 kg of starter daily (typically 12.5 MJ ME/kg DM, 18% crude protein). Offer good-quality forage; ensure no other stresses within two weeks before or after weaning.

---

### General husbandry

The consistency of husbandry routines when feeding and managing the environment of pre-weaned replacement heifers is a vital aspect of husbandry. The herd health advisor should work with farm staff to develop operating procedures for all routine tasks (e.g. feeding and disbudding) and those for identification of sick animals. Animals should be individually inspected at least twice daily for signs of disease; a thermometer should always be available to check the rectal temperature if a calf is thought to be unwell.

Young calves are most at risk of acquiring disease from older cattle, either directly or indirectly. Ideally, calf-rearing units should be separate biosecure units either with separate staff (large units), separate over-clothes and boots (including for visitors) or good-quality washing and disinfection facilities. At a very minimum, calf feeding and husbandry should be performed before any contact is made with older cattle or with sick calves. Equipment should be washed at least once daily and ideally after every feed. The use of numbered buckets and pens, to limit the sharing of equipment between animals, is recommended.

The isolation of any high-risk or clinically infected calves, as soon as they are identified, is an essential component of the management of infectious disease such as neonatal diarrhoea and respiratory disease. The main reservoirs of infection are infected animals: calves with diarrhoea shed pathogens

---

**Box 3.11.** Aspects of environmental management during the pre-weaning period affecting calf health.

- Type of housing: from a disease management perspective, it is preferable to rear calves in individual pens until 7–10 days of age. After this, calf hutches are the preferred form of calf housing because these are easily cleaned and disinfected between groups and generally provide good air quality (see Box 3.12). If calves are grouped in pens, we recommend group sizes of no greater than 4–6 calves.
- Space allowances: for calves housed individually, reducing the level of airborne bacteria means increasing the area of the pen and a minimum of 3 m² per calf is recommended. For calves in groups, a volume of airspace of 6 m³ per calf is recommended. Stocking density has a large impact on air quality: a tenfold increase in ventilation has been found to be needed for a twofold increase in stocking density (Wathes *et al.*, 1983).
- Grouping of calves: calves should be grouped according to size and age group and an 'all-in, all-out' policy adopted to create a logical flow of animals from youngest to oldest through the housing system. Mixing of calves from different sources and of different ages must be avoided. A maximum of 30 calves in a single air space is recommended.
- Ventilation: See Box 3.12.
- Bedding and cleaning: the accommodation must provide a clean, dry, free-draining, comfortable bed (the frequency of re-bedding required will depend on the type of housing and the bedding used); the amount of bedding is sufficient when the calf's legs are not visible when recumbent. The accommodation must be easily and regularly cleaned and disinfected (at least between each calf or group).
- Disinfection must be incorporated into a routine; it is suggested that a combination of surface cleaner, disinfectant and steam-cleaning is most effective (see Box 3.9). A recommended procedure for routine cleaning and disinfection of accommodation between batches of animals is:
  - Remove all fittings and equipment and disinfect or sterilize in steam.
  - Remove all bedding.
  - Clean roof and structural supports.
  - Clean walls and floors with pressure washer and detergent/disinfectant.
  - Apply broad-spectrum disinfectant to all surfaces.
- Partitions: the presence of a solid panel between single-housed calves has been shown to reduce the risk of respiratory disease, although this may interfere with the overall ventilation of the barn by blocking external wind forces and disturbance of the stack effect.
- Temperature: the lower critical temperature for neonatal calves is ~12°C. Older calves are able to remain comfortable at low temperatures (down to zero; Wathes *et al.*, 1983), provided they have deep straw beds and are able to 'nest' in deep bedding. Increasing the amount of bedding is recommended over reducing shed ventilation during the colder months, as long as direct draughts are excluded.

---

in huge numbers compared with clinically normal animals.

Stressful events such as mixing of calves, dietary changes, removal of horn buds/supernumary teats and vaccination should be kept to a minimum and, where they are necessary, should not be carried out together. Disbudding should take place as early as practically possible while buds are still small.

*Preventive treatments*

Oocysts of *Cryptosporidium* and *Eimeria* spp. are resistant to many commonly used farm disinfectants and their removal can be difficult to achieve through management of the environment alone, particularly in more intensive continuous rearing systems. The use of chemotherapeutic agents therefore becomes an option as part of disease control. Unfortunately, the research literature on the benefits of using halfuginone lactate to control *Cryptosporidium* is equivocal. A systematic review on its prophylactic use concluded that treatment delays shedding and resulted in a lower prevalence of oocysts in the first week of life, but a higher prevalence at three weeks of age compared with untreated controls (Silverlås *et al.*, 2009). A second study demonstrated that it was effective at reducing the clinical signs of cryptosporidiosis and environmental contamination, although

---

**Box 3.12.** Practical assessment of ventilation and air quality in calf housing.

---

*Indicators of poor ventilation, moisture management and/or air quality*

- incidence rate of calf pneumonia above target (see monitoring and targets);
- smell – the air smells stale on entering the calf accommodation;
- poor cleanliness of the calves;
- presence of cobwebs in the roof area indicating lack of air movement;
- condensation and discoloration of roof panels caused by excessive water vapour production. This may be higher in summer due to a reduced ability of calves to lose heat by radiation and an increased loss of heat through respiration;
- excessive requirement for bedding in the calf accommodation to combat moisture; and
- temperature of the accommodation is too hot in summer months.

*Assessment of ventilation, adequacy of air quality*

- Check the size of the air 'inlet' and air 'outlet' areas and inlet sizes. The following figures are useful as a general guide.
  - The area of outlet required per animal housed is a function of bodyweight and floor area per animal, and for pre-weaned calves is usually in the region of $0.03\,m^2$. For 100 kg calves with $2\,m^2$ of floor space an outlet area of $\sim0.04\,m^2$ is required. Later in the rearing period, 200 kg animals with $3\,m^2$ of floor space would require an outlet area per animal of $\sim0.06\,m^2$.
  - Inlet: the total inlet area should be at least twice the outlet area.
- Avoid wall areas with no inlet at all.
- Avoid draughts (inlets that allow high air speed at animal height).
- Consider mechanical ventilation if inlets or outlets cannot be made adequate or signs of poor air quality remain (see above).
- Use a smoke emitter to assess air flow within the building.
- Monitor house temperature and relative humidity.
- Consider monitoring $CO_2$ and $NH_3$ levels using a meter.

---

treatment did not affect the timing of the onset of diarrhoea or reduce the risk of infection in groups of calves housed together in a contaminated environment (De Waele *et al.*, 2010). Finally, a third study reported that heifers treated orally daily for the first 7 days of life were significantly less likely to shed oocysts during the 3-week study period, although no association was reported between treatment and incidence rate of diarrhoea (Trotz-Williams *et al..* 2011). The data suggest that if halfuginone lactate is used as a preventive treatment for cryptosporidiosis, it should be combined with hygiene measures and improved environmental management.

Vaccinations are available to enhance immunity against many of the major organisms responsible for calf pneumonia. It should be recognized, however, that vaccines should be viewed as an addition to excellent management, not a replacement for it. The aim of a vaccination programme is to enhance acquired immunity, either in advance of the expected occurrence of disease or in the face of an outbreak. The former generally requires a primary course of vaccinations administered two to four weeks apart, while the latter is usually achieved by using modified live or attenuated vaccines presented to mucosal surfaces in order to stimulate a rapid IgA and IgM response at the epithelial level (24–48 h) ahead of the slower IgG response (10–14 days). Multivalent intranasal vaccines are available against a wide variety of respiratory disease pathogens (Xue *et al.*, 2010), and offer an opportunity to boost immunity before the expected risk period for disease. However, again we stress that these should be considered as a supplement to excellent management; in many cases, when management is improved, vaccines should not be required.

The use of metaphylactic antibiotics to control calf pneumonia through the pre-weaning period should not be necessary if other husbandry measure are adequate. While a range of antibiotics are licensed for the prevention of calf pneumonia, disease control programmes that are reliant on blanket prophylactic antibiotic administration are not sustainable and are likely to come under increasing societal and government pressure in the future. The prevention of calf pneumonia is an excellent example of the importance of environmental and nutritional management to minimize challenge and maximize host immunity.

## Disease control and fertility management in the post-weaning period

### Feeding

Feeding of growing heifers from weaning to first calving encompasses many possible feeds and management systems. The overall aim during this period is to sustain growth rates at required levels (see section on monitoring) and maintain good health. It is important that growth rates are maintained at a high level before service, particularly to allow for breeding between 400 and 462 days (13–15 months). Previous research has suggested that rapid rates of growth may compromise future milk yield (Foldager and Sejrsen, 1982) but more recent evidence suggests that bodyweight and age of the heifer are the most important factors affecting mammary development, rather than the rate of growth (Daniels *et al.*, 2009). Therefore rapid rates of growth (800–900 g/day) are recommended prior to breeding but this must not result in heifers becoming over conditioned. Key principles of feeding management to minimize disease during the post-weaning period are set out in Box 3.13.

### Environment

HOUSING.  It is preferable where possible to rear heifers in small groups when housed, ideally with no more than 10–20 animals per group. This will help to minimize the spread of infectious agents between animals. We highlight key principles of environmental management during the post-weaning period in Box 3.14.

Suggested space allocations for young-stock are given in Table 3.13.

PASTURE.    Good pasture management is based on sustaining the required growth rates (see section on monitoring and targets) and managing the sward (see Chapter 8). In terms of health, a critical feature of the grazing period is the prevention of parasitic gastroenteritis and other parasitic diseases. Providing clean grazing at the start of the season can avoid anthelmintic treatments altogether, and it may also be possible to avoid treatments by moving youngstock to clean grazing from higher-risk pastures from mid-July onwards. Further details on the prevention of parasitic disease are provided in subsequent sections.

### Specific disease prevention

PARASITIC GASTROENTERITIS. Gastrointestinal nematode infections have been linked to loss of appetite, decreased nutrient intake, disrupted digestive function, loss of tissue fluids and a decrease in immune function (Stromberg and Gasbarre, 2006). Animals treated with anthelmintic drugs tend to have increased growth rates (Elsener *et al.*, 2001), an advancement in the onset of ovarian function (Mejía *et al.*, 1999) and a reduction in the faecal shedding of nematode eggs and pasture contamination. Cattle can be infected by many different species of gastrointestinal nematode, but the most important species is *Ostertagia ostertagi*. The other species are of lesser importance but *Cooperia oncophora*, which is commonly found in younger cattle in their first grazing season, may contribute the majority of eggs found in faecal worm egg counts (WEC) and may be associated with mild clinical signs. An outline of key features of the epidemiology of *O. ostertagi* is given in Box 3.15.

**Box 3.13.** Principles of feeding management for dairy heifers in the post-weaning period.

*Reasons for concern (see sections on monitoring and targets)*

- not achieving target growth rates through the post-weaning period;
- insufficient bodyweight at service;
- insufficient height at the withers at service; and
- body condition score at 1st calving: fewer than 10% of heifers should be either <2.5 or >3.5.

*Principles of feeding growing heifers*

- In the immediate period post-weaning, concentrate (typically 12.5 MJ ME/kg DM, 18% crude protein) should be fed ad lib to compensate for the lack of milk nutrients and ensure that growth checking does not occur.
- From 12 to 16 weeks, concentrate should be restricted depending on quality of the forage; for example, a suitable ration could consist of 3–4 kg of 16% crude protein concentrate with ad lib straw or 2 kg of 16% crude protein concentrate with ad lib grass silage.
- Forages should be of good quality and palatable (e.g. a well-made grass silage of 30% DM and 10.8–11.0 MJ ME/kg DM).
- For heifers at grass, the sward height during the 1st season should be 5–6 cm in spring, 7–8 cm in summer and 9–10 cm in the autumn to avoid under-nutrition. Older heifers (2nd season) should be maintained on a sward height of 6–8 cm at a stocking rate of 6–7 animals/ha.
- Supplementary feeding with concentrates and forage may be required in the immediate period after turnout depending on weather and stocking density, and should be offered towards the end of the grazing season.
- Energy density should be increased around the time of service (e.g. an additional 20 MJ ME/day for 12 weeks, commencing 6 weeks prior to expected service). Crude protein requirement is reduced to 13–14% for post-pubertal heifers.
- Pregnant heifers fed high-quality silage and barley straw should only require a mineral and vitamin supplementation.
- Mineral and vitamin requirements: see Table 3.12.
- Feed space required by growing heifers is typically 0.35 m per heifer from 4 months of age to 0.60 m per heifer at 22 months of age; all heifers should be able to eat at the same time.

**Table 3.12.** Mineral and vitamin requirements for growing Holstein heifers (mature bodyweight 680 kg, calving at 24 months; from the National Research Council).

|  | 6 months old (200 kg) BCS[a] 3.0 | 12 months old (300 kg) BCS 3.0 | 18 months old (450 kg) 90 days pregnant BCS 3.0 |
|---|---|---|---|
| Vitamin A (IU/day) | 16,000 | 24,000 | 36,000 |
| Vitamin D (IU/day) | 6,000 | 9,000 | 13,500 |
| Vitamin E (IU/day) | 160 | 240 | 360 |
| Dietary calcium (%)[b] | 0.41 | 0.41 | 0.37 |
| Copper (mg/kg)[c] | 10 | 10 | 9 |
| Cobalt (mg/kg)[c] | 0.11 | 0.11 | 0.11 |
| Selenium (mg/kg)[c] | 0.3 | 0.3 | 0.3 |
| Iodine (mg/kg)[c] | 0.27 | 0.3 | 0.3 |
| Manganese (mg/kg)[c] | 22 | 20 | 14 |
| Zinc (mg/kg)[c] | 32 | 27 | 18 |

[a] BCS, body condition score. [b] % dry matter intake. [c] mg/kg dry matter intake.

**Box 3.14.** Aspects of environmental management influencing health during the post-weaning period.

**Type of housing**: semi-covered straw yards are common and allow regular removal of manure and application of fresh bedding. Slatted flooring may be used for animals >250 kg. The feed areas and water sources should be kept clean and situated so that contamination with faeces is minimal.

**Space allowances**: see Table 3.10.

**Grouping of heifers**: after 4 months of age, heifers should be housed with other heifers of the same age and in groups of similar size (for example, <100 kg of weight variation within the group and between 2 and 4 months of age variation). An 'all-in, all-out' system should be used, with a unidirectional flow of cattle (i.e. always moving heifers to housing containing older animals rather than younger animals). Fewer than 30 animals in a single airspace is recommended and no contact with adult stock allowed.

**Ventilation**: see Box 3.12.

**Hygiene**: the accommodation must provide a clean, dry, free-draining, comfortable bed; deep straw yards must not become wet. Fresh bedding should be applied at least every other day and straw yards cleaned out monthly.

**Disinfection should be incorporated into the cleaning routine** (see Boxes 3.9 and 3.11).

**Isolation**: facilities should be made available for the treatment and nursing of sick or poorly performing animals away from the main group.

**Temperature**: the lower critical temperature for older heifers may range from 0 to 10°C, depending on feed consumption and exposure to moisture in the form of rain or snow. The upper critical temperature is ~25°C. Provision must be given to additional bedding in winter or increased ventilation/measures to cool heifers in summer.

**Table 3.13.** Suggested dimensions for housing heifer calves during the post-weaning period (after Menzi, 1995).

| | Age (months) | | | | |
|---|---|---|---|---|---|
| | 3–4 | 5–8 | 9–12 | 13–15 | 16–25 |
| Bedded lying area (m²/animal) | 1.8 | 2.3 | 2.6 | 2.9 | 3.7 |
| Outside lot (m²/animal) | 2.7 | 3.2 | 3.7 | 4.1 | 4.6–6.9 |
| Solid floor (total confinement, m²/animal) | 1.8 | 2.3 | 2.7 | 3.7 | 5.5 |
| Slatted floor (total confinement, m²/animal) | 1.0 | 1.1 | 1.2 | 1.6 | 2.3 |
| Cubicle dimensions (m) | 0.6 × 1.4 | 0.75 × 1.50 | 0.9 × 1.65 | 1.1 × 2.0 | 1.1 × 2.0 |
| Minimum width of manure alley (m) | 1.5 | 2.7 | 2.7 | 2.7 | 2.7 |

It is becoming increasingly well recognized that excessive treatment with anthelmintics leads to a reduction in the proportion of the worm population 'in refugia' (i.e. the population of worms not exposed to anthelmintics, either in untreated animals or from eggs that are deposited on to pasture prior to treatment). This exacerbates selection pressure in the population, increasing the risk of anthelmintic resistance developing, and wastes money (Coles *et al.*, 2010). This topic is described below and the reader is directed to the current Control of Worms Sustainably (COWS) guidelines (Taylor, 2010) for further details. In Box 3.16 we provide a strategy for the use of anthelmintics in replacement heifers. Heifers should only be treated during their first grazing season and the majority of nematodes (i.e. those in older animals) should be left untreated to ensure that resistant worms are 'diluted' by eggs passed by untreated animals. The herd health advisor should make sure they are aware of any anthelmintic resistance issues in their locality.

---

**Box 3.15.** Important features of the epidemiology of *Ostertagia ostertagi*.

- The life cycle of *Ostertagia ostertagi* takes about three weeks to complete under favourable conditions, but can last as long as 6 months if L4 larval stages become dormant (see below).
- Adult worms produce eggs that are passed in faeces; these eggs develop into infective larvae (L3) within two weeks and migrate out of the faecal pat on to pasture and are ingested by cattle. The L3 larvae then exsheath in the rumen and invade the abomasal glands where they moult to the L5 stage. Emergence of L5 on to the abomasum mucosal surface takes around 18 days.
- The number of infective larvae is low in spring but increases rapidly to a peak in summer months as calves in the 1st season at grass are infected by larvae remaining on pasture from the previous year.
- Wet summers will cause an earlier peak in numbers of infective larvae; dry summers result in a delayed build-up of infection as infective larvae are locked into the faecal pat.
- *Ostertagia ostertagi* infections tend to affect first-season/yearling grazing animals and are classified according to when the larvae that cause clinical disease were ingested. For example, in the UK clinical signs seen from mid-July onwards due to larvae ingested 3–4 weeks previously are classified as type I, and those seen in late winter or early spring due to the emergence of larvae ingested in the autumn that then become dormant (hypobiotic state) are classified as type II.
- The main clinical sign in both types of infection is a profuse, watery diarrhoea which is generally persistent in type I infections and often intermittent in type II. There is often marked weight loss associated with both types of disease, which may be up to 20% after 7–10 days. Morbidity is high with type I disease but mortality is usually low, provided effective treatment is instituted swiftly, whereas with type II disease morbidity is generally low but the mortality rate can be high.
- Young cattle will slowly acquire immunity to *O. ostertagi* over the first grazing season. This will wane slightly by turnout the following year but is rapidly re-established following exposure. By the second and third years, a high degree of immunity is usually achieved and hence such animals play little role in the epidemiology of the disease. Clinical disease is sometimes seen, however, in peri-parturient animals – particularly heifers – due to the natural wane in immune function around that time.

---

LIVER FLUKE. The liver fluke (*Fasciola hepatica*) causes disease (fasciolosis) due to the migration of large numbers of immature fluke through the liver and from the presence of adult fluke in the bile ducts. The life cycle is complex, involving an intermediate host, the mud snail *Galba truncatula*, several free-living stages (miracidium larvae, cercariae and metacercariae) and is summarized in Box 3.17. The hatching of fluke eggs and subsequent development within the snail is dependent on environmental conditions being warm and wet (e.g. the months May–October usually offer the best conditions in the UK).

Clinical signs of liver fluke include anaemia and hypoalbuminaemia (which may manifest as submandibular oedema). Diarrhoea is not normally a symptom in cattle. Cattle do develop partial immunity over time, which is affected by the age of the host, previous exposure of the host and the current level of parasite exposure (Kaplan,

2001). Most studies agree that treatment/ control is likely to be economically beneficial given the improvements seen in growth rates, feed conversion efficiency and conception rates (Oakley *et al.*, 1979).

A liver fluke control plan should therefore be developed based on farm history, geography and the prevailing weather, combined with post-mortem, serology and WEC results. Control is often on the targeted use of flukicides and so ideally a herd should be monitored to confirm the presence of fluke before such measures are instigated (adult cows can be monitored using bulk milk antibody tests). If the farm is deemed to be at risk of fasciolosis, then treatment with a flukicide for larval or adult forms, at the correct time of year, is required (see Box 3.17). In high-risk scenarios, cattle can be treated again in the spring to remove burdens and reduce the contamination of pastures by fluke eggs. There have been no reported

---

**Box 3.16.** Anthelmintic treatments to avoid resistance: suggested strategies (from Taylor, 2010).

---

**Work out a control strategy**: using the principles below, results of faecal egg counts (FEC – see section on monitoring) and post-mortem examinations.

**Administer anthelmintics effectively**: avoid under-dosing by dosing at the rate recommended for the heaviest animal in a group. Ensure dosing equipment is working correctly and maintain it carefully. Ensure operators are trained in correct dosing technique.

**Administer anthelmintics only when necessary**: the treatment of calves at turnout should not be necessary when calves have been born and reared indoors over the winter. A long-acting preparation such as a sustained-release bolus or a persistent macrocyclic lactone (ML) may be considered if the calves are being turned out on to high-risk pastures, to prevent both disease and further pasture contamination. When calves are at grass, a 'dose and move' strategy is considered to be highly selective for resistant worms and is not recommended. If monitoring of FEC at the beginning of the grazing season indicates an increased worm burden, strategic dosing (3-week, 8-week and 13-week strategy using ivermectin or the 0- and 8-week strategy using doramectin) may be used. Boluses would also provide an effective means of control in this situation. Calves dosed in this strategic manner should remain set-stocked on the same fields for maximum effect. Adult cattle have usually acquired a strong immunity to internal parasites by the end of their second grazing season. Despite some evidence in the literature of increased milk yields and improved conception rates as a response to anthelmintic treatments, it is unlikely to be cost-effective in many herds and the added selection pressure caused by this sort of treatment makes it hard to justify. We do not recommend routine treatment of adult cows.

**Select the appropriate anthelmintic**: there are many different anthelmintics available for the treatment of cattle. A narrow-spectrum product should be used where possible (e.g. using levamisole for the treatment of *Ostertagia* and *Cooperia* spp. rather than a broader-spectrum ML); avoid unnecessary use of combination products (particularly applies to combination flukicide and broad-spectrum anthelmintic products when treatment for fluke only is required); and reduce the use of long-acting preparations and boluses as these may delay the onset of immunity, leaving animals exposed when drugs concentrations wane.

**Rotation of anthelmintic class**: this is a contentious issue as there is a lack of evidence in the current literature that rotating the class of anthelmintic will delay the development of resistance. The practice of using a different class of wormer at each treatment has been shown to be highly selective for resistance (Barnes *et al.*, 1995); one class should be used until it fails, at which point a different class should be selected (Craig, 2006). The report by Taylor (2010) suggests that the rotation of wormers could delay the appearance of ML resistance on farms where the gene for resistance is either absent or present at very low levels. We therefore suggest that rotation of treatment class is not as important as the other issues above.

**Preserve susceptible worms on the farm**: the two main strategies to help maintain a population of susceptible parasites on the farm are targeted selective treatments (TSTs) and delay of movement. The practice of TST aims to target treatments based on FEC and leave a proportion of the group (the healthiest-looking animals) untreated, allowing a pool of unselected parasites to compete with the selected ones. Delay of movement after the dose allows time for the calves to become lightly reinfected, so when they are moved on to 'clean' pasture they will pass eggs from susceptible worms as well as resistant ones, thus helping to dilute the resistant population.

---

incidences of resistance to flukicides in cattle to date, but resistance to triclabendazole has been reported in sheep. The widespread use of triclabendazole (due to its efficacy against immature fluke) makes it a prime target for resistance; any opportunity to avoid its use is advisable.

LUNGWORM. *Dictyocaulus viviparus* is an important nematode in growing cattle and causes parasitic bronchitis (lungworm or 'husk'). Clinical disease due to infestation with *D. viviparus* tends to occur in first-year grazing animals on permanent or semi-permanent pasture in late summer or early autumn; however, in recent years clinical disease has been seen in adults that have either failed to develop sufficient immunity from exposure or have simply been overwhelmed by large numbers of infective larvae. An outline of key features of the epidemiology of *Dictyocaulus viviparus* is given in Box 3.18.

---

**Box 3.17.** Outline of the life cycle of *Fasciola hepatica*.

- Eggs passed in the faeces of cattle and sheep develop into motile miracidium larvae after 9 days at the optimal temperature range of 22–26°C. The ideal conditions are therefore warm and wet (e.g. the majority of fluke infections occur between May and October in the UK).
- The snail population increases rapidly with summer rainfall and the miracidium larvae penetrate and infect intermediate snail hosts, developing via sporocyst and redial stages to a final cercarial stage.
- These cercariae are passed from the snail and on to pasture where they encyst, forming metacercariae which are infective to ruminant hosts.
- The development from miracidia to metacercariae normally takes around 7 weeks, and a single miracidium is able to produce 600 metacercariae; therefore if conditions remain warm and wet, snails will shed massive numbers of metacercariae on to pasture. In the UK, this means cows can be challenged from August onwards or earlier if overnight temperatures are above 10°C allowing miracidium development earlier in the season.
- Metacercariae that are ingested excyst in the small intestine and penetrate the liver capsule, after migrating through the gut wall and across the peritoneal cavity.
- Immature fluke migrate through the liver parenchyma before invading small bile ducts and undergoing maturation to adult liver fluke.
- The period between ingestion of metacercariae to the passage of eggs in the faeces (i.e. patent infection) is between 10 and 12 weeks, and therefore the entire life cycle takes around 17–19 weeks in total. This means that subclinical disease is normally seen in young cattle from October onwards in the UK.

---

Clinically, animals with lungworm often present with a cough and may show signs of tachypnoea, which may progress to dyspnoea in the more severe cases. A small proportion of animals will die following sudden-onset dyspnoea during the pre- or post-patent period. Cattle rapidly develop immunity to *D. viviparus*, which is why parasitic bronchitis is mostly seen in young, naïve animals. This immunity will, however, wane in the absence of re-exposure, making it possible for adults to suffer from clinical disease once more.

Lungworm is a sporadic but devastating disease when it occurs. Vaccination is extremely effective against *D. viviparus* and is recommended for all dairy replacement heifers in regions at risk. Animals that become immune following vaccination or natural exposure are highly resistant to subsequent challenge, although if not reinforced immunity declines over ~12 months. Reinforcement of immunity through exposure to worms from carrier animals is an essential component of ongoing protection, and the practice of aggressive anthelmintic treatment strategies in the second grazing season and into adult life will result in minimal challenge of lungworm larvae and the development of a naïve population of animals. Background levels of exposure to the parasite will vary enormously depending on weather conditions and rainfall – dry summers will mean decreased exposure and therefore field infection cannot be relied upon to maintain immunity within the herd. 'Reinfection husk' syndrome is seen when a large larval challenge occurs in an immune or partially immune animal; development to the L4 stage takes place but patent infection does not occur.

*Fertility management*

Fertility management in nulliparous heifers is an important part of a herd health programme, and monitoring of the fertility indices outlined in the earlier sections of this chapter is essential. The general aims of reproductive management in nulliparous heifers are that they calve at the right time (particularly in terms of age at first calving (AFC)) and that the first calving occurs without dystocia or health problems.

Full details of herd reproductive management are described in Chapter 4, but

---

**Box 3.18.** Important features of the epidemiology of *Dictyocaulus viviparus*.

- The life cycle of *Dictyocaulus viviparus* is similar to that of other netamodes but has characteristic features, as outlined below.
- Female *D. viviparus* worms are ovo-viviparous: they produce eggs containing fully developed larvae. The larval output is enormous, reaching levels of $10^6$ larvae shed per day in natural infections. The L1 larvae hatch almost immediately and migrate up the trachea, are subsequently swallowed and passed out in the faeces.
- Development to the L3 stage is reached at around 5 days. L3 larvae migrate out of the faecal pat and climb on to surrounding herbage (periods of heavy rainfall will assist this process) or utilize the *Pilobolus* fungus found growing on faecal pats for windborne dispersal.
- The infective dose required for disease is small compared with other nematode infections.
- After ingestion, the L3 larvae pass through the intestinal mucosa into the lymphatic system and travel via lymph and blood to the lungs as L4 larvae. This process takes about one week.
- A final moult to L5 occurs in the small bronchioles a few days after the L4 emerge from capillaries into the alveoli.
- The young adult worms then emerge from the bronchioles and move up to the bronchi to mature. The entire life cycle takes around 21–28 days in total.
- Small numbers of adult worms can persist in the bronchi of young cattle and may act as a reservoir of infection for the next grazing season; these 'carrier' animals may explain outbreaks of disease in the absence of overwintering infection on pasture.
- A mild climate with high rainfall means outbreaks of disease may occur for many months of the year, making parasitic bronchitis increasingly difficult to predict, and vaccination is therefore an essential element of control.

---

additional key areas, pertinent for heifers, are highlighted in Box 3.19.

Where heat detection in nulliparous heifers is problematic or when the herd calving pattern has to be carefully controlled, the use of fertility synchronization protocols can be useful. While these are described in Chapter 4, a few details related to nulliparous heifers are worth emphasis here.

- Heifers can be successfully synchronized using a single injection of prostaglandin (with visual oestrus detection), two injections of prostaglandin 11 days apart or intra-vaginal progesterone applications.
- Heifers tend to respond poorly to an 'Ovsynch' protocol (see Chapter 4); heifers are more likely to show premature oestrus before a timed AI (Rivera *et al.*, 2004).
- Treatment of dairy heifers with prostaglandin every 14 days until insemination

has been reported to provide an optimal economic return compared with oestrus detection alone, oestrus detection with timed AI using intra-vaginal progesterone or timed AI using gonadotropin-releasing hormone (GnRH) (Stevenson *et al.*. 2008).

## Summary

The culling and replacement of dairy cows is an important element of a herd health programme. Replacement heifers are the future of the dairy herd, and a successful rearing period improves the chances of a long and productive life. It is essential to have in place methods to monitor the health and well-being of replacement heifers, and to take corrective action when needed. Establishing a herd health programme for youngstock will prove beneficial for farm finances and cow welfare.

---

**Box 3.19.** Areas of reproductive management relevant for nulliparous heifers.

---

**Essential components of reproductive management apply equally to nulliparous and multiparous cows**: these are described in detail in Chapter 4.

**Artificial insemination or natural service**

Natural service is often considered for nulliparous heifers because it avoids the need for oestrus detection and removes the cost of semen. However, artificial insemination (AI) is recommended because it offers more in terms of genetic progress and thus long-term economic gain. Other advantages of AI include removal of feeding and housing costs for a stock bull; reduced risk of introducing infectious disease associated with bull movements; reduced risk of dystocia in heifers (if semen is selected from bulls with low calving difficulties); removal of risk of injury to farm staff from handling the bull; and removal of the risk of severe pregnancy rate reductions due to an injured, lame or sick bull.

**Age at first calving**

Weight and age at first calving are closely related to lifetime milk production, reproductive performance, health and longevity (Ettema and Santos, 2004; Haworth *et al.*, 2008). The optimal age is generally 24–26 months: nulliparous heifers that calve into the herd on time return more profit compared with heifers that calve later. AFC can have an important influence on the occurrence of dystocia – if the heifer is too young (immature body size) or too old (with excessive body condition score, >3.5) the probability of dystocia is increased.

**Care during the service period**

It is particularly important that management changes (e.g. cow groupings, feed types, daily routines) and other stressors (e.g. overcrowding, erratic handling) are avoided during the service period. Reaching target body weight at first service is critical (see earlier section on targets) and heifers should maintain a weight gain of around 0.80 kg/day throughout the service period. It is often beneficial to feed 1–2 kg of a high-energy concentrate feed during the service period, depending on forage quality, and heifer rations should be fully mineralized throughout the rearing period (see Chapter 8).

---

# References and Further Reading

Abeni, F., Calamari, L., Stefanini, L. and Pirlo, G. (2000) Effects of daily gain in pre- and postpubertal replacement dairy heifers on body condition score, body size, metabolic profile and future milk production. *Journal of Dairy Science* 83, 1468–1478.

Andrews, A.H., House, A. and Hill, M. (2000) Calf pneumonia costs! *Cattle Practice* 8, 109–114.

Bach, A. (2011) Associations between several aspects of heifer development and dairy cow survivability to second lactation. *Journal of Dairy Science* 94, 1052–1057.

Bach, A. and Ahedo, J. (2008) Record keeping and economics of dairy heifers. *Veterinary Clinics of North America (Food Animal Practice)* 24, 117–138.

Barkema, H., Schukken, Y., Lam, T., Beiboer, M., Benedictus, G. and Brand, A. (1999) Management practices associated with the incidence rate of clinical mastitis. *Journal of Dairy Science* 82, 1643–1654.

Barnes, E., Dobson, R. and Barger., I. (1995) Worm control and anthelmintic resistance: Adventures with a model. *Parasitology Today* 11, 56–63.

Beaudeau, F., Ducrocq, V., Fourichon, C. and Seegers, H. (1995) Effect of disease on length of productive life of French Holstein dairy cows assessed by survival analysis. *Journal of Dairy Science* 78, 103–117.

Bell, M., Wall, E., Russell, G., Roberts, D. and Simm, G. (2010) Risk factors for culling in Holstein-Friesian dairy cows. *Veterinary Record* 167, 238–240.

Besser, T. and Gay, C. (1994) The importance of colostrum to the health of the neonatal calf. *Veterinary Clinics of North America (Food Animal Practice)* 10, 107–117.

Besser, T., Szenci, O. and Gay, C. (1990) Decreased colostral immunoglobulin absorption in calves with postnatal respiratory acidosis. *Journal of the American Veterinary Medical Association* 196, 1239–1243.

Besser, T., Gay, C. and Pritchett. L. (1991) Comparison of three methods of feeding colostrum to dairy calves. *Journal of the American Veterinary Medical Association* 198, 419–422.

Bielmann, V., Gillan, J., Perkins, N., Skidmore, A., Godden, S. and Leslie, K. (2010) An evaluation of Brix refractometry instruments for measurement of colostrum quality in dairy cattle. *Journal of Dairy Science* 93, 3713–3721.

Brickell, J.S., McGowan, M.M. and Wathes, D.C. (2008) Aspects of heifer rearing. *Cattle Practice* 16, 183–187.

Brickell, J., Bourne, N., McGowan, M. and Wathes, D. (2009) Effect of growth and development during the rearing period on the subsequent fertility of nulliparous Holstein-Friesian heifers. *Theriogenology* 72, 408–416.

Caraviello, D., Weigel, K., Fricke, P., Wiltbank, M., Florent, M., Cook, N. *et al.* (2006) Survey of management practices on reproductive performance of dairy cattle on large US commercial farms. *Journal of Dairy Science* 89, 4723–4735.

Charlier, J., Claerebout, E., Duchateau, L. and Vercruysse, J. (2005) A survey to determine relationships between bulk tank milk antibodies against *Ostertagia ostertagi* and milk production parameters. *Veterinary Parasitology* 129, 67–75.

Charlier, J., Dorny, P., Levecke, B., Demeler, J., von Samson-Himmelstjerna, G., Höglund, J. *et al.* (2011) Serum pepsinogen levels to monitor gastrointestinal nematode infections in cattle revisited. *Research in Veterinary Science* 90, 451–456.

Chebel, R.C., Guagnini, F.S., Santos, J.E., Fetrow, J.P. and Lima, J.R. (2010) Sex-sorted semen for dairy heifers: Effects on reproductive and lactational performances. *Journal of Dairy Science* 93, 2496–2507.

Coles, G.C. (2003) Strategies to minimise anthelmintic resistance in large animal practice. *In Practice* 25, 494–499.

Coles, G.C., Watson, C.L., and Anziani, O.S. (2001) Ivermectin-resistant Cooperia in Cattle. *Veterinary Record* 148, 283–284.

Coles, G.C., Stafford, K.A. and Morgan, E.R. (2010) Anthelmintic resistant worms of cattle - a common problem? *Cattle Practice* 18, 139–141.

Cornelissen, A.W., Verstegen, R., van den Brand, H., Perie, N.M., Eysker, M., Lam, T.J. *et al.* (1995) An observational study of *Eimeria* species in housed cattle on Dutch dairy farms. *Veterinary Parasitology* 56, 7–16.

Craig, T.M. (2006) Anthelmintic resistance and alternative control methods. *Veterinary Clinics of North America (Food Animal Practice)* 22, 567–581.

Cringoli, G., Rinaldi, L., Maurelli, M.P. and Utzinger, J. (2010) FLOTAC: new multivalent techniques for qualitative and quantitative copromicroscopic diagnosis of parasites in animals and humans. *Nature Protocols* 5, 503–515.

Crouch, C.F., Oliver, S. and Francis, M.J. (2001) Serological, colostral and milk responses of cows vaccinated with a single dose of a combined vaccine against rotavirus, coronavirus and *Escherichia coli* F5 (K99). *Veterinary Record* 149, 105–108.

Daniels, K.M., McGilliard, L.M., Meyer, M.L., Van Amburgh, M.E., Capuco, A.V. and Akers, R.M. (2009) Effects of body weight and nutrition on histological mammary development in Holstein heifers. *Journal of Dairy Science* 92, 499–505.

Daugschies, A. and Najdrowski M. (2005) Eimeriosis in cattle: Current understanding. *Journal of Veterinary Medicine. B, Infectious Diseases and Veterinary Public Health* 52, 417–427.

De Vries, A., Olson, J.D. and Pinedo, P.J. (2010) Reproductive risk factors for culling and productive life in large dairy herds in the eastern United States between 2001 and 2006. *Journal of Dairy Science* 93, 613–623.

De Waele, V., Speybroeck, N., Berkvens, D., Mulcahy, G. and Murphy, T.M. (2010) Control of cryptosporidiosis in neonatal calves: Use of halofuginone lactate in two different calf rearing systems. *Preventive Veterinary Medicine* 96, 143–151.

Dechow, C.D. and Goodling, R.C. (2008) Mortality, culling by sixty days in milk, and production profiles in high- and low-survival Pennsylvania herds. *Journal of Dairy Science* 91, 4630–4639.

Donovan, G.A., Dohoo, I.R., Montgomery, D.M., and Bennett, F.L. (1998) Calf and disease factors affecting growth in female Holstein calves in Florida, USA. *Preventive Veterinary Medicine* 33, 1–10.

Donovan, G.A., Bennett, F.L. and Springer F.S. (2003) Factors associated with first service conception in artificially inseminated nulliparous Holstein heifers. *Theriogenology* 60, 67–75.

Dorny, P., Shaw, D.J. and Vercruysse, J. (1999) The determination at housing of exposure to gastrointestinal nematode infections in first-grazing season calves. *Veterinary Parasitology* 80, 325–340.

Drew, B. and Pointer, C.G. (1977) The effect of level of nutrition on fertility in Friesian heifers in autumn and early winter. In: *EAAP 28th Annual Meeting*, Brussels, 22–27 August. *Commission on Animal Health and Production*, paper 77/8, 1–3.

Elsener, J., Villeneuve, A. and DesCôteaux, L. (2001) Evaluation of a strategic deworming programme in dairy heifers in Quebec based on the use of moxidectin, an endectocide with a long persistency. *Canadian Veterinary Journal* 42, 38–44.

Epe, C., von Samson-Himmelstjerna, G., Wirtherle, N., von der Heyden, V., Welz, C., Beening, J. *et al.* (2005) Efficacy of toltrazuril as a metaphylactic and therapeutic treatment of coccidiosis in first-year grazing calves. *Parasitology Research* 97(Suppl. 1), S127–S133.

Esslemont, R.J. (1992) Measuring dairy herd fertility. *Veterinary Record* 131, 209–212.

Esslemont, R.J. and Kossaibati, M.A. (1996) Incidence of production diseases and other health problems in a group of dairy herds in England. *Veterinary Record* 139, 486–490.

Esslemont, R.J. and Kossaibati, M.A. (1997) Culling in 50 dairy herds in England. *Veterinary Record* 140, 36–39.

Esslemont, R.J. and Kossaibati, M.A. (2002) DAISY Research Report No. 5, University of Reading, UK.

Ettema, J.F. and Santos, J.E. (2004) Impact of age at calving on lactation, reproduction, health, and income in first-parity Holsteins on commercial farms. *Journal of Dairy Science* 87, 2730–2742.

Faulkner, P.M. and Weary, D.M. (2000) Reducing pain after dehorning in dairy calves. *Journal of Dairy Science* 83, 2037–2041.

Foldager, J. and Sejrsen, K. (1982) Nutrition of replacement heifers affects mammary development and their ability to produce milk. In: *World Congress on Diseases of Cattle*, The Netherlands, vol. I, 45.

Frank, N.A. and Kaneene, J.B. (1993) Management risk factors associated with calf diarrhoea in Michigan dairy herds. *Journal of Dairy Science* 76, 1313–1323.

Fuerst-Waltl, B. and Sørensen, M.K. (2010) Genetic analysis of calf and heifer losses in Danish Holstein. *Journal of Dairy Science* 93, 5436–5442.

Gasbarre, L.C. and Canals, A. (1989) Induction of protective immunity in calves immunized with adult *Oesophagostomum radiatum* somatic antigens. *Veterinary Parasitology* 34, 223–238.

Godden, S.M., Smith, S., Feirtag, J.M., Green, L.R., Wells, S.J. and Fetrow, J.P. (2003) Effect of on-farm commercial batch pasteurization of colostrum on colostrum and serum immunoglobulin concentrations in dairy calves. *Journal of Dairy Science* 86, 1503–1512.

Gross, S.J., Ryan, W.G. and Ploeger, H.W. (1999) Anthelmintic treatment of dairy cows and its effect on milk production. *Veterinary Record* 144, 581–587.

Grove-White, D. (2000) Resuscitation of the newborn calf. *In Practice* 22, 17–23.

Gulliksen, S.M., Lie, K.I. and Østerås, A. (2009) Calf health monitoring in Norwegian dairy herds. *Journal of Dairy Science* 92, 1660–1669.

Gundelach, Y., Essmeyer, K., Teltscher, M.K. and Hoedemaker, M. (2009) Risk factors for perinatal mortality in dairy cattle: Cow and fetal factors, calving process. *Theriogenology* 71, 901–909.

Guy, M.A., McFadden, T., Cockrell, D. and Besser, T. (1994) Regulation of colostrum formation in beef and dairy cows. *Journal of Dairy Science* 77, 3002–3007.

Hadley, G.L., Wolf, C.A. and Harsh, S.B. (2006) Dairy cattle culling patterns, explanations, and implications. *Journal of Dairy Science* 89, 2286–2296.

Haworth, G.M., Tranter, W.P., Chuck, J.N., Cheng, Z. and Wathes, D.C. (2008) Relationships between age at first calving and first lactation milk yield, and lifetime productivity and longevity in dairy cows. *Veterinary Record* 162, 643–647.

Hoedemaker, M., Ruddat, I., Teltscher, M.K., Essmeyer, K. and Kreienbrock, L. (2010) Influence of animal, herd and management factors on perinatal mortality in dairy cattle - a survey in Thuringia, Germany. *Berliner und Munchener Tierarztliche Wochenschrift* 123, 130–136.

Hoffman, P.C. (1997) Optimum body size of Holstein replacement heifers. *Journal of Animal Science* 75, 836–845.

Hultgren, J., Svensson, C., Maizon, D. and Oltenacu, P.A. (2008) Rearing conditions, morbidity and breeding performance in dairy heifers in southwest Sweden. *Preventive Veterinary Medicine* 87, 244–260.

Kaplan, R.M. (2001) *Fasciola hepatica*: A review of the economic impact in cattle and considerations for control. *Veterinary Therapeutics* 2, 40–50.

Kertz, A.F., Barton, B.A. and Reutzel, L.F. (1998) Relative efficiencies of wither height and body weight increase from birth until first calving in Holstein cattle. *Journal of Dairy Science* 81, 1479–1482.

Kuhn, M.T., Hutchison, J.L. and Wiggans, G.R. (2006) Characterization of Holstein heifer fertility in the United States. *Journal of Dairy Science* 89, 4907–4920.

Lago, A., McGuirk, S.M., Bennett, T.B., Cook, N B. and Nordlund, K.V. (2006) Calf respiratory disease and pen microenvironments in naturally ventilated calf barns in winter. *Journal of Dairy Science* 89, 4014–4025.

Larsson, A., Dimander, S.O., Rydzik, A., Uggla, A., Waller, P.J. and Höglund, J. (2006) A 3-year field evaluation of pasture rotation and supplementary feeding to control parasite infection in first-season grazing cattle: Effects on animal performance. *Veterinary Parasitology* 142, 197–206.

López-Gatius, F. (2000) Short synchronization system for estrus cycles in dairy heifers: A preliminary report. *Theriogenology* 54, 1185–1190.

Lucy, M.C., Billings, H.J., Butler, W.R., Ehnis, L.R., Fields, M.J., Kesler, D.J. *et al.* (2001) Efficacy of an intravaginal progesterone insert and an injection of PGF2alpha for synchronizing estrus and shortening the interval to pregnancy in postpartum beef cows, peripubertal beef heifers, and dairy heifers. *Journal of Animal Science* 79, 982–995.

MAFF (1986) *Manual of Veterinary Parasitological Laboratory Techniques*. Her Majesty's Stationery Office, London.

Martin, S.W., Schwabe, C.W. and Franti, C.E. (1975) Dairy calf mortality rate: The association of daily meteorological factors and calf mortality. *Canadian Journal of Comparative Medicine* 39, 377–388.

Matjila, P.T. and Penzhorn, B.L. (2002) Occurrence and diversity of bovine coccidia at three localities in South Africa. *Veterinary Parasitology* 104, 93–102.

McCoy, M.A., Smyth, J.A., Ellis, W.A. and Kennedy, D.G. (1997) Stillbirth/perinatal weak calf syndrome. *Cattle Practice* 5, 31–34.

McDougall, S., Parker, K.I., Heuer, C. and Compton, C.W. (2009) A review of prevention and control of heifer mastitis via non-antibiotic strategies. *Veterinary Microbiology* 134, 177–185.

McGuirk, S.M. (2008) Disease management of dairy calves and heifers. *Veterinary Clinics of North America (Food Animal Practice)* 24, 139–153.

Mee, J.F. (2007) Perinatal calf mortality: Risk factors and prevention in dairy cows. *Cattle Practice* 15, 290.

Mejía, M., Gonzalez-Iglesias, A., Díaz-Torga, G.S., Villafañe, P., Formía, N., Libertun, C. *et al.* (1999) Effects of continuous ivermectin treatment from birth to puberty on growth and reproduction in dairy heifers. *Journal of Animal Science* 77, 1329–1334.

Menzi, W. (1995) Heifer housing system for improved performance. In: *AABP Specialty Seminars. Seminar 13, Optimizing Dairy Heifer Replacement Programs*, San Antonio, Texas, 12–13.

Mohammed, H.O., Shearer, J.K. and Brenneman, J.S. (1991) Transfer of immunoglobulins and survival of newborn calves. *Cornell Veterinarian* 81, 173–182.

Mohammed, H.O., Wade, S.E. and Schaaf, S. (1999) Risk factors associated with *Cryptosporidium parvum* infection in dairy cattle in southeastern New York State. *Veterinary Parasitology* 83, 1–13.

Morin, D.E., Nelson, S.V., Reid, E.D., Nagy, D.W., Dahl, G.E. and Constable, P.D. (2010) Effect of colostral volume, interval between calving and first milking, and photoperiod on colostral IgG concentrations in dairy cows. *Journal of the American Veterinary Medical Association* 237, 420–428.

Mourits, M.C., Dijkhuizen, A.A., Huirne, R.B. and Galligan, D.T. (1997) Technical and economic models to support heifer management decisions: Basic concepts. *Journal of Dairy Science* 80, 1406–1415.

Muller, L.D. and Ellinger, D.K. (1981) Colostral immunoglobulin concentrations among breeds of dairy cattle. *Journal of Dairy Science* 64, 1727–1730.

Oakley, G.A., Owen, B. and Knapp, N.H. (1979) Production effects of subclinical liver fluke infection in growing dairy heifers. *Veterinary Record* 104, 503–507.

Parker, K.I., Compton, C., Anniss, F.M., Weir, A., Heuer, C. and McDougall, S. (2007) Subclinical and clinical mastitis in heifers following the use of a teat sealant precalving. *Journal of Dairy Science* 90, 207–218.

Parker, K.I., Compton, C., Anniss, F.M., Weir, A., Heuer, C. and McDougall, S. (2008) Quarter-level analysis of subclinical and clinical mastitis in primiparous heifers following the use of a teat sealant or an injectable antibiotic, or both, precalving. *Journal of Dairy Science* 91, 169–181.

Passchyn, P., Piepers, S., Schmitt-Van de Leemput, E., Guidarini, C. and De Vliegher, S. (2010) Concentration of penicillin G in mammary tissue and secretion of end-term dairy heifers following systemic prepartum administration of penethamate hydriodide. *Journal of Dairy Research* 77, 33–36.

Peeler, I.D., Nebel, R.L., Pearson, R.E., Swecker, W.S. and Garcia, A. (2004) Pregnancy rates after timed AI of heifers following removal of intravaginal progesterone inserts. *Journal of Dairy Science* 87, 2868–2873.

Petrie, L. (1984) Maximising the absorption of colostral immunoglobulins in the newborn dairy calf. *Veterinary Record* 114, 157–163.

Pilarczyk, B. (1999) Economical consequences of coccidia infection in calves. *Wiadomosci Parazytologiczne* 45, 199–205.

Pinedo, P.J., De Vries, A. and Webb, D.W. (2010) Dynamics of culling risk with disposal codes reported by Dairy Herd Improvement dairy herds. *Journal of Dairy Science* 93, 2250–2261.

Potgieter, L.N. (1997) Bovine respiratory tract disease caused by bovine viral diarrhea virus. *Veterinary Clinics of North America (Food Animal Practice)* 13, 471–481.

Prichard, R.K., Hall, C.A., Kelly, J.D., Martin, I.C. and Donald, A.D. (1980) The problem of anthelmintic resistance in nematodes. *Australian Veterinary Journal* 56, 239–251.

Pritchett, L.C., Gay, C.C., Besser, T.E. and Hancock, D.D. (1991) Management and production factors influencing immunoglobulin G1 concentration in colostrum from Holstein cows. *Journal of Dairy Science* 74, 2336–2341.

Pursley, J.R., Wiltbank, M.C., Stevenson, J.S., Ottobre, J.S., Garverick, H.A. and Andeson, L.L. (1997) Pregnancy rates per artificial insemination for cows and heifers inseminated at a synchronized ovulation or synchronized estrus. *Journal of Dairy Science* 80, 295–300.

Quigley, J.D., Strohbehn, R.E., Kost, C.J. and O'Brien, M.M. (2001) Formulation of colostrum supplements, colostrum replacers and acquisition of passive immunity in neonatal calves. *Journal of Dairy Science* 84, 2059–2065.

Raboisson, D., Cahuzac, E., Sans, P. and Allaire, G. (2011) Herd-level and contextual factors influencing dairy cow mortality in France in 2005 and 2006. *Journal of Dairy Science* 94, 1790–1803.

Ridpath, J. (2010) The contribution of infections with bovine viral diarrhea viruses to bovine respiratory disease. *Veterinary Clinics of North America (Food Animal Practice)* 26, 335–348.

Rivera, H., Lopez, H. and Fricke, P.M. (2004) Fertility of Holstein dairy heifers after synchronization of ovulation and timed AI or AI after removed tail chalk. *Journal of Dairy Science* 87, 2051–2061.

Rivera, H., Lopez, H. and Fricke, P.M. (2005) Use of intravaginal progesterone-releasing inserts in a synchronization protocol before timed AI and for synchronizing return to estrus in Holstein heifers. *Journal of Dairy Science* 88, 957–968.

Rivera, H., Sterry, R.A. and Fricke, P.M. (2006) Presynchronization with gonadotropin-releasing hormone does not improve fertility in Holstein heifers. *Journal of Dairy Science* 89, 3810–3816.

Roberts, A.J., Geary, T.W., Grings, E.E., Waterman, R.C. and MacNeil, M.D. (2009) Reproductive performance of heifers offered ad libitum or restricted access to feed for a one hundred forty-day period after weaning. *Journal of Animal Science* 87, 3043–3052.

Rocha, A., Martins, A. and Carvalheira, J. (2010) Fertility time trends in dairy herds in northern Portugal. *Reproduction in Domestic Animals* 45, 896–899.

Sampimon, O.C., De Vliegher, S., Barkema, H.W., Sol, J. and Lam, T.J. (2009) Effect of prepartum dry cow antibiotic treatment in dairy heifers on udder health and milk production. *Journal of Dairy Science* 92, 4395–4403.

Sanchez, J. and Dohoo, I. (2002) A bulk tank milk survey of *Ostertagia ostertagi* antibodies in dairy herds in Prince Edward Island and their relationship with herd management factors and milk yield. *Canadian Veterinary Journal* 43, 454–459.

Sejrsen, K., Huber, J.T. and Tucker, H.A. (1983) Influence of amount fed on hormone concentrations and their relationship to mammary growth in heifers. *Journal of Dairy Science* 66, 845–855.

Sejrsen, K., Purup, S., Vestergaard, M. and Foldager, J. (2000) High body weight gain and reduced bovine mammary growth: Physiological basis and implications for milk yield potential. *Domestic Animal Endocrinology* 19, 93–104.

Selim, S.A. and Cullor, J.S. (1997) Number of viable bacteria and presumptive antibiotic residues in milk fed to calves on commercial dairies. *Journal of the American Veterinary Medical Association* 211, 1029–1035.

Silva del Río, N., Stewart, S., Rapnicki, P., Chang, Y.M. and Fricke, P.M. (2007) An observational analysis of twin births, calf sex ratio, and calf mortality in Holstein dairy cattle. *Journal of Dairy Science* 90, 1255–1264.

Silverlås, C., Björkman, C. and Egenvall, A. (2009) Systematic review and meta-analyses of the effects of halofuginone against calf cryptosporidiosis. *Preventive Veterinary Medicine* 91, 73–84.

Snodgrass, D.R. (1986) Evaluation of a combined rotavirus and enterotoxigenic *Escherichia coli* vaccine in cattle. *Veterinary Record* 119, 39–42.

Stafford, K. and Coles, G.C. (1999) Nematode control practices and anthelmintic resistance in dairy calves in the south west of England. *Veterinary Record* 144, 659–661.

Stevenson, J.L., Rodrigues, J.A., Brage, F.A., Bitente, S., Dalton, J.C., Santos, J.E. *et al.* (2008) Effect of breeding protocols and reproductive tract score on reproductive performance of dairy heifers and economic outcome of breeding programmes. *Journal of Dairy Science* 91, 3424–3438.

Stromberg, B.E. and Gasbarre, L.C. (2006) Gastrointestinal nematode control programmes with an emphasis on cattle. *Veterinary Clinics of North America (Food Animal Practice)* 22, 543–565.

Svensson, C., Lundborg, K., Emanuelson, U. and Olsson, S.O. (2003) Morbidity in Swedish dairy calves from birth to 90 days of age and individual calf-level risk factors for infectious diseases. *Preventive Veterinary Medicine* 58, 179–197.

Svensson, C., Hultgren, J. and Oltenacu, P.A. (2006) Morbidity in 3–7-month-old dairy calves in southwestern Sweden, and risk factors for diarrhoea and respiratory disease. *Preventive Veterinary Medicine* 74, 162–179.

Swanson, E.W., Bearden, B.J., Culvahouse, E.W. and Miles J.T. (1967) Restricting growth of cattle without depressing lactation. *Journal of Dairy Science* 50, 863–869.

Taylor, M.A. (2010) COWS – Control of Worms Sustainably. A technical manual for veterinary surgeons and advisors. Agriculture and Horticulture Development Board, Kenilworth, UK.

Taylor, M.A., Catchpole, J., Marshall, J., Marshall, R.N. and Hoeben, D. (2003) Histopathological observations on the activity of diclazuril (Vecoxan) against the endogenous stages of *Eimeria crandallis* in sheep. *Veterinary Parasitology* 116, 305–314.

Tenhagen, B.A., Kuchenbuch, S. and Heuwieser, W. (2005) Timing of ovulation and fertility of heifers after synchronization of oestrus with GnRH and prostaglandin F(2alpha). *Reproduction in Domestic Animals* 40, 62–67.

Tozer, P.R. and Heinrichs, A.J. (2001) What affects the cost of rearing replacement dairy heifers: a multiple component analysis. *Journal of Dairy Science* 84(8), 1836–1844.

Trotz-Williams, L.A., Martin, S.W., Martin, D., Duffield, T., Leslie, K.E., Nydam, D.V. *et al.* (2005) Multiattribute evaluation of two simple tests for the detection of *Cryptosporidium parvum* in calf faeces. *Veterinary Parasitology* 134, 15–23.

Trotz-Williams, L.A., Jarvie, B.D., Peregrine, A.S., Duffield, T.F. and Leslie, K.E. (2011) Efficacy of halofuginone lactate in the prevention of cryptosporidiosis in dairy calves. *Veterinary Record* 168, 509.

Uhde, F.L., Kaufmann, T., Sager, H., Albini, S., Zanoni, R., Schelling, E. *et al.* (2008) Prevalence of four enteropathogens in the faeces of young diarrhoeic dairy calves in Switzerland. *Veterinary Record* 163, 362–366.

USDA (2010) USDA Dairy 2007. *Management* (January).

Vasseur, E., Borderas, F., Cue, R.I., Lefebvre, D., Pellerin, D., Rushen, J. *et al.* (2010) A survey of dairy calf management practices in Canada that affect animal welfare. *Journal of Dairy Science*, 93, 1307–1315.

Villarroel, A., Dargatz, D.A., Lane, V.M., McCluskey, B.J. and Salman, M.D. (2007) Suggested outline of potential critical control points for biosecurity and biocontainment on large dairy farms. *Journal of the American Veterinary Medical Association* 230, 808–819.

Virtala, A.M., Mechor, G.D., Gröhn, Y.T. and Erb, H.N. (1996) The effect of calfhood diseases on growth of female dairy calves during the first 3 months of life in New York State. *Journal of Dairy Science* 79, 1040–1049.

Waltner-Toews, D., Martin, S.W. and Meek, A.H. (1986) The effect of early calfhood health status on survivorship and age at first calving. *Canadian Journal of Veterinary Research* 50, 314–317.

Warnick, L.D., Erb, H.N. and White, M.E. (1997) The relationship of calfhood morbidity with survival after calving in 25 New York Holstein herds. *Preventive Veterinary Medicine* 31, 263–273.

Wathes, C.M., Jones, C.D. and Webster, A.J. (1983) Ventilation, air hygiene and animal health. *Veterinary Record* 113, 554–559.

Weaver, D.M., Tyler, J.W., VanMetre, D.C., Hostetler, D.E. and Barrington, G.M. (2000) Passive transfer of colostral immunoglobulins in calves. *Journal of Veterinary Internal Medicine* 14, 569–577.

Webster, K.A., Smith, H.V., Giles, M., Dawson, L. and Robertson, L.J. (1996) Detection of *Cryptosporidium parvum* oocysts in faeces: comparison of conventional coproscopical methods and the polymerase chain reaction. *Veterinary Parasitology* 61, 5–13.

Wells, S.J., Dee, S. and Godden, S. (2002) Biosecurity for gastrointestinal diseases of adult dairy cattle. *Veterinary Clinics of North America (Food Animal Practice)* 18, 35–55.

Whitaker, D.A., Kelly, J.M. and Smith, S. (2000) Disposal and disease rates in 340 British dairy herds. *Veterinary Record* 146, 363–367.

Windsor, P.A. and Whittington, R.J. (2010) Evidence for age susceptibility of cattle to Johne's disease. *Veterinary Journal* 184, 37–44.

Xue, W., Ellis, J., Mattick, D., Smith, L., Brady, R. and Trigo, E. (2010) Immunogenicity of a modified-live virus vaccine against bovine viral diarrhoea virus types 1 and 2, infectious bovine rhinotracheitis virus, bovine parainfluenza-3 virus, and bovine respiratory syncytial virus when administered intranasally in young calves. *Vaccine* 28, 3784–3792.

Yang, C., Gibbs, H.C. and Xiao, L. (1993) Immunologic changes in *Ostertagia ostertagi*-infected calves treated strategically with an anthelmintic. *American Journal of Veterinary Research* 54, 1074–1083.

Young, G.B., Lee, G.J., Waddington, D., Sales, D.I., Bradley, J.S. and Spooner, R.L. (1983) Culling and wastage in dairy cows in East Anglia. *Veterinary Record* 113, 107–111.

Yusuf, M., Nakao, T., Yoshida, C., Long, S.T., Fujita, S., Inayoshi. Y. *et al.* (2010) Comparison in effect of Heatsynch with heat detection aids and CIDR-Heatsynch in dairy heifers. *Reproduction in Domestic Animals* 45, 500–504.

# 4 Managing Herd Reproduction

**Chris Hudson,[1] Mike Kerby,[2] Jonathan Statham[3] and Wendela Wapenaar[1]**
[1]*School of Veterinary Medicine and Science, University of Nottingham, Sutton Bonington Campus, Leicestershire LE12 5RD, UK;* [2]*Delaware Veterinary Group, Fulford House, Torbay Road, Castle Cary, Somerset BA7 7DT, UK;* [3]*Bishopton Veterinary Group, Mill Farm, Studley Road, Ripon, North Yorkshire HG4 2QR, UK*

## Introduction

Reproductive inefficiency influences herd milk production, culling rate, calving pattern, genetic progress and profitability, and is estimated to cost the major dairy economies hundreds of millions of euros per year. Milk production in the average dairy herd has risen enormously over the past 20 years, as the result of increased genetic merit through widespread adoption of AI and significant advances in nutrition and management. For example, the US dairy cattle population peaked in 1944 at an estimated 25.6 million animals with a total annual milk production of approximately 53.1 billion kg (USDA, 1961). By 1997, dairy cattle numbers had declined to 9.2 million animals and total annual production was estimated at 70.8 billion kg (USDA, 1998): a 369% increase in milk yield for the average dairy cow in a little under 50 years. One apparent consequence of this huge change has been a negative impact on reproductive efficiency (Washburn *et al.*, 2002). Reversing this decline in reproductive performance is a priority for the industry.

The role of the veterinary surgeon in dairy herd fertility has changed radically in recent years. There has been a gradual shift away from treatment of individual animals towards management of fertility performance at herd level. More recently the role of the veterinary surgeon has evolved further, with more emphasis on using farm data to monitor the performance of the herd and the design of appropriate strategies to improve performance. Reproductive herd health in this sense appears to be a medium- to long-term activity for veterinary practitioners. Since fertility can be affected by a wide range of factors, it is important to ensure that herd management is tailored specifically to each individual herd. The herd's veterinary surgeon is ideally placed at the hub of the farm team to help monitor reproductive performance and develop appropriate solutions. In this chapter we describe the key activities involved in managing reproductive herd health. We start by providing background information, including that on economics and current levels of fertility performance. We then provide details on how to measure and monitor herd fertility and finally how to manage and enhance reproductive performance in a dairy herd.

### The economics of fertility

Reproductive performance has an influence on the profitability of dairy herds through two main routes:

- it affect the number of days between successive calvings; and

- it affect the proportion of the herd culled annually because of failure to re-conceive.

In addition to these two principal routes, specific reproductive diseases (such as endometritis, abortion and retained fetal membranes) add further financial cost. It is accepted that in the majority of cases, extending the interval between successive calvings (the calving interval) above a certain level will result in a decrease in profitability (Gonzalez-Recio et al., 2004; Evans et al., 2006; LeBlanc, 2007). Cows in late lactation (or with extended dry periods) are less profitable, both because they are producing less milk per day (and are earning less margin over feed cost per day than a cow in early lactation) and because feed conversion efficiency decreases over the course of the lactation (Britt et al., 2003; Cook, 2010).

The length of calving interval at which a further reduction does not improve profitability has historically been considered to be 365 days (Esslemont, 2003), but this has been subject to recent debate. Extended lactations have attracted a large amount of interest, possibly due in part to the gulf between an 'ideal' 365-day calving interval and level of performance in the vast majority of herds (see 'Current levels of reproductive performance'). While there has been research published suggesting that intentionally extended lactations (and therefore calving intervals) can be more profitable, this has often been conducted on cows in very high-producing herds which conceived within a specific time window (Arbel et al., 2001). In the majority of cases, the absolute optimum value for calving interval is not critical, as it is likely to be well below the current level of achievement.

It is important to remember when evaluating the economic impact of reproductive performance on a herd that both calving interval and excess culling represent sources of loss, so it is critical to evaluate both together to provide an estimate of the overall lost profit due to fertility. The unit costs for both of these can vary substantially between farms, and it is difficult to calculate standard figures that will be applicable across a range of circumstances. For this reason, cost calculations should ideally be tailored to a specific herd: use of 'average' figures can lead to disengagement with farm owners and managers. It is important to have an understanding of the factors that will alter the cost of a day added to the calving interval (see Box 4.1 and Table 4.1) or an unplanned cull.

There are a number of methods for calculation of cost of a cull, but at the simplest level this can be estimated by the cost of purchasing a similar replacement animal at the point of calving minus the sale value of the culled cow. Even where homebred replacements are used this is a valid concept, as each cow culled requires a homebred replacement which could otherwise be sold. It is useful to combine losses from extended calving intervals and culling into a single figure, with a recognized method for this being the FERTEX score (Esslemont and Kossaibati, 2002), or modifications thereof. This provides an estimate of the total lost profit per year due to suboptimal reproductive performance by adding together losses from calving interval, culling and service costs.

## Current levels of reproductive performance

Although a detailed comparison of fertility performance worldwide is difficult, there is substantial evidence that reproductive performance has been in decline over the past 20–30 years. Reproductive performance also varies markedly between nations, due in part to variation in farming systems throughout the world. Performance generally tends to be poorer in high-input, high-output systems whereas more extensive systems tend to achieve better fertility. There is also increased necessity for good reproductive performance in herds that depend on seasonal 'block' calving. A summary of reproductive performance from a variety of major dairying nations is shown in Table 4.2. The different indices used to monitor fertility in different areas make direct comparisons difficult, and this is compounded by the different balances between calving interval and culling driven by the economics of different farming systems (e.g. calving interval in intensively managed herds in the USA will often be extended in order to minimize culling, while extensive herds in New Zealand are more likely to maintain their calving index, and so calving pattern, at the expense of culling). Added to these factors, there is an element of selection bias in studies reporting fertility performance, because measurement of this relies on farmer data recording (thus the results of such studies may reflect fertility performance in herds with relatively good data recording).

---

**Box 4.1.** Factors affecting the cost of an increase in calving interval.

- **Milk yield and lactation curve shape:** the main component of economic loss by extending a cow's calving interval comes from lost milk production, as extending the interval is effectively 'postponing' her next lactation, and replacing it with an extra day on the end of her current lactation. Lost milk production can therefore be represented as the predicted mean daily yield for the next lactation minus the predicted mean yield at the end of the current lactation. This will partly depend on the degree of persistency of yield during lactation.
- **Degree of extension of calving interval:** as calving interval increases, the yield at the end of the current lactation diminishes. The cost per day of extension will therefore increase with increasing calving interval.
- **Margin over purchased feed (cost per litre):** margin over purchased feed is a term used to represent the cost of lost milk sales offset by the reduction in feed costs. A decrease in milk production, as outlined above, will result in a decrease in feed requirement to support the lower yield. It is therefore not the absolute value of milk sales lost that is important but the margin associated with that loss.
- **Calf value:** a cow calving less frequently will produce fewer calves during her lifetime, i.e. another source of lost profit. Calf value can be extremely variable from herd to herd, depending on sire selection (especially proportion of dairy and beef sires used) and market calf prices.
- **Cost of extra serves and veterinary interventions:** again, this can be very variable between herds and should be estimated for each situation.
- **Gains through decreased chance of calving-associated disease and increased early lactation yield in non-pregnant cows:** it is important to note that because fewer calvings occur when calving interval is extended, there is often a cost saving from the associated reduction in peri-parturient disease. An additional decrease in yield for pregnant cows early in lactation is also reported. Again, these should be estimated for each farm; typical gains of 43 pence and 13 pence per day, respectively have been reported (Esslemont and Kossaibati, 2002).

---

**Table 4.1.** Example calculation of the cost of a one-day increase in calving interval. This is a sample calculation for a herd with a 9000 l average 305-day yield and a relatively flat lactation curve shape (reflected in the relatively high estimated yields at drying off). For example, additional days added to a cow's calving interval in the region of 396–425 days effectively entails postponing the cow's next lactation (estimated average yield 29.5 l/day) and adding extra days at the end of this lactation (estimated yield 21.1 l/day). This loss of 8.4 l/day of production will lead to a loss of £1.31/day in margin over purchased feed. If an average calf is worth around £200 and the herd's target calving interval is 380 days, the value of lost calf sales is around £0.53/day (£200/380 days). Inclusion of the additional costs and gains at the bottom of the table result in an estimated lost profit of around £1.98/day.

| Calving interval range (days) | 365–395 | 396–425 | 426–455 |
|---|---|---|---|
| Likely days in milk at drying off | 330 | 360 | 390 |
| Estimated daily yield at drying off (l) | 22.5 | 21.1 | 20.4 |
| Estimated daily yield in next lactation (l) | 29.5 | 29.5 | 29.5 |
| Lost production (l/day) | 7.1 | 8.4 | 9.1 |
| Margin over purchased feed (£ cent/l) | 15.6 | 15.6 | 15.6 |
| Cost of lost margin over feed (£/day) | 1.1 | 1.31 | 1.41 |
| Cost of lost calf production (£/day) | 0.53 | 0.53 | 0.53 |
| Cost of extra serves/vet. spend (£/day) | 0.7 | 0.7 | 0.7 |
| Gain by reducing disease risk (£/day) | 0.43 | 0.43 | 0.43 |
| Gain in yield for empty cows (£/day) | 0.13 | 0.13 | 0.13 |
| Total cost (£/day) | 1.77 | 1.98 | 2.08 |

**Table 4.2.** Levels of reproductive performance reported in studies from a variety of major dairying nations.

| Parameter | Country | Year(s) | Value | Reference |
|---|---|---|---|---|
| Calving index (days) | USA | 2000 | 429 | deVries and Risco (2005) |
| | Ireland | 2000 | 395 | Mee (2004) |
| | Norway | 2005 | 383 | Refsdal (2007) |
| | USA | 2006 | 422 | Norman et al. (2009) |
| | UK | 2007 | 418 | Hudson et al. (2010) |
| | UK | 2009 | 426 | National Milk Records plc (2009) |
| Failure to conceive (%) | Ireland | 2000 | 14 | Mee (2004) |
| | New Zealand | 2002–2004 | 9.0–10.2 | Compton and McDougall (2010) |
| | Norway | 2005 | 6 | Refsdal (2007) |
| | UK | 2007 | 10 | Hudson et al. (2010) |
| 8-week in-calf rate (%)[a] | New Zealand | 2002–2004 | 78–83 | Compton and McDougall (2010) |
| 6-week in-calf rate (%)[b] | Australia, seasonal | 1996–1998 | 63 | Morton (2003) |
| 100-day in-calf rate (%)[c] | Australia, year-round | 1996–1998 | 53 | Morton (2003) |
| | UK | 2007 | 34 | Hudson et al. (2010) |
| Calving to first service interval (days) | USA | 2001 | 104 | deVries and Risco (2005) |
| | Norway | 2005 | 86 | Refsdal (2007) |
| | USA | 2006 | 86 | Norman et al. (2009) |
| Pregnancy rate (%)[d] | USA | 2006 | 30 | Norman et al. (2009) |
| | UK | 2007 | 37 | Hudson et al. (2010) |
| First service pregnancy rate (%) | Australia | 1996–1998 | 49 | Morton (2003) |
| | USA | 2006 | 31 | Norman et al. (2009) |

[a] Defined as percentage of cows eligible for service at the start of the breeding season that had conceived by 8 weeks into the breeding season. [b] Defined as percentage of cows eligible for service at the start of the breeding season that had conceived by 6 weeks into the breeding season. [c] Defined as percentage of cows eligible for service that had conceived by 100 days into lactation. [d] Defined as percentage of serves leading to a pregnancy.

## Welfare and ethics of reproductive herd health

There are a number of ways in which reproduction can have an impact on cow welfare, and management of reproductive performance raises ethical dilemmas. We shall now highlight the areas we consider most important.

The time around calving is a period of risk in terms of dairy cow welfare. The key elements to address are a suitable calving environment, appropriate supervision at calving and minimizing the risks of calving problems. It is a legal requirement in the UK that cows that calve when housed are kept in an area of sufficient size to permit access to provide aid with calving and that they are separate from other livestock. Size of calving accommodation is particularly important, as

this can also have health and safety implications for staff supervising calving (especially where mechanical calving aids are to be used). A minimum of 15 m² per cow should be provided where cows calve in a communal pen, and ideally more than 25 m² per cow in individual pens. Cleanliness and depth of bedding are also very important, and in a straw yard environment these elements can be particularly challenging to manage simultaneously. Freshly cleaned out and re-bedded calving accommodation often provides lower levels of comfort and underfoot grip (as this is usually supplemented by manure under the clean surface of the bed). Fresh straw should be added to calving pens at least once daily, and yards should be cleaned out at least once every four weeks. In addition, individual calving pens should be cleaned out and/or disinfected between cows. Use of a sand base under the straw pack can be helpful in providing grip, and also aids drainage.

Supervision should be provided at calving, whilst ensuring that calving cows are not disturbed unless there are indications that the birth process is not proceeding normally. Enough space should be available to allow cows to exhibit their normal behaviour at calving. If space is limited, heifers should not be housed with older cows, as the cows may dominate feeding and lying areas. Stock-keepers in charge of calving should be familiar with the signs that a cow is about to calve and well trained in caring for calving cows and their calves (including the use of mechanical calving aids).

There are several steps that can be taken to minimize the risk of dystocia, including ensuring that cows are at the correct condition at calving (see Chapter 8). It is also critical to ensure that heifers calve for the first time in appropriate body condition and with sufficient body size (see Chapter 3). Sire selection is very important in the prevention of dystocia. This involves ensuring that an appropriate breed of sire is selected (for example, avoidance of continental beef breeds associated with high birth-weight offspring in dairy heifers), but there is also substantial variation within breeds. In many countries (including the UK), calving ease indices are available as part of bull proofs, and should be considered in all sire selection decisions. Induction of calving has also been associated with dystocia, and should therefore be avoided where possible and should only be carried out under veterinary supervision.

It is also important to consider the welfare and ethical considerations of fertility management in herd health. Whilst other areas of herd health management (such as lameness, mastitis and infectious disease) have direct welfare implications, the welfare implications of inadequate reproductive management are often less clear. However, there are welfare consequences for extending a cow's calving interval, not least that she is likely to gain body condition in late lactation and calve over-fat at the next calving. This will increase the risk of dystocia, as well as having severe implications for

peri-parturient energy balance (see Chapter 8). Additionally, whilst culling itself should not impair welfare, there are ethical and environmental reasons to minimize failure-to-conceive culling rates.

Another ethical dilemma in reproductive management comes from the use of synthetic reproductive hormones. This has become increasingly popular in recent years, as fertility performance has declined. Use of hormone treatments to treat pathological ovarian and uterine conditions (such as cystic ovarian disease or endometritis) may raise few ethical concerns, but hormones are more commonly used for other reasons. For example, it is common in normal, cycling cows that are treated with hormonal products to see a reduction in the time to the animal's next oestrus. More recently, there has been increasing use of synchronization with a variety of hormone-based protocols to allow insemination at a fixed time without detection of oestrus. Whilst use of such treatments is considered to pose no threat to food safety or animal health, consumers may find the use of hormones for routine manipulation of breeding undesirable. An assessment of the ethics of this situation requires, amongst other things, consideration of whether it is acceptable to use hormonal products to help overcome management problems, and the balance to be struck between using hormonal products in normal cows and an increase in the number of fertility culls that would be expected if such treatments were withdrawn. Whilst the need for such treatments will vary widely between units, reduction in use of hormonal manipulation of reproduction would seem a prudent long-term aim of a herd health programme.

## Public health and reproduction

*Zoonotic diseases of reproductive importance*

Various zoonotic diseases of cattle are considered to be primarily of reproductive importance, and these are briefly outlined below.

BRUCELLOSIS.      Whilst the UK has been officially free of this infectious cause of abortion since 1985, it remains of great importance in other countries. In cattle it causes abortion (normally in the last third of gestation), and is often seen as explosive herd outbreaks. Infection of humans can occur either by direct contact with aborted material (fetus and placenta) or via consumption of unpasteurized dairy products. Symptoms in humans include intermittent fever, joint pain and headache; onset can be acute or insidious.

LEPTOSPIROSIS.    Leptospirosis is a group of conditions caused by a variety of serovars of the bacterium *Leptospira interrogans*, which is discussed in more detail in Chapter 7. Whilst the serovars commonly causing reproductive disease in cattle are different to those considered most pathogenic in humans, occupational exposure to cattle is a recognized route of infection and risk factor for human disease. Urine is the main source of infection, and in dairy herds exposure of milking personnel in the parlour is a major risk. Clinical signs in humans include flu-like symptoms, muscle pain and fever. Severe complications follow in a small proportion of cases.

Q FEVER.    This is a potential cause of abortion in cattle caused by the bacterium *Coxiella burnetii*. It can be spread to humans by either direct or indirect contact (the spore-like form of the organism is very resilient in the environment, and the organism can also be present in milk from infected individuals). Infection in humans is characterized by fever, headaches and muscle pain. Some cases are complicated by pneumonia, and chronic disease is also a feature.

## Underlying Principles of Dairy Cow Reproduction

### Reproductive physiology and hormonal control of the oestrous cycle

Although the focus of this book is not on the individual animal, we provide a brief outline of some reproductive physiology to give context to hormonal control of the oestrous cycle. We emphasize our belief that improved herd management is the preferred route to improved reproductive performance, rather than through hormonal treatments, but it should be acknowledged that often both approaches are used.

Important features of the hormonal basis for follicular development and oestrus control are summarized in Fig. 4.1. The main principles of therapeutic manipulation of the oestrous cycle and synchronization of oestrus are provided in Box 4.2.

## Monitoring Reproduction in Herd Health

### The practicalities of data recording

The first step in monitoring of reproductive performance is the acquisition of data. Accurate recording of calving and service events, in conjunction with a source of basic cow data (including identity and parity number) and regular pregnancy diagnosis (see next section) are the bare minima required to conduct a successful reproductive programme. However, if more data are collected, this will allow a greater depth and accuracy of analysis and ultimately better decision making. In Box 4.3 we present data that we recommend are collected in regard to reproductive herd health.

There are a number of ways in which data can be captured, and below we highlight three main methods.

1. On-farm software: a wide variety of software packages exist that can be used to capture information on the farm. These may be linked to the milking plant, or may be stand-alone. Responsibility for keeping data up to date lies with the farmer, who is usually also able to access an assortment of extra management aids through the software.
2. Bureau recording systems: these rely on an outside organization holding data from the farm on a dedicated computer system. Typically, farmers are provided with data capture forms, which they fill in as events occur and which are then returned to the bureau for input to the computer system.

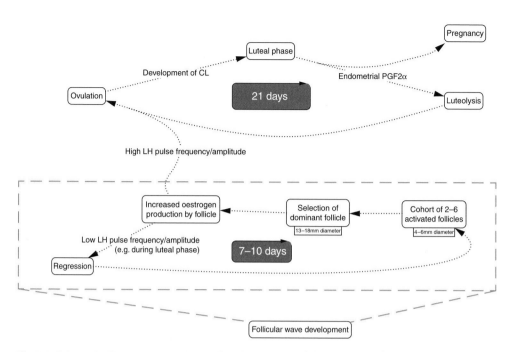

**Fig. 4.1.** Schematic diagram representing the functional events of the oestrous cycle. CL, corpus luteum; LH, luteinizing hormone; PG, prostaglandin.

---

**Box 4.2.** Outline of hormonal control and manipulation of the oestrous cycle.

The functional corpus luteum (CL) plays a pivotal role in the physiological control of the oestrous cycle, because the lifespan of the CL effectively determines the length of the cycle. The CL is therefore key to therapeutic approaches to manipulating the cycle. The two commonest approaches are:

- Use of exogenous synthetic prostaglandin analogues, leading to luteolysis of a CL from around day 5–day 17 post-oestrus. This effectively shortens the lifespan of the CL, cutting the cycle short and reducing number of days to the subsequent oestrus.
- Use of exogenous progestagen (usually via a sustained-release intravaginal device) to mimic the luteal phase of the cycle. Ovulation normally follows withdrawal of the progestagen source (provided that a functional CL is not present at the same time – this is often ensured using prostaglandin).

These approaches are often combined in programmes for synchronization of oestrus, and these are discussed in more detail later in the chapter.

---

Veterinary businesses are the most common agencies to offer this type of recording. It was popular in the UK in the early and mid-1990s, but has declined in prevalence with the falling cost of computing power and the general rise in computer literacy amongst the farming population.

**3.** Milk recording organizations: this is effectively an alternative type of bureau recording, where the data are collected and held by a milk-recording organization.

The main differences from method 2 are that data are usually only collected at each milk recording test day (normally monthly), and that the range of events and details that can be recorded is limited. Some milk-recording organizations offer a facility whereby farmers can enter event data directly into the central database via a web portal.

In many respects the first option is preferable, because it usually offers more flexibility

---

**Box 4.3.** Data recording required for fertility monitoring.

Each of the following events should be recorded (for each event, cow ID, date and any further specified details should be captured).

- calving (including occurrence of dystocia, Caesarean, stillbirth);
- oestrus (where no serve occurs, e.g. during the voluntary waiting period (VWP));
- service (including sire, AI/natural service, inseminator, observed oestrus/fixed-time AI);
- pregnancy diagnosis (including result);
- other veterinary fertility examinations (including diagnosis and treatment);
- retained fetal membranes (including treatment);
- metritis (including treatment);
- endometritis (including treatment); and
- abortion (including treatment).

(NB: we exclude here other important health-related data such as body condition score and mobility score, which are described in other chapters).

---

in data entry and allows the greatest level of detail to be captured. It is also the least likely to suffer from 'data drift', where the database slowly becomes less representative of the situation on the farm (e.g. as cows are culled or join the herd without these events being recorded). However, this option does not suit all farmers.

Whatever the source of the data, it is important to be aware of the potential impact of poor data quality, which often arises simply from missing events (especially services). It should be remembered that since the final (i.e. successful) service in a lactation is often the most reliably recorded, analysis of data sets with missing service information tends to reveal poorer submission and better pregnancy rates than is actually the case. Some software systems provide an estimation of data quality, but it is always important to treat data critically. In particular, very high pregnancy rates should be viewed with suspicion. It is easy to check the efficiency of service (artificial insemination, AI) recording by counting the services carried out in a time period using the farm's paper records (e.g. artificial insemination chart or calendar) and comparing this with the same period in the data file.

A multiplicity of software systems provide analysis of fertility performance, each with strengths and weaknesses, and it is not our intention to review software systems here. More important is the way in which

reproductive monitoring is provided by the veterinary practitioner, and this is often done in one of two ways:

**1.** Intermittent data analysis and production of a written report, often performed away from the farm.
**2.** Regular data analysis using a computer with the client (e.g. during routine visits to the farm).

The second of these approaches is recommended, as it allows the most rapid detection of trends, as well as being easy to integrate into a routine. The two methods can of course be combined, with occasional written reports supplementing more regular 'live' monitoring sessions. We again emphasize the importance of establishing a transparent fee structure for the delivery of agreed herd health services, as described in Chapter 1. Larger herds will merit more frequent monitoring because a larger number of cows means that trends can be reliably evaluated over shorter time periods. As a rule, it is useful to evaluate the key indicators of fertility performance on at least a monthly basis.

### Monitoring reproductive data on the farm

*Routine fertility visits*

Routine veterinary visits are common on dairy farms and vary in frequency, depending on seasonality of breeding period and herd size. Visits often work best at weekly (large herds) or fortnightly intervals. Visits at three-weekly intervals are difficult to manage successfully because the interval does not fit easily with strategies for hormonal intervention. Reproductive visits should be a regular event because this will provide regular pregnancy diagnosis for monitoring purposes, and is also often a good route into other areas of herd health.

An action list summarizing cows that need attention at a routine fertility visit is advisable, and a suggested list of cows to be included is given below.

- post-natal checks of all (or high-risk) cows at around 21 days post-partum;
- vulval discharge: any cows where abnormal vaginal discharge has been observed;
- oestrus not observed (ONO, also known as not seen bulling); cows not observed in oestrus by a specified stage of lactation. In herds recording reference heats (during the voluntary waiting period), it is useful to examine all cows that have not demonstrated an oestrus during the voluntary waiting period. In herds where this information is not reliably recorded, cows reaching 24 days after the end of the voluntary waiting period without being served are often examined;
- pregnancy diagnosis from 25–35 days in gestation onwards dependent on use of ultrasound and experience of the practitioner;
- repeat breeder cows, served more than 5 times with regular service intervals; and
- cows overdue to calve or with no recorded event in the previous 250 days.

It is important to record veterinary findings and the use of medicines in a way that facilitates easy data entry and analysis. It is also wise to ensure that all farm staff and veterinary colleagues record data using the same coding structure, to maximize data reliability.

While examination and treatment of cows on an action list is likely to be of great benefit to the profitability of the farm business and is an important element of a reproductive visit, the clinician's involvement should extend far beyond this. Regular evaluation of performance data and inspection of the cows and their environment during the visit are critical, and the visit should include feedback on the data collected and a review of previous recommendations. This discussion should cover how specific changes and recommendations are to be implemented, and include all members of the farm team. Facilitating change in dairy herd health is considered in detail in Chapter 2.

When conducting routine fertility visits for a herd, setting goals is important. These goals will differ from farm to farm and it is worthwhile setting aside some time to make a list of medium- and long-term goals with regard to reproductive performance. Further details of this are provided in later sections, but it is important to appreciate that trends over time are often more important than reaching a preset target. Long-term goals should be reviewed on a yearly basis and are essential to guide the vet and farmer and to prioritize actions. It is important to look at previous and current performance when setting achievable goals for the future.

*Herds with limited data*

If no records are available it is impossible to monitor the herd's reproductive performance. Routine visits will still have value but it is important to realize that interventions made will be more problem-based, and focused on the findings during every visit. In this instance, an important step is to raise awareness that monitoring performance is one of the main benefits of routine veterinary involvement in fertility management, and that this should be put in place.

When data are very limited, a guide to reproductive performance can be obtained from the number of pregnancies expected at each visit. In year-round calving herds this is calculated by simply dividing the number of cows in the herd by the number of veterinary visits per year (under the assumption that each cow would ideally become pregnant once a year). In block-calving herds, the number of cows eligible is divided by the number of visits planned through the season (although in these herds more pregnancies are expected towards the start of the breeding season). Suggested measures of performance for herds where few data exist are shown in Table 4.3.

### Routine performance monitoring

*Pros and cons of calving interval and related indices*

A number of methods have been proposed for monitoring reproductive performance in dairy herds. When considering the relative merits of these methods, it is important to remember why fertility is important in a dairy herd: as discussed in 'The Economics of fertility' section, it will affect profitability primarily by determining the time between a cow's successive calvings (and so the length of lactation) and by contributing to the herd's cull rate. There is some logic in using these outcomes as a way to evaluate fertility performance in a herd. This is easily done: the average of the calving intervals in the herd is known as the herd calving index, and is a commonly used measure of overall

performance. While calving index provides a useful indicator of long-term performance in a herd, there are a number of reasons why it is a poor monitor when used alone:

- It is extremely retrospective: the end point of each calving interval is the cow's next calving, so a cow that conceives today will not alter the calving interval of the herd until she calves in around 280 days' time.

- It is dramatically influenced by culling strategy: herds where it is important that a short calving interval is maintained (e.g. those with a tight seasonal calving pattern, where long calving intervals will rapidly result in cows calving outside the season) will tend to cull cows not conceiving sufficiently quickly after calving, and thereby maintain a tight calving interval even in the face of poor reproductive performance.

Therefore, it is essential that calving interval is viewed in the context of the degree of fertility-related culling in a herd. Unfortunately, the proportion of the herd culled each year due to failure to conceive can be very difficult to calculate. Recording of reasons for culling in dairy herds is generally poor, and cows are often culled for more than one reason (a first-lactation heifer with a low somatic cell count (SCC) is likely

**Table 4.3.** Parameters for measuring fertility performance for use in herds in which few data are available.

| Parameter | Gives an indication of | Suggested target(s) |
|---|---|---|
| Number of positive pregnancy diagnoses at each visit | Overall fertility performance | Cows in herd/number of visits per year (year-round calving herds) Cows to breed/number of visits planned during breeding season (seasonal calving herds) |
| Proportion of pregnancy diagnoses that are positive | Predominantly detection of returns to service, but also affected by pregnancy rate | > 80% (in herds where pregnancy rate is at least 40%) |
| Number of normally cycling cows presented as ONO at each visit | Heat detection, especially in cows due for first service | < (0.5 × herd size)/number of visits per year (i.e. around 50% of cows examined over a year) |
| Number of cases of reproductive disease diagnosed at each visit | Incidence rates of endometritis, anoestrus, etc. | < (target lactational incidence of disease concerned as a fraction × herd size)/number of visits per year |

to be allowed a longer time to conceive than an older, high-SCC cow in the same herd). Proxy measures (such as the proportion of cows receiving a first serve during a lactation but ultimately not conceiving and ending the lactation as a cull) have some use, but there are many situations in which they provide an inaccurate picture of fertility culling. Thus it is ultimately very difficult to assess wastage due to poor fertility in a herd where reasons for culling are not accurately and reliably recorded. This in turn reduces the usefulness of calving interval in many herds.

In an attempt to improve the usefulness of the calving index, a variety of related measures have been developed. These generally comprise breaking down a calving index into its component parts (such as the calving to first service and calving to conception intervals: see Fig. 4.2), and summarizing these across the herd. Calving to conception interval provides similar information to the calving index, but in a less retrospective manner as the end point of the interval is a successful service (usually confirmed by pregnancy diagnosis), which clearly occurs some time before the subsequent calving. Calving to first service interval and first service to conception interval provide information about specific parts of the reproductive process, in contrast to the measures of overall performance described thus far.

However, these interval-based measures have a number of inherent limitations (Box 4.4). One of these is the difficulty in selecting a denominator (or 'at-risk') population for acquiring the interval data. This is often done by selecting a cohort of cows that calved over a specified period. This is problematic in that not all cows in the cohort may yet have reached the end point for the interval (e.g. may not have received a first serve); indeed, it is important to select a cohort such that the outcome (or end point) is known for every cow included. The problem of interval-based fertility indices is demonstrated using the examples in Box 4.4 and Table 4.4.

Summarizing interval data for a herd by calculating a single number can also be problematic. Traditionally, the mean has been used for this, but analysis of the distribution of intervals within the majority of herds reveals positively skewed distributions (i.e. there is a heavy 'tail' of longer intervals, see Fig. 4.3). Since outliers have a relatively strong influence on the value of the mean, alternative measures of a herd average are often considered. The median value is the most useful alternative, being less influenced by outliers and producing a more representative measure of general herd performance. However, this value provide no indication of the dispersion of the data (i.e. how widely the intervals are spread on either side of the

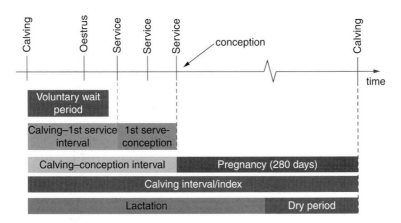

**Fig. 4.2.** Illustration of the construction of intervals during a lactation cycle.

---

**Box 4.4.** A herd example to illustrate the problems with the interpretation of interval-based fertility data.

**This example relates to the fertility data presented in Table 4.4.** Cows calving over the most recent months (to the right of the table) have had limited opportunities to be served: the mean calving to first service interval for cows calving in August 2009 was 59 days but this is based on just 9% of the cows calving in that month (i.e. only one of the 11 cows calving had been served at the date when the report was produced). Similarly, the interval for July is based on two of the four cows that calved in that month. This is clearly using incomplete data, but more problematically the intervals contributed for those months will not reflect those of the other cows calved in the same month still to contribute an interval – the majority of the other ten cows calved in August 2009 are likely to receive a first serve at some point, so we are likely to be including the shortest of the intervals for this month (introducing systematic bias into the analysis). Clearly this is relatively easily resolved by ensuring that a large majority of the cows in the cohort have had a first serve (in this example, perhaps by ending the analysis with cows calving in April 2009), but this often results in very historical results. This problem becomes even more marked when evaluating calving to conception interval (as this tends to be more variable between cows): in this example it would be very difficult to choose a sensible end point for the analysis, but it would seem unwise to rely on results for cows calving in any of the months in 2009 (as for each month a sizeable percentage of cows in the cohort has yet to conceive or be culled). If the time frame is pushed back to finish in December 2008, this problem will be much less important, but cows calving over the previous 9 months will contribute no information to the analysis.

Another related problem is that improvements in performance can be reflected in paradoxical increases in intervals to first service or conception: an increase in heat detection rates after a period of poor detection will lead to service of more cows in the herd, many of which may have calved a long time ago but failed to be detected in oestrus during the period of poor detection. When heat detection improves and these cows are finally served, their (highly extended) intervals to first service become available for analysis and can increase the herd average.

---

**Table 4.4.** Difficulty in choosing cohorts for interval analysis. This fertility summary report was run in October 2009 using cows calving from September 2008 to August 2009.

| Parameter | Total | Month of calving | | | | | | | | | | | |
| --- | --- | --- | --- | --- | --- | --- | --- | --- | --- | --- | --- | --- | --- |
| | | Sep 08 | Oct 08 | Nov 08 | Dec 08 | Jan 09 | Feb 09 | Mar 09 | Apr 09 | May 09 | Jun 09 | Jul 09 | Aug 09 |
| Number of cows calved | 113 | 16 | 18 | 11 | 8 | 13 | 8 | 7 | 6 | 4 | 7 | 4 | 11 |
| % served | 84 | 100 | 100 | 100 | 88 | 85 | 100 | 100 | 83 | 50 | 100 | 50 | 9 |
| % conceived | 57 | 94 | 78 | 64 | 88 | 62 | 88 | 43 | 0 | 50 | 14 | 0 | 0 |
| % re-calved | 11 | 44 | 28 | 0 | 0 | 0 | 0 | 0 | 0 | 0 | 0 | 0 | 0 |
| % culled or died | 10 | 6 | 16 | 18 | 0 | 15 | 0 | 0 | 17 | 0 | 0 | 0 | 18 |
| % not re-calved/ culled/died | 80 | 50 | 56 | 82 | 100 | 85 | 100 | 100 | 83 | 100 | 100 | 100 | 82 |
| Calving to first serve interval (days) | 83 | 77 | 84 | 93 | 84 | 74 | 79 | 80 | 115 | 68 | 85 | 76 | 59 |
| Calving to conception interval (days) | 115 | 119 | 120 | 119 | 121 | 114 | 105 | 121 | | 68 | 54 | | |
| First serve to conception interval (days) | 34 | 43 | 35 | 22 | 37 | 39 | 31 | 32 | | 0 | 0 | | |
| Calving interval (days) | 355 | 360 | 349 | | | | | | | | | | |

median value). For these reasons, it is essential to examine the distribution of the intervals (Fig. 4.3) as well as the mean and median.

## Monitoring herd fertility using rates

An alternative way to assess fertility data is by calculating rates. Rates provide a proportion of cases in which a specified criterion is

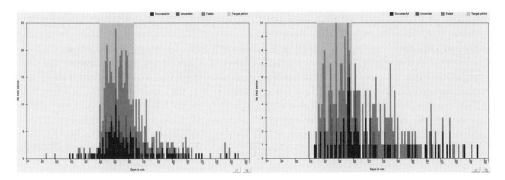

**Fig. 4.3.** Interval data taking a relatively symmetrical distribution (left) and a heavily positively skewed distribution (right) (Total Vet™; QMMS/SUM-IT software). Days in milk at first service are shown on the x-axis, with frequency on the y-axis.

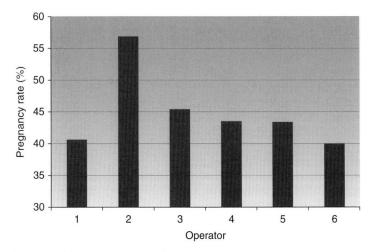

**Fig. 4.4.** Estimating the likely importance of difference between inseminators on pregnancy rate. Although operator 2 has a pregnancy rate that may be considered to be 'clinically' different to those of the other operators, the use of a statistical test helps us to make a meaningful comparison between groups because differences between groups can occur simply due to random variation. The most appropriate statistical test to use will depend on the data. As an example, a chi-squared test would be appropriate for the data presented in this figure, where we want to test the null hypothesis, 'The pregnancy rate achieved is the same between the operators' versus the alternative hypothesis, 'The pregnancy rate is not the same between the operators'. (NB: to apply this test to the data provided in this figure requires the expected number of pregnancies in each group to be > 5). The chi-squared test here produced a $p$-value of 0.65, which means that there is a low weight of evidence to reject the null hypothesis that the pregnancy rate is the same between operators (i.e. the probability of finding these data is quite high even if there is no real difference between inseminators). Thus, while it may be tempting at first glance to conclude that operator 2 is achieving a pregnancy rate that is different from the other operators, the current data do not support this. Furthermore, potential confounding factors are often forgotten here: for example, is operator 2 inseminating predominantly heifers?

met (e.g. the proportion of cows receiving a first serve within 24 days of becoming eligible, proportion of serves leading to a pregnancy) in a given time period. It is usually straightforward to define a denominator population for rate-based indices, and these usually do not need to be calculated in a retrospective fashion. However, there are also potential problems with summarizing data as rates: they provide only limited information about the population as a whole (e.g. a low first service submission rate is less damaging if most cows not served within 24 days of becoming eligible receive a first serve within the next few days after this), and great care has to be taken that the denominator population doesn't become too small. The latter issue is often countered by using three-month rolling average rates, but it is always wise to consider the size of the denominator population along with the rate.

When deciding which parameters are most useful in terms of measuring fertility performance, a useful framework is provided by evaluating the components of success in fertility management. Broadly speaking, there are only three things required in order to manage fertility successfully:

- submission for service: this encompasses oestrus expression and detection, as well as post-partum return to ovarian cyclicity;
- establishment of pregnancy: i.e. the likelihood of a pregnancy resulting from a given serve; and
- minimizing reproductive disease: effective management of diseases such as endometritis, abortion and retained fetal membranes is important in its own right.

*Measuring submission rates and oestrus detection*

Monitoring oestrus detection is a complex and very important area, as this will often be the main determinant of overall fertility performance in a herd. There are two main aspects of heat detection to evaluate: the proportion of heats being detected and the proportion of inaccurately detected heats. In some ways, these are analogous to the sensitivity and specificity of heat detection in the herd. It is useful to evaluate heat detection separately in cows being submitted for first service, and those returning to service.

MONITORING FIRST SERVICES. We can evaluate how effectively cows are being submitted for first service using the first service submission rate. This is defined as the proportion of cows receiving a first service within 24 days of becoming eligible. Eligibility is usually determined by stage of lactation (i.e. the cow is considered to be eligible for first service after the voluntary wait period is over). As the vast majority of normally cycling cows will have an oestrus within 24 days of the voluntary wait period (VWP) ending, irrespective of the stage of their cycle at the end of the VWP, the first service submission effectively reflects the proportion of cows receiving a first serve at the first opportunity.

First service heat detection can also be measured using the calving to first service interval, although it is more helpful to view the distribution of intervals within the herd than to summarize this as a single number (e.g. median or mean). First service submission rate is generally more useful than calving to first service interval for ongoing monitoring because it will respond more quickly to changes and more effectively show trends over time. However, periodic examination of calving to first service interval data is also useful as this provides information about cows not receiving a first serve 'on time' (are they generally served in the next 24 days, or is there a very positively skewed distribution where a number of cows have very long intervals?), as well as allowing evaluation of the actual VWP being observed. It is important to remember that measures of first service efficiency can also be affected by post-partum disease: if a substantial number of cows are anoestrous or have uterine bacterial infection when they reach the end of the VWP, then this will depress first-service submission rate and extend calving to first service intervals.

MONITORING RETURNS TO SERVICE. It is also possible to use submission rates to measure heat detection in cows returning to service. Return to service submission rate is normally calculated as the proportion of failed serves (i.e. serves not leading to a pregnancy) in which a subsequent serve occurs 18–24 days later. It is usual for return to service submission rates to be slightly lower than first service submission rate, as late embryonic death accounts for a proportion of failed serves. Cows experiencing late embryonic death will often be pregnant at 24 days post-service but return at an irregular interval after this time – although these cows do not represent a true failure to detect an oestrus, they will reduce the apparent return to service submission rate. Partly for this reason, it is also instructive to look at interval-derived data to assess heat detection in returns to service. In this case, the intervals between successive serves (inter-service intervals) are used. Again, it is more useful to look at the distribution of these intervals than to attempt to summarize them with a single statistic (e.g. the mean or median). Since there is an expected biological norm for the length of the oestrous cycle, it is logical to examine the distribution of intervals relative to this: typically intervals are grouped into categories of <18 days, 18–24 days, 25–35 days, 36–48 days and >48 days. Likely explanations of intervals falling into these categories are given in Table 4.5.

Examining the distribution of these categories across the cows in the herd over a specified period of time provides information not only about the sensitivity of heat detection for returns to serve, but gives an indication of the frequency of late embryonic death and the specificity of heat detection. Herds where detection is inaccurate (i.e. cows are being served when not in oestrus) will tend to have higher proportions of intervals outside of the 18–24 and 36–48 day categories; this is often particularly noticeable as a large proportion of intervals at less than 18 days. Target ranges for the distribution of inter-service intervals are given later in the section 'Summary of key targets'.

*Measuring service success*

The other critical component of fertility management is ensuring that as many services as possible lead to a pregnancy. This is relatively straightforward to measure, using the proportion of serves that leads to a pregnancy, a term we define here as pregnancy rate. This measurement is also known as the conception rate, a term which is potentially confusing in suggesting that the outcome being measured is conception rather than pregnancy. Pregnancy rate, like submission rate, is usefully measured on a month-to-month basis, and three-month rolling averages can be used where denominator populations (in this case the number of serves) are small. The outcome of a serve is usually determined by pregnancy diagnosis, so regular and early pregnancy diagnosis means that the pregnancy rate can be measured without an excessive time lag. Where pregnancy diagnosis data are not available, the analyst is left with the choice of non-return to service after a specified period of time (commonly 50–60 days) or subsequent calving as an outcome measure. The former is clearly heavily affected by return to service submission rate (as herds

**Table 4.5.** Interpretation of inter-service intervals.

| Interval | Description |
|---|---|
| < 18 days | Often indicates cows served when not truly in oestrus, as it is very unusual for true heats to occur less than 18 days apart; can also be produced by cows with follicular cysts |
| 18–24 days | Normal cycle length – likely to represent correctly detected heats with no missed oestrus in between |
| 25–35 days | Return at an extended interval – may represent late embryonic death, incorrectly identified/missed heats or the use of prostaglandin after an early negative pregnancy diagnosis |
| 36–48 days | Double the normal cycle length – likely to represent correctly identified heats with a missed oestrus in between |
| > 48 days | Could represent more than one missed heat, or fetal death/abortion |

where ability to detect returns to service is poor will have a higher non-return rate), while the latter makes analysis extremely retrospective.

It is common to compare pregnancy rates between different groups: for example, different inseminators, observed oestrus versus fixed-time AI, etc. This is often a useful exercise, but it is important to be aware of shortcomings. Pregnancy rate tends to vary over a relatively limited range (the majority of UK herds are between 32 and 41% (Hudson *et al.*, 2010)), and we are apt to see relatively small differences between groups as 'clinically meaningful'. When using this technique, it is important to be aware of random variation (and thus that different pregnancy rates in different groups may be due to random variation rather than to a true difference between groups). This is illustrated in Fig. 4.4.

### *Monitoring reproductive performance using three-week time periods*

One of the most useful and least retrospective methods of monitoring herd fertility is to measure the proportion of eligible cows that become pregnant every 21 days. This is known as 'fertility efficiency' in UK software (Breen *et al.*, 2009) and 'pregnancy rate' in software from the USA (Cook, 2010). An excellent summary is obtained by plotting two overlying parameters: (i) the proportion of eligible cows that are served in the three-week period (an indicator of submission rate) and (ii) the proportion of cows served that become pregnant (an indicator of pregnancy rate). In this way, the key elements of reproductive performance are monitored over time with a minimum time lag. The eligible population (determined separately for each 21-day block) is defined as cows intended for breeding that have passed through the VWP and that are not yet pregnant. This three-weekly summary provides an early indication of whether submission or establishment of pregnancy is currently the main limiting factor, and works well in both seasonal and block-calving herds (where other measures can be biased by

the existence of a non-breeding period). Examples of this concept are shown in Fig. 4.5.

### *Monitoring reproductive disease*

Certain reproductive diseases merit monitoring in their own right. These include uterine bacterial disease (metritis and endometritis), retained fetal membranes, dystocia and abortion. Monitoring the incidence of these diseases is relatively straightforward, and follows the principles of disease monitoring described in other chapters. Target values for incidence rates of these conditions is provided in a later section of this chapter; however, there are some points that are important to keep in mind:

- Many of these events are only likely to occur around the time of calving. Therefore, although incidence rate targets are commonly given in cases per 100 cows per year, strictly the denominator for this calculation should be calvings (i.e. cases per 100 calvings). This allows for the effect of calving interval on the incidence rate, and makes evaluation of disease incidences in seasonal calving herds much easier to interpret.

- The same phenomenon is important in distinguishing new and repeat cases. For the majority of reproductive diseases, a new case will occur only around calving – any repeat cases recorded later in the lactation are best considered as recurrences of the initial case.

- As with many other diseases, there may be problems with definition of a clinical case. Retained fetal membranes are a good example here, because treatment may not be advocated earlier than five days post-partum, whereas membranes are considered retained if still present at 24 h. Therefore, recording a disease event does not necessarily correspond with a treatment. The definition of vulval discharge can also be variable, and a recommended system to record vulval discharge is provided in Box 4.5.

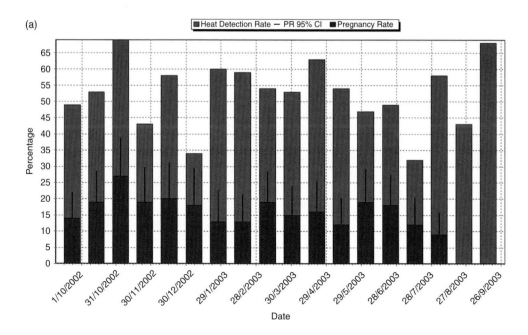

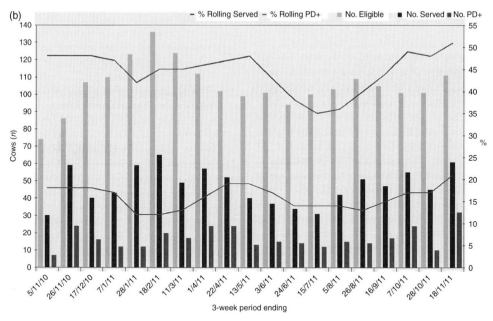

**Fig. 4.5.** Examples of the fertility efficiency concept. (a) The x-axis represents time split into 21-day blocks, the light grey bars representing the proportion of eligible cows served in each block while dark grey bars represent the proportion of eligible cows becoming pregnant in each block (DairyComp305, Valley Ag Software). (b) The x-axis represents time split into 21-day blocks, the light grey bars representing the number of cows eligible to serve in each block, the dark grey bars the number served and the medium grey bars the number becoming pregnant. The upper and lower lines represent the proportion of eligible cows being served and becoming pregnant, respectively, in each block. In this herd, an improvement in submission for service over the previous 5–6 blocks had led to an improvement in overall performance (Total Vet™; QMMS/SUM-IT software).

---

**Box 4.5.** Suggested definitions of clinical syndromes presenting as vulval discharge (from Sheldon *et al.*, 2009).

- puerperal metritis: acute systemic illness characterized by fetid, red–brown uterine discharge and pyrexia, within 21 days of calving (although these cases usually occur within the first 10 days in milk);
- clinical metritis: purulent uterine discharge with an abnormally enlarged uterus within 21 days of calving, but no other clinical signs; and
- clinical endometritis: purulent or mucopurulent uterine exudate in the vagina at 21 or more days after calving, in the absence of systemic signs.

---

### Measuring overall fertility performance

Monitoring of overall reproductive performance in a herd can be carried out in a variety of ways, and there are advantages and disadvantages of each. Traditionally, herd calving index alongside failure to conceive culling rate have been used (problems with these have been described earlier), and these can be combined into a single measure using the fertility economic score (FERTEX; Esslemont and Kossaibati, 2002). This is a very useful long-range, historical measure of the impact of fertility on the profitability of a dairy enterprise, but is of limited use in regular routine monitoring.

Alternatives include measuring herd calving to conception interval (although this is affected by the problems with using interval-derived data described earlier), or 100-day in-calf rate. The latter parameter represents the proportion of eligible cows becoming pregnant by 100 days after calving. However, the 100-day in-calf rate is a measure of the success of the 'front' end of the fertility process (i.e. success early in lactation), and can be heavily affected by herd VWP policy. For example, in a herd with a VWP of 35 days, the 100-day in-calf rate measures the proportion of cows becoming pregnant over the course of about three oestrous cycles (100–35 = 65 days). In a herd where the VWP is 60 days, the 100-day in-calf rate measures the proportion of cows becoming pregnant over the course of two cycles (100–60 = 40 days). Clearly we would expect very different results for these two herds, but this difference derives from farm policy rather than fertility performance per se. Performance at the later stages of lactation

can also be measured using the same concept. Use of 200 and 300 day in-calf rates (sometimes alternatively presented as not-in-calf rates) is common here, and provides useful extra detail.

We recommend the fertility 'survival curve' (Wapenaar *et al.*, 2008; Breen *et al.*, 2009), which allows more complete visualization of performance, effectively 'filling in the gaps' between the point measures at 100, 200 and 300 days in milk (DIM). Using this approach, all cows calving within a specified period of time are considered as the eligible population, and survival curves are used to describe the cumulative proportion of cows that receive a first service or become pregnant at different times after calving. This is illustrated in Fig. 4.6.

While fertility efficiency (described above) is a good way to monitor changes over time on a regular basis, the survival curve can be used periodically for a detailed performance evaluation of a cohort of cows. These two methods together provide an excellent framework to gain a regular overview of herd reproductive performance.

### Summary of key targets

It is wise to be cautious when comparing the performance of one farm with that of another. Whilst benchmarking can often be a highly useful way to motivate farmers and encourage sharing of best practice, goals of different farm businesses may be very different. The same principle applies when setting targets and intervention levels: it is more useful to evaluate trends over

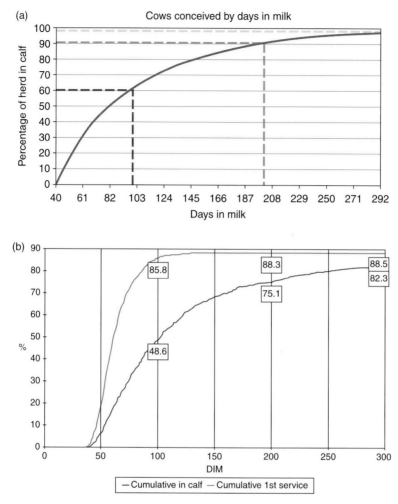

**Fig. 4.6.** Example of the use of a survival curve to monitor fertility. (a) Predicted illustration for a herd with a first service submission rate of 75%, returns submission rate of 60% and pregnancy rate of 42% (i.e. excellent performance). The broken lines show approximate 100-day (around 60%), 200-day (around 90%) and 300-day (almost 100%) in-calf rates. (b) Example of the application of this approach to actual data – the upper line shows the proportion of cows receiving a first serve and the lower line the proportion in calf (y-axis) by days in milk (DIM; x-axis) (Total Vet™; QMMS/SUM-IT software).

time rather than become too focused on a certain target value. As with assessment of levels of achievement across different nations, parameters used and reported vary considerably between different countries, and in some instances different names are used for the same parameter, or the same name may have different meanings (e.g. pregnancy rate, which is used for the proportion of serves leading to a pregnancy in

the UK but the proportion of eligible cows becoming pregnant over a 21-day period in the USA).

It is important to set specific time-related targets for each herd that are achievable and realistic. It can be helpful to think in terms of long-term goals (for example, a herd with a 100-day in-calf rate of 25% may aspire to increase this to 50%), with interim targets used as time-related milestones (such as initial target of increasing a 100-day in-calf rate to 35% within the next year). It is vital to keep in mind the retrospective nature of the parameters being monitored when setting goals: calving interval in particular is an inappropriate choice for short-term target-setting. Aiming for a measurable reduction in calving interval within 12 months in response to altered management is unwise – even if the new strategy resulted in an immediate increase in performance, this would not begin to be reflected in calving interval for at least another 280 days.

In the literature a variety of different targets are reported (Fetrow *et al.*, 1990; Morton, 2003; Wapenaar *et al.*, 2008). These references provide a thorough description of the different parameters used, as well as their strengths and weaknesses. There is a wide geographical variation in the target values considered to be appropriate; this is often related to different breeding patterns (areas where seasonal or year-round predominate), different breed characteristics (long calving intervals in tropical breeds) and management differences (grazing compared with more intensive systems). Differences between countries (and also in many cases within countries) make common targets very difficult to set. However, proposed achievable target ranges for key parameters are provided in Table 4.6.

## Control of Herd Fertility: Enhancing Reproductive Performance

When herd targets or aspirations are not met, areas in which performance can be improved need to be identified. The principles of this process are outlined in the previous sections, and this should ideally be carried out through regular monitoring rather than as a one-off 'investigation' when performance is unsatisfactory. Commonly,

**Table 4.6.** Guide to reproductive performance targets for year-round calving and seasonal calving herds.

| Parameter | Year-round calving herds | Seasonal calving herds |
|---|---|---|
| Age at first calving (months) | 22–26 | 22–24 |
| Calving to first service interval (days) | 50–70 | N/A[a] |
| Calving to conception interval (days) | 85–115 | N/A[a] |
| Submission rate (first service, %) | >75 | >75–90 |
| Submission rate (returns to service, %) | >60 | >65 |
| 100-day in-calf rate (%)[b] | >50 | >75 |
| 200-day in-calf rate (%) | >85 | >90 |
| 300-day in-calf rate (%) | >95 | >95 |
| Fertility efficiency (%)[c] | >20–25 | >30–35 |
| Calving index (days) | 375–385 | 365 |
| Failure to conceive culling rate (%/year) | <5–10 | <5–10 |
| Pregnancy rate (%)[d] | >40–45 | >40–45 |
| Inter-service interval (%) | >60 at 18–24 days; <10 at <18 days | |
| Incidence rate of abortion (%/year) | <3–5 | <3–5 |
| Incidence rate of retained fetal membranes (% of calvings) | <3–5 | <3–5 |
| Incidence rate of endometritis (% of calvings) | <10–15 | <10–15 |

[a] Calving to first service and calving to conception intervals are less meaningful in seasonal-calving herds, because cows (and often first-lactation heifers) calving early in the calving season will often be well into lactation before the breeding season begins: this can create a misleading impression of performance (especially in herds where a good breeding season the previous year led to the majority of cows calving at the beginning of the season!). [b] The target for a 100-day in-calf rate in seasonal herds will also be dependent on the proportion of cows calving early in the season – where this is high there may be large numbers of cows having limited opportunity to become pregnant before 100 days in milk. In-calf rate targets are defined as the proportion of the cows intended for breeding (i.e. excluding any marked for cull from the start of the lactation). [c] Defined as the proportion of eligible cows becoming pregnant every 21 days (often referred to as 'pregnancy rate' in North America). [d] Defined as the proportion of serves leading to a pregnancy (often referred to as 'conception rate').

one of the following three areas will be suboptimal.

- submission rate (encompassing expression and detection of oestrus);
- pregnancy rate;
- reproductive disease.

Use of the monitoring techniques described in the preceding sections makes choice between these areas relatively straightforward, and often entails simply evaluating which aspect of performance is furthest below an achievable target level. At a more sophisticated level, use of sensitivity analysis can be extremely useful; this process includes a variety of different approaches to predict the effect on overall reproductive performance (or its economic impact) of specified changes in management. This is especially relevant in herds where neither submission nor pregnancy rate is obvious as the limiting factor (e.g. where both are moderately below target). A variety of commercially available tools offer this function, and such analyses are likely to become more sophisticated in future.

Having selected an area to address, the development of an action plan is dependent on understanding the factors influencing performance in that area. These are discussed in detail in the following sections, and Fig. 4.7 outlines an approach to improving herd fertility performance.

### Improving accuracy and rate of oestrus detection

In the majority of situations, creating more chances for cows to become pregnant through improved submission rates is more important to overall fertility performance than the success rate of a single service (Mawhinney

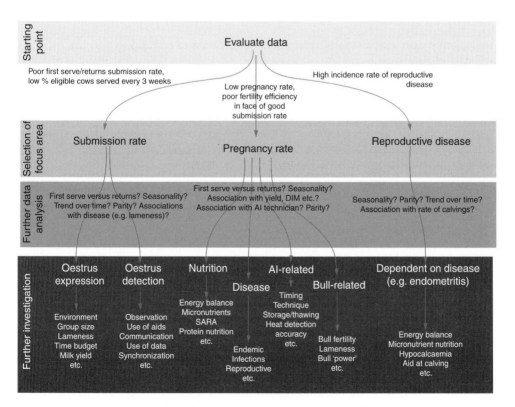

**Fig. 4.7.** Outline of an approach to improving herd fertility performance. More details on factors affecting each area and strategies for improvement are provided in subsequent sections. DIM, days in milk. SARA, subacute ruminal acidosis.

and Biggadike, 1998). Oestrus detection has been described as the central event in the success of dairy cow reproduction, particularly when AI is used. Traditionally, oestrus detection has been conducted using visual observation of behaviours linked to oestrus. For visual oestrus detection to be effective, it requires a skilled observer, sufficient observation time and for cows to show overt signs of oestrus (Van Vliet and Van Eerdenburg, 2006). The trend towards larger herds has increased the number of cows per herdsperson, and tended to decrease the amount of time available for observations (Peter and Bosu, 1986).

Achieving a high accuracy and rate of oestrus detection requires that cows sufficiently express signs of oestrus and that the oestrus is detected. Factors that influence oestrus expression and detection are described below.

### Factors affecting oestrus expression

Poor behavioural expression of oestrus ('suboestrus') may contribute to infertility, and will clearly compound the effects of decreased observation time on submission rates. There is substantial evidence that the duration and intensity of oestrus expression has been declining over the past 20 years, which has been summarized by Yoshida *et al.* (2009). In a study combining serial ultrasound scanning with intensive observation in a single Holstein-Friesian herd, Roelofs *et al.* (2005) demonstrated that 44% of cows either failed to express standing oestrus or showed behavioural signs for only a brief period or overnight. There is controversy over the extent to which a decline in oestrus expression is caused by genetic rather than environmental (management/disease) factors, but it is likely that in most instances both play a role.

A large number of factors relating both to the cow and to the environment will affect the degree to which oestrus is expressed. It is vital to ensure that the influence of factors suppressing expression of heat is minimized, and these are discussed below.

COW FACTORS.    It has been proposed that neuroendocrine factors link pain and stress with reduced oestrus expression (Sheldon and Dobson, 2003). Pain and stress can be associated with management factors such as stocking density and handling methods, as well as with diseases such as lameness, mastitis and metritis.

Severe lameness has been associated with a reduction in the intensity of behavioural oestrus (Collick *et al.*, 1989; Walker *et al.*, 2008a, b), although the association between a lower level of lameness (as detected by mobility scoring) and oestrous behaviour is less clear (Gomez *et al.*, 2003; Walker *et al.*, 2008a, b). It seems logical that improved foot health will maximize expression of behavioural oestrus and certainly lameness should be addressed (see Chapter 6). It can be useful to evaluate the effect of lameness at herd level, by comparing submission rates in lame versus sound cows, with care taken over the potential confounding effects of milk yield and nutritional status (both of which could influence expression of oestrus).

It is likely that milk yield has an effect on expression of oestrus, with higher-yielding animals usually considered to express heat less intensely or for a shorter period (Lopez *et al.*, 2004). It is contentious that this relationship is largely mediated by energy balance (i.e. cows with higher milk yields are more likely to be in or have experienced more severe negative energy balance, and that this could be responsible for the decrease in intensity of oestrus expression). Despite negative energy balance commonly being implicated as a cause of poor oestrus expression (Ferguson, 2005; Roelofs *et al.*, 2010), many studies have failed to find convincing evidence that body condition score or energy balance has a significant effect on oestrous expression (Knutson and Allrich, 1988; Wilson *et al.*, 2008), and this relationship remains unclear.

ENVIRONMENTAL FACTORS.    Housing design has a particularly important effect on the expression of oestrus behaviour. Floor surface is important, and there is evidence that non-slip, comfortable flooring will encourage mounting behaviour (Britt *et al.*, 1986; Platz *et al.*, 2008). Ensuring a non-slip surface can be achieved by a variety of methods, including grooving of concrete and use of rubber matting. Housing layout is also important, especially the provision of sufficient loafing area. This is defined as an area to which cows have access during housing, which is outside of the cubicle passageways and feed area. Pennington *et al.* (1985) found that 80% of mounting behaviour occurred in an outdoor loafing and feeding area when cows were housed in cubicle accommodation. Lack of appropriate loafing area is a common reason for poor expression of oestrus when cows are housed. It is important to ensure that the layout of the housing minimizes stress and the opportunity for bullying. Ambient temperature may also have an effect on the intensity of oestrus expression, with high temperatures usually considered to have a negative impact on expression; this appears to be a more consistent finding where maximal temperatures are in excess of 30°C. This may be more important in coming years, with increasing numbers of herds being housed through the summer months. A summary of factors that can contribute to poor oestrus expression is given in Box 4.6.

THE OPPORTUNITY FOR OESTRUS EXPRESSION.  It is also important to ensure that cows have maximum opportunity to express oestrus. This will be influenced by the time budget: for example, there will be less opportunity for oestrous behaviour in herds milking three times daily where milking times are long, because the cows will spend a large proportion of the time in the collecting yard (where they are less likely to be able to express oestrus). Another opportunity factor is the number of other sexually active cows in the group (i.e. those in or close to oestrus). Hurnik *et al.* (1975) found that the number and duration of mounts increased significantly when more than one cow was in oestrus at one time. One advantage of block-calving herds can be that a large proportion of the cows are non-pregnant at the same time, and thus there are relatively more sexually active cows in the group compared with a year-round calving herd of the same size. Low numbers in the sexually active group can be a particular problem in small herds that calve all year round. The presence of a bull can be useful to encourage oestrus expression where the sexually active group size is small.

### Factors affecting oestrus detection

In order to optimize the submission rate, it is clearly critical to maximize the efficacy of oestrus detection for a particular farm system.

DETECTION BY OBSERVATION.  The efficacy of heat detection by observation is mainly influenced by the duration and timing of periods of observation and the ability of the observer to detect signs. Appropriate training in the signs of a cow in oestrus is vital, and a written protocol detailing signs of oestrus can be useful in herds where several members of staff are

---

**Box 4.6.** Areas of housing and related management that contribute to poor oestrus expression.

- lack of sufficient loafing area (>2–3m²/cow required);
- poor flooring surface;
- factors affecting expression of natural behaviour (especially in subdominant animals):
  - poor housing layout – this would include dead-ends in cubicle passageways and poor access to resources (see Chapter 6);
  - cubicle passageways of insufficient width (>3 m required); and
  - inadequate feedspace (see Chapter 8).
- poor ventilation leading to excessive ambient temperatures;
- poor stockmanship (e.g. excessive force or hurrying when moving cows); and
- lack of space and time when being moved to and from milking.

involved in heat detection. A scoring system for oestrus detection is described by Van Vliet and Van Eerdenburg (1996), which attributes scores to different primary and secondary signs of oestrus and suggests that oestrus should be diagnosed when the total score reaches a threshold level. This provides a standardized way to diagnose oestrus in cows showing only secondary signs of oestrus (i.e. not standing to be mounted). This is presented in Table 4.7.

Van Vliet and Van Eerdenburg (1996) found that only 37% of cows studied were observed standing to be mounted during oestrus, despite observation of small herds for 30 min every 2 h. The same study reported a heat detection rate of over 70% with 100% accuracy where the scoring system was used for two observation periods of 30 min daily, and that after milking and feeding were the optimum times for observation. However, scoring systems can be very difficult to implement effectively when detecting oestrus in large groups of cows.

In addition, the effect of the cows' environment on the observer's ability to detect cows in heat should always be considered; simple practical problems such as poor animal identification or poor lighting in housing during the winter can have a major impact on submission rate.

HEAT MOUNT DETECTORS.    Perhaps the most common type of oestrus detection aid is based on the principle of detecting pressure or friction over the tail head area in a cow standing to be mounted. This concept is implemented by a variety of different commercially available products. One of the least expensive (although often highly effective) is the use of tail paint or chalk. This is cheap and simple, although frequent inspection and reapplication is often required for accurate detection. Extending this principle, proprietary adhesive devices are slightly more expensive, although more durable and in some situations more reliable. These are usually based either on a capsule of coloured dye within a white paste (where rupture of the capsule when the cow is mounted causes an observable colour change) or a 'scratch-card' system, where a brightly coloured sticker is covered with a layer of grey latex which is cumulatively rubbed off with successive mounts. By trial and error, it is often found that one will be more effective than another on a particular unit. At the more sophisticated end of the market, radiotelemetric heat mount detectors are available in some countries (Dransfield *et al.*, 1998).

The proportion of heats detected with the use of heat mount detectors varies widely between different studies, ranging from 35% (Holman *et al.*, 2011) to 95% (Xu *et al.*, 1998). Evidence comparing specific devices is less compelling. Holman *et al.* (2011) compared a capsule-based heat mount detector with a scratch-card system and found

**Table 4.7.** Scoring system for oestrus detection (after Van Vliet and Van Eerdenburg, 1996). Where observation is carried out two or three times per day, a total threshold score of 50 points is recommended for diagnosis of oestrus.

| Signs of oestrus | Score |
| --- | --- |
| Mounting signs | |
|     Mounted by another cow but not standing | 10 |
|     Mounting (or attempting to mount) other cows | 35 |
|     Mounting head end of another cow | 45 |
|     Standing to be mounted | 100 |
| Other signs | |
|     Mucous vaginal discharge | 3 |
|     Cajoling | 3 |
|     Restlessness | 5 |
|     Sniffing the vulvas of other cows | 10 |
|     Chin-resting on other cows | 15 |

that the latter method detected significantly fewer heats, although this was in a single herd. It should be remembered that housing and management conditions have a substantial effect on the relative usefulness of different heat mount detectors, and it is usually worthwhile trialling a variety of different methods on a particular farm.

ACTIVITY METERS. Automated technologies are targeted on detecting the occurrence of physiological or behavioural changes that correlate with ovulation (Senger, 1994). One such change is an increase in motor activity as measured by a pedometer or other activity meter. Such devices measure cow activity, and are usually attached either to the distal limb (pedometers) or worn as a neck collar. It has been demonstrated that motor activity increases during oestrus in the dairy cow (Moore and Spahr, 1991; Redden et al., 1993), and activity monitors work by comparing activity on the day in question against a baseline consisting of one or more previous days using either a simple ratio, or a complex

algorithm. A threshold value is then set, and increases in activity exceeding this threshold are recorded as 'alerts'. Figure 4.8 shows an example of an output trace from an activity monitor system (Heatime™; SCR Technologies), showing raw activity data (upper), and 'standardized' activity (lower), corrected for the individual cow's baseline activity and day-to-day variability.

Firk et al. (2003) evaluated the use of thresholds of between 40 and 120% increase in daily activity for the detection of oestrus. This study found that sensitivity ranged from 94.2% (at a 40% threshold) to 71.0% (at a 120% threshold) and error rates were 53.2 and 21.5%, respectively. Statham (2011) showed that at activity threshold >5 'Heatime units' (HTU), sensitivity of identification of low milk progesterone was 75%, with a specificity of 29% and a positive predictive value of 95%. When activity threshold was set at >10 HTU, sensitivity fell to 62% but specificity rose to 68% and positive predictive value to 97%. Roelofs et al. (2005) compared the number of steps taken

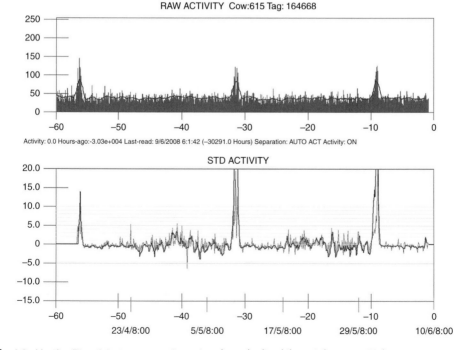

**Fig. 4.8.** Heatime™ activity traces: raw (upper) and standardized (lower) data over 60 days.

in a 2 h time period with the number of steps taken in the same time period during the 10 preceding days using a median or a mean to calculate the baseline activity. Thresholds of the mean plus 2.5, 3.0 and 3.5 standard deviations (SD) resulted in high percentages of correct pedometer oestrus alerts (87, 83 and 79%, respectively) and relatively low percentages of false pedometer oestrus alerts (17, 8 and 5%, respectively). Holman *et al.* (2011) found that neck-mounted activity monitors and leg-mounted pedometers performed similarly in a single dairy herd, with both systems detecting in the region of 60% of heats when used alone. However, this was not significantly different from the proportion of heats detected by observation for 10 minutes six times per day.

These studies suggest that activity meters can play a useful role in oestrus detection (particularly in herds in which observation is poor), but that the methods are not perfect. It is likely that with rapid progress in technology and computer modelling, these systems will continue to become more effective.

EFFECTIVE USE OF INFORMATION. As in many areas of herd health management, making the best use of the information available is extremely useful in maximizing submission rates. Perhaps most importantly, it is useful to make the most of predicted oestrus dates. For a cow that has had an oestrus in the current lactation, it is simple to predict the time frame within which her next oestrus is likely to fall. This allows increased focus on any cows due into oestrus at any specific point, and can be a very useful adjunct to other methods (Firk *et al.*, 2003). Where reference heats (heats during the VWP) are consistently recorded, this method can be applied to animals eligible for first serve, as well as to those already served, and this is strongly recommended. Recording of reference heats also allows identification of cows that have not shown oestrus by the time they become eligible for first service, allowing these cows to be examined and managed as appropriate. In order for this to work effectively, there needs to be good communication of information between members of the farm team.

OTHER AIDS TO HEAT DETECTION. A number of other oestrus detection aids can be adopted. A vasectomized bull, fitted with a chin harness (marking cows that are in oestrus) can be an effective aid to heat detection. This can improve submission rates substantially in some circumstances (Foote, 1975), but there are practical and safety implications of running a bull with a dairy herd, so care is required.

Another useful tool in heat detection is the use of milk progesterone assays. Regression of the corpus luteum at the end of the preceding cycle is normally accompanied by a decrease in circulating progesterone concentration, which results in a decrease in the level of progesterone in milk. This can be tested using a variety of simple assays (including cow-side tests), usually giving a 'high' or 'low' progesterone result (often shown as a colour change). This is especially useful in assessing the accuracy of heat detection (i.e. the frequency with which cows are being served outside of oestrus). Where inaccurate detection is suspected, milk progesterone testing on a series of cows to be served can provide evidence to support or refute this. While a high milk progesterone result is strong evidence that a cow is not in oestrus, a low milk progesterone result does not definitively confirm oestrus, or allow for accurate timing of service. Despite this, milk progesterone testing has been used as a method of oestrus detection (Foulkes *et al.*, 1982), although the frequency of testing required for this is high and thus the practice is not currently widespread in the UK. A major potential future development in this area is the automation of milk progesterone testing, which would provide a variety of opportunities to extend use of this information and improve submission rates.

It is possible to use an external specialist provider to supply a service to detect oestrus in the herd (often in association with artificial insemination). Such schemes commonly rely on the use of heat mount detectors (often tail paint), in conjunction with detailed herd records. The technician employed is generally present on the farm for only a short period of time each day, and thus the opportunities for observation of oestrus behaviour are limited. Such services can be useful, especially where farm labour is a limiting factor, but are highly dependent on the skill and commitment of the individual technician.

RETURN TO CYCLICITY AND OESTRUS SYNCHRONIZATION.    First service submission rates will be affected by the stage at which cows are returning to cyclicity after calving: if postpartum anoestrus is a problem then there may be a high proportion of cows not cycling at the end of the VWP. It is important to rule this out as a contributory factor where submission rates are poor. There are a number of approaches that can be taken, including the use of milk progesterone assays during the VWP, but in herds where routine veterinary visits are in place, the incidence rate of treatment for anoestrus can be a useful indicator. Similarly, in herds where endometritis is a problem, there may be cows that remain affected at the end of the VWP, and which are therefore not served even where signs of oestrus are observed. Causes and control of post-partum anoestrus and endometritis are discussed later in this chapter.

Oestrus synchronization can improve submission rates. Targeted breeding programmes have become established in larger dairy herds, where systematic treatments offer huge efficiencies of labour and consistency of delivery (Nebel and Jobst, 1998). Various programmes have been proposed, most notably the Ovsynch regime and its variations Cosynch, Heatsynch, Selectsynch and PreSynch (Cavalieri et al., 2006). Inclusion of progesterone-releasing devices has offered an alternative approach (Stevenson, 2008). De Rensis et al. (2008) showed that inclusion of human chorionic gonadotropin (hCG) in place of the second gonadotropin-releasing hormone (GnRH) treatment of the standard Ovsynch programme could produce significant improvements in plasma progesterone levels and improve fertility in dairy cows during the warmer months of the year. A summary of synchronization protocols is given in Fig. 4.9.

Pregnancy rates to synchronized services tend to be lower than those to observed oestrus. In many situations this is outweighed by the benefit of increased submission rates, but it is important to be aware of the possibility of reduced pregnancy rate, and to monitor

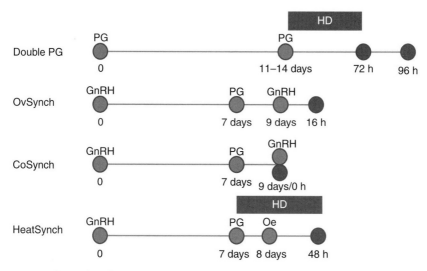

**Fig. 4.9.** Commonly used synchronization protocols featuring fixed-time AI. Treatments are denoted by light gray circles (with days post-enrolment beneath in light gray), and fixed-time AI by dark gray circles (with timing after last treatment in dark gray). PG, prostaglandin $F_2\alpha$ analogue; GnRH, gonadotropin-releasing hormone analogue; Oe, oestrogen analogue (not for use in the EU); HD, heat detection with AI to any observed heats (after Cavalieri et al., 2006).

the outcomes of synchronized serves when implementing a programme on the farm. Consumer attitudes to the routine use of hormones in synchronization programmes can be negative. Some of the systems described above cannot be used in the European Union (EU) as they involve hormones that are not licensed for use in food animals (e.g. the Heatsynch protocol, which involves the use of oestradiol benzoate).

### A multifaceted, dedicated approach to oestrus detection

Several studies have demonstrated improved heat detection by using a combination of methods (Firk *et al.*, 2003; Peralta *et al.*, 2005; Holman *et al.*, 2011) and, in a herd health programme, a multifaceted approach is often required. Using a combination of methods will also allow detection of different oestrous behaviours and this should be beneficial; for example, a combination of activity monitors and tail paint can be used to detect an increase in activity and also in mounting behaviour.

The difficulty, as well as the importance, of oestrus detection in modern, high-producing dairy cows should not be underestimated. Oestrus detection requires skill, dedication and hard work on a continuous basis. Whilst new technology will undoubtedly have an increasingly important role to play, currently traditional methods that require good stockmanship remain a vital component of oestrus detection. A checklist for the investigation of poor submission rates is provided in Box 4.7.

### Improving pregnancy rates

Royal *et al.* (2000) reported that over the previous 25 years, pregnancy rates (the proportion of serves leading to a pregnancy) in UK dairy herds had fallen from about 50% to around 35%, and this appears to reflect a global trend. It has been suggested that up to 90% of cows accurately identified in heat and correctly inseminated will be in calf and carrying live embryos seven days after insemination (Diskin and Morris, 2008).

This is supported by Sheldon (1997), who reported that events around the time of insemination and fertilization account for only 10% of observed reproductive wastage. The main constraint on pregnancy rate in the dairy herd is the rate of early and late embryonic death that occurs post-insemination (Humblot, 2001). It is predominantly for this reason that the term 'pregnancy rate' is preferred to represent the proportion of serves leading to a pregnancy: the alternative term 'conception rate' suggests that the outcome being measured is conception, and it would appear that this step of the process is often successful even where a pregnancy does not result.

Key factors influencing pregnancy rate include nutrition, infectious disease, concurrent disease, timing of insemination, semen quality and AI technique. These are discussed in the following sections and, while many dairy herds rely mostly on AI, we also briefly discuss the use of natural service.

### Nutrition

In many situations, nutrition has a major effect on pregnancy rate, and nutritional causes should always be considered as a differential diagnosis when investigating poor pregnancy rates. Probably the most important nutritional influence on pregnancy rate is energy balance. A variety of mechanisms exist whereby negative energy balance (NEB) over a prolonged period of early lactation can exert an influence on the success of subsequent serves.

Energy balance during transition and early lactation is extremely important in determining pregnancy rate to serves through lactation. Mechanisms for this long-lasting effect include the effects of exposure of developing follicles to NEB (Leroy *et al.*, 2005) and the increase in pregnancy rate seen with increasing numbers of oestrous cycles prior to service. Villa-Godoy *et al.* (1988) found that levels of progesterone during the luteal phase increased over the course of the first three ovulatory cycles after calving, but that this increase was less marked in cows experiencing greater levels of NEB.

---

**Box 4.7.** Quick checklist for investigation of poor submission rate.

- Oestrus detection
  - Correct signs used for detection?
  - Duration/timing of observation periods?
  - Observation during other activities?
  - Is cow identification easy? Lighting?
  - Training required to identify oestrus?
  - Communication between staff?
- Aids
  - Activity monitors
    - How are they being used?
    - Display/alerts easily accessible?
    - Proactive evaluation of activity traces?
    - Sufficient number of collars/pedometers?
    - Correct application of collars/pedometers?
  - Heat mount detectors
    - Which cows? What stage?
    - Who applies them? Correct application? How often?
    - Who checks them/when?
    - What type (appropriate to environment)?
  - Any use of milk progesterone, vasectomized bull, other aids?
- Using management data
  - Method of recording?
  - Recording of all heats including those in voluntary waiting period?
  - System for determining cows due in oestrus?
- Oestrus expression
  - Environment?
    - Loafing area
    - Flooring
    - Housing design (stress/bullying)
  - Cow factors?
    - Lameness
    - Yield and energy balance
  - Opportunity?
    - Sexually active group size
    - Time budget
- Others
  - Routine vet. visits
    - Frequency?
    - Which cows are being seen?
  - Use of synchronization? Protocol? Which cows?

---

Levels of progesterone post-service have a major influence on embryonic survival (Butler, 2001). The length of the post-partum anovulatory period is strongly associated with NEB in early lactation (Garnsworthy et al., 2008), and this provides a further mechanism for poor fertility (because cows experiencing a greater degree of early-lactation NEB will tend to have delayed return to cyclicity and so are likely to be served to an earlier cycle number post-calving). NEB can also delay post-partum endometrial repair (Wathes et al., 2007), again potentially influencing subsequent pregnancy rate.

Energy balance around the time of service is also important. Many of the effects here appear to be mediated by insulin-like growth factor 1 (IGF-1), which is present at lower levels under conditions of NEB. The effects of low IGF-1 include a decrease in the responsiveness of the ovary to gonado-tropins (Butler, 2003) and changes in the micro-environment of the oviduct and uterus that are potentially detrimental to embryo survival (Fenwick *et al.*, 2008).

Maximizing dry matter intake is one of the key strategies for avoiding NEB in early lactation, and is vital in minimizing body condition loss in high-yielding cows at peak lactation. However, high dry matter intakes tend to increase blood flow to the liver, which in turn tends to increase the rate at which endogenous steroid hormones are broken down (Sangsritavong *et al.*, 2002). These include both oestrogen and proges-terone, so cows in this state of high meta-bolic turnover are at greater risk of perturbation of ovarian cyclicity and embryo loss (Roche, 2006).

A final potential mechanism by which NEB can influence pregnancy rate is through its influence on the levels of peri-parturient disease. NEB is recognized as a risk factor for retained fetal membranes, metritis, endometritis, ketosis, displaced abomasum and a variety of other diseases, many of which are in turn recognized as having a detrimental effect on pregnancy rate. Moni-toring and management of energy balance is described in detail in Chapter 8.

High blood urea levels have also been associated with poor pregnancy rates, with the predominant mechanisms proposed being through alteration in uterine environment and compromised embryo survival (Butler, 1998). This may be due to an excess of dietary crude protein (Butler, 1998), but can also be associated with a relative deficit in fermenta-ble metabolizable energy (Whitaker, 1998).

Subacute ruminal acidosis has also commonly been linked with poor pregnancy rates (Grove-White, 2004), and while this is plausible, solid research evidence is cur-rently lacking. Micronutrient nutrition can also be important in determining pregnancy rate. Copper-responsive disorders in partic-ular have classically been associated with poor pregnancy rates (Phillippo *et al.*, 1987), although the prevalence, diagnosis and pathogenesis of such disorders remain con-troversial (further details of mineral nutri-tion are provided in Chapter 8).

*Infectious disease and embryonic mortality*

Several infectious diseases of cattle are associated with a decrease in pregnancy rate. The most commonly implicated dis-eases include bovine viral diarrhoea (BVD), infectious bovine rhinotracheitis (IBR) and leptospirosis. McGowan *et al.* (1993) found that seroconversion to BVD around the time of insemination was associated with a sig-nificantly lower pregnancy rate; this is most likely to be due to the effect of BVD on embryo survival. There is also strong *in vitro* evidence that *in utero* exposure to IBR or BVD virus has a negative effect on surviv-ability of embryos (Vanroose *et al.*, 1997, 1998). The effects of leptospirosis are less clear: although serological evidence of exposure to the causal agent has been asso-ciated with lower pregnancy rates (Dhaliwal *et al.*, 1996), evidence for a causal link is not comprehensive.

Diagnosis of an infectious disease as the primary cause for a poor pregnancy rate at herd level can be challenging, because the dynamics of infection within herds tends to be complex. In a situation where a novel infectious agent has entered a naïve herd, dramatic decreases in pregnancy rate are often seen, generally followed by steady recovery as the majority of the animals develop immunity. A much more common scenario is a poor or steadily declining pregnancy rate in a herd with evidence of long-standing circulating disease. In this situation it can be extremely difficult to evaluate the effect of the disease on the problem. A decision is often made to vacci-nate for the disease under suspicion, but results, in terms of pregnancy rates, are often disappointing (see Chapter 7 for more details on the control of infectious disease).

Other less common pathogens have also been associated with reduced preg-nancy rates. These include *Ureaplasma* spp. (Doig *et al.*, 1979; Kreplin *et al.*, 1987), *Histophilus somni* (van der Burgt *et al.*, 2007), *Trichomonas fetus* and *Campylobacter fetus* subsp. *venerealis*. Subclinical Johne's dis-ease is associated with poor fertility per-formance (Merkal *et al.*, 1975), although this may simply be due to a negative effect on energy balance. Neosporosis is sometimes considered as a potential contributor to poor pregnancy rate, but studies have failed to find an effect of *Neospora caninum* infection status on either pregnancy rate or embryo/early fetal loss (López-Gatius *et al.*, 2004, 2005).

### Concurrent disease

Endemic, non-infectious disease can also play a major role in herds with poor pregnancy rates. Disease of the reproductive tract itself is important, and there is comprehensive evidence that cows experiencing retained fetal membranes (Holt *et al.*, 1989; McDougall, 2001), metritis and endometritis (LeBlanc *et al.*, 2002; Gilbert *et al.*, 2005) tend to have lower pregnancy rates in the same lactation. When evaluating the impact of these diseases at a herd level, it can be useful to compare pregnancy rate (especially to first serve) in affected and unaffected cows. Control of these diseases is discussed in the 'Controlling reproductive disease' section. As well as having a possible direct effect on pregnancy rate via the uterine environment, these diseases are all associated with delayed return to ovarian cyclicity and abnormal oestrous cycles (Sheldon, 2004), which may represent a further mechanism whereby pregnancy rates are decreased. More recently, it has been recognized that cows with subclinical endometritis also tend to have poorer pregnancy rates, both to first serve and to all serves (Kasimanickam *et al.*, 2004). The impact of this can be very difficult to appreciate at herd level, but it is likely that the effect of subclinical endometritis is more significant in herds where the incidence rate of clinical endometritis is high.

Other concurrent endemic disease can have an impact on pregnancy rate. Lameness during early lactation has been associated with a negative impact on pregnancy rate to first service (Melendez *et al.*, 2003), and the presence of lameness lesions in the foot pre-calving has been associated with decreased overall fertility performance (Machado *et al.*, 2010). It is possible that the majority of the apparent effect of lameness on pregnancy rate is

mediated by a decrease in dry matter intake and consequently in energy balance in lame cows. Clinical mastitis (Hertl *et al.*, 2010) and subclinical mastitis (Pinedo *et al.*, 2009) have also been associated with decreased pregnancy rates. Again, when evaluating the effects of these diseases on pregnancy rate in a particular herd, it can be instructive to compare pregnancy rates in affected and unaffected cows.

### Timing of insemination

Timing of insemination during oestrus is important in determining success of a service. Premature insemination may result in aged sperm that cannot achieve fertilization by the time of ovulation (Hawk, 1987). Delayed insemination may result in failed fertilization, or formation of a less viable embryo due to ageing of the oocyte (Hunter and Greve, 1997). Trimberger (1948) found the highest pregnancy rates when cows were inseminated 13–18 h before ovulation. Insemination time should ideally be based on ovulation time, and accurate prediction of timing of ovulation is a key aim of oestrus detection. However, prediction of time to ovulation from signs of oestrus is problematic (Roelofs *et al.*, 2005) and in practice ovulation cannot always be predicted with sufficient accuracy to minimize the negative effects of aged gametes on embryo quality and embryonic death.

Various studies have used activity monitors to estimate the timing of onset of oestrus to allow determination of optimal timing of subsequent insemination. Roelofs *et al.* (2005) found that ovulation occurred approximately 29 h (range, 22–39) after onset of pedometer-detected oestrus. Maatje *et al.* (1997) found that pregnancy rates were highest when insemination occurred at an estimated interval of 11.8 h after onset of pedometer-detected oestrus. Humblot *et al.* (2009) found lower pregnancy rates in cows inseminated early (<6 h) or late (>24 h) relative to the first observed signs of oestrus.

Traditionally, advice has been to serve cows 12 h after they are first observed in oestrus, with the intention that this will coincide with the end of standing oestrus. However, as the typical duration of standing oestrus has decreased over the years, this advice has been questioned. One large study found that optimal pregnancy rates occurred where insemination took place 4–12 h after the first standing mount, which is in agreement with traditional advice (Dransfield *et al.*, 1998). However, the same study found that the average cow had been in oestrus for 6 h when first visually observed by herd staff, suggesting that insemination 12 h after first observed oestrus might be too late for optimum pregnancy rates. Further research demonstrated comparable pregnancy rates in once- versus twice-daily insemination programmes (Nebel *et al.*, 1994).

In the light of current research, a sensible recommendation is that cows detected in oestrus should be inseminated at the next opportunity, but no later than 10–12 h after detected oestrus. Where appropriate insemination timing is in question, early insemination is less likely to compromise conception (DeJarnette *et al.*, 2004).

It is also important to minimize the number of cows inseminated while not truly in oestrus. The percentage of non-oestrous cows presented for AI has been estimated to be as high as 18–25%, and was determined to be a significant cause for low pregnancy rates (Nebel *et al.*, 1987; Sturman *et al.*, 2000). This issue is particularly relevant with respect to previously inseminated cows, where studies have indicated that inseminations may cause embryonic or fetal loss in as many as 17% of cases, dependent on AI technique (Weaver *et al.*, 1989; Sturman *et al.*, 2000). This is potentially important as a cause for poor pregnancy rates, and a useful initial evaluation can be achieved using inter-service intervals (see 'Routine performance monitoring' section). Follow-up investigation can include the use of milk progesterone testing to measure the proportion of cows served that are outside of oestrus (as demonstrated by a high milk progesterone concentration).

### Semen quality, storage, thawing and insemination technique

With the rise and predominance of artificial insemination (AI) in dairy herds, there has been a substantial reduction in focus on the male elements of reproduction. However, even where AI is extensively or exclusively used, there is still potential for insemination-related factors to depress pregnancy rates. Although reputable genetics companies have stringent quality control measures in place, this still leaves scope for variation in fertility between bulls meeting the 'acceptable' criteria; for example, substantial variation in fertility between 'high-demand' AI sires has been reported in Australia (Phillips *et al.*, 2004). Large differences in pregnancy rate between different bulls can be a clue that this is important, and examination of thawed straws can be useful. Methods for evaluation of thawed semen are described elsewhere (Phillips *et al.*, 2004).

It is important to store and thaw semen correctly before insemination. One of the most important factors here is to retain straws below the frost line in the liquid nitrogen storage tank. The viability of frozen sperm that is re-cooled after partial thawing has been shown to be extremely low (this may occur when straws not immediately required are lifted above the frost line and replaced; DeJarnette, 1999). This is implicated as an important semen handling error. Control of this is achieved through good flask organization; straws should be easily identifiable within the flask (then only the straw required for use needs to be removed) and liquid nitrogen should always be maintained at the correct level.

Thawing must also be carried out correctly. Since optimum thaw rate is affected by the exact pre-freezing processing methods used, it is important to follow any specific recommendations from the semen suppliers. However, thawing in water at 35°C for at least 45 s is generally recommended. Hygiene and temperature control of the thaw bath is important, and is worth checking as part of an investigation. Although there is conflicting evidence regarding the maximum number of straws that can be thawed together without depressing pregnancy rate (DeJarnette *et al.*, 2004), it is logical to suggest that no more straws should be thawed in one batch than can be used within 10–15 min. Maintenance of straw temperature until the time of insemination is vital, as is maintaining strict hygiene.

There is controversy surrounding the optimum technique for semen deposition. Traditionally, advice has been to deposit semen in the uterine body, just cranial to the cervix, and this remains the method taught as standard in most AI courses. More recently, however, there has been increased interest in techniques where deposition is more cranial, such as uni- or bilateral cornual. The evidence supporting different techniques is summarized by DeJarnette et al. (2004), but there is currently a lack of convincing data to demonstrate that cornual deposition is associated with higher pregnancy rates, even where low sperm doses are used (as in sexed semen). Insemination technique may vary between inseminators, and this can provide a useful clue that technique is an important factor in herds where more than one person is responsible for carrying out AI. Where this is not the case but there is suspicion that poor AI technique is contributing to a poor pregnancy rate, it can be useful to institute a trial period where cows are randomly assigned to be inseminated either by the normal member of farm staff or by a professional technician. Care must be taken here to ensure that randomization is carried out properly.

*Other factors affecting pregnancy rate*

Negative genetic correlations exist between milk production traits and fertility variables (Veerkamp et al., 2001), and it appears that cows with high milk index are less fertile than females with lower genetic merit *after* adjustment for milk production. Information obtained from different countries supports the role of genetics in declining cow fertility. Selection for milk production has been particularly implicated in inadvertently breeding less fertile cows (Royal et al., 2000; Lucy, 2001). Wall and Coffey (2005) describe how a fertility index can help to reverse the long-term decline in the fertility of dairy cattle and how genetic indices, based on reproductive performance, are becoming

more widely used. Whilst genetics may be playing some role in the long-term decline in pregnancy rate, it is likely that other factors related to nutrition, disease and management are also important. At herd level, it is clearly unwise to attempt to control reproductive performance solely or mainly through genetic manipulation.

Extreme ambient temperatures have also been associated with poor pregnancy rates. This has been implicated as one of the reasons why pregnancy rates tend to be lower in the summer months in herds that are housed year-round. Heat stress is much more likely to become a problem than cold stress in most situations, with modern dairy cows showing physiological evidence of this at ambient temperatures above 20°C. There is a wide variety of potential mechanisms for this link, but it is worth investigating temperature and relative humidity during summer housing when a seasonal pregnancy rate problem is observed in a herd where early-lactation cows are housed through the year. The level at which heat stress is likely to affect pregnancy rate is not simple to predict, partly because of the interaction of ambient temperature and relative humidity. The temperature–humidity index (THI) is often used to represent the combination of these two effects: this is described in more detail by Ravagnolo and Misztal (2002), who found that a THI of >70 was negatively associated with pregnancy rate.

Decreased pregnancy rates have also been associated with the presence of mycotoxins in cattle rations (Whitlow and Hagler, 1999). The most likely causal agent is generally considered to be zearalenone, an oestrogenic fungal toxin that can be found in maize silage or grain products. Mycotoxin-related disorders are notoriously challenging to diagnose, as signs are often intermittent (toxins are not uniformly distributed through feedstuffs) and vague (Wilde, 2005). In terms of poor pregnancy rate, this is often a diagnosis of exclusion, and it is possible to advise inclusion of an adsorbent in the ration where pregnancy rates are poor and other causes have been excluded. In this instance, it is extremely important to monitor the outcome of the intervention, since this will provide evidence for or against mycotoxins being the original cause of the problem.

*Pregnancy rate in herds using natural service*

Although many dairy herds rely predominantly on AI, there are still a number where bulls play an important part. A normal fertile bull is expected to get 90% of a group of 50 normal, cycling, disease-free females pregnant within 9 weeks, and 60% of these in the first 3 weeks (McGowan, 2004). However, of 319 bulls examined in a UK survey, around one third were sub-fertile (Eppink, 2005). Reasons included lameness, poor scrotal circumference, scrotal enlargement, poor semen quality (motility or morphology) and impaired ability to serve cows.

A bull pre-breeding evaluation (PBE) performed prior to the service period in seasonally breeding herds allows a proactive approach to screening out sub-fertile bulls (McGowan, 2004; Penny, 2005, 2009). Furthermore, a judgement as to how many cows may be served by a bull can be attempted, rather than proceeding with no assessment of likely performance. Evaluation of bull fertility is also encouraged in year-round calving herds, especially where there is heavy reliance on natural service.

The structure of the PBE should be modular, as follows:

- history and disease status;
- physical examination (including palpation of testes and measurement of scrotal circumference);
- semen collection (using an artificial vagina or electro-ejaculator) and examination of motility and morphology;
- serving assessment (using synchronized heifers or cows from farmer observation of oestrus prior to visit); and
- special diagnostics (e.g. testicular ultrasound).

A detailed description of the procedure and a specimen record form is provided by Penny (2009).

Semen collection from bulls by artificial vagina (AV) can be tedious and potentially dangerous. Electro-ejaculation (EEJ) is the standard method of semen collection used in the field in North America and Australasia, and has allowed the development of the PBE as a routine procedure. However, approximately two-thirds of sub-fertile bulls can be detected by physical examination alone. Careful examination, including palpation of the testes and measurement of the scrotal circumference, may determine the presence of any abnormalities, and allow an indication of fertility of an individual bull. An estimate of the likely effect of bull fertility on overall pregnancy rate can be obtained by measuring pregnancy rate to natural service compared with that to AI, or by comparing pregnancy rates between different bulls. The need to account for potential confounding factors is important here: in many cases AI is used for the first few serves of lactation, and natural service reserved for animals not conceiving to these serves, with the latter possibly representing a biased selection of problem cows.

There are a number of specific reproductive diseases that are spread by natural service. After notifiable or zoonotic diseases (such as brucellosis), perhaps the most important of these is venereal campylobacteriosis, caused by *Campylobacter fetus* subsp. *venerealis*. The aetiology, clinical signs and diagnosis of infectious causes of reproductive diseases spread by natural service are provided in Box 4.8.

### Controlling reproductive disease

Most diseases of dairy cows can have a deleterious impact on reproductive performance, either directly or indirectly. Following disease, damage to the reproductive system can occur through altering nutrition/metabolism, affecting ovarian or uterine function and modifying inflammatory mechanisms. Therefore, to optimize herd reproduction it is essential to maximize general herd health.

Monitoring, diagnosis and control of major infectious diseases (including infectious bovine rhinotracheitis, BVD and leptosporosis) are discussed in detail in

---

**Box 4.8.** Outline of the infectious causes of reproductive diseases spread by natural service.

---

- **Venereal campylobacteriosis and _Trichomonas fetus_ infection:** although these diseases are caused by quite different agents, they share many clinical features. Both are generally carried by asymptomatic bulls, introduced at natural service and cause an inflammatory process in the uterus, often resulting in loss of the embryo or fetus at a variable period post-service. The infection will normally subsequently be eliminated, although the timescale for this is variable, and the cow is likely to remain sub-fertile during this period (and may or may not cycle). Vulval discharge is sometimes observed. Diagnosis is by microbiological/immunological examinations of the bull, but generally test sensitivity is limited and serial tests are often recommended. Sampling and transport requirements should be discussed with the chosen laboratory before sampling. In the UK, diagnosis of campylobacteriosis is usually by fluorescent antibody testing or bacterial culture of a preputial wash.
- **Mycoplasmae and ureaplasmae:** these organisms have been isolated from both the male and lower female genital tract, and have also been associated with endometritis, poor pregnancy rates and fetal loss/abortion. However, it is likely that clinical disease is rare and diagnostic testing is not commonly performed (again, sampling requirements should be discussed with a laboratory first).
- **IBR and BVD:** although spread by other means (e.g. aerosol) is more common, both of these viruses can be spread by natural service. This can occur in a variety of situations, but bulls that are persistently infected with BVD or are latent carriers of IBR (in which periods of stress can lead to recrudescence and shedding) can be major sources of reproductive losses. Venereal spread can also be a feature of genital lesions caused by bovine herpesvirus (for further details on IBR and BVDV see Chapter 7).

---

Chapter 7. Nutrition-related diseases that can affect reproduction, such as hypocalcaemia and ketosis, are discussed in Chapter 8. Here we concentrate on the major diseases of the reproductive tract that affect reproductive performance, and briefly discuss abortion. Parturition is probably the single most important event in determining whether subsequent reproductive disorders occur. Avoidance of dystocia and excellent management of the cow during calving are paramount.

### Retained fetal membranes

Expulsion of fetal membranes in a timely manner after parturition is important in allowing clearance of the uterine bacterial contamination that occurs at calving, thus ensuring normal uterine involution. Membranes are generally considered to be 'retained' for an abnormally prolonged time if they are still present at more than 24 h after parturition (Paisley _et al._, 1986). This can present problems in terms of recording, as treatment is not normally instituted until a later stage, so the farmer is being asked to record a disease incidence that will not necessarily be associated with treatment (the condition may spontaneously resolve before the stage at which treatment would be considered). For this reason, incidence of retained fetal membranes (RFM) is commonly under-recorded.

Control of RFM centres around prevention of predisposing factors, and these are outlined in Box 4.9.

Recently, there has been a change in the perceived relative importance of the factors listed in Box 4.9. Traditionally, uterine contractility has been considered to be key, but more recent research has suggested greater importance of prompt immune-mediated breakdown of the cotelydon–caruncle attachment (Frazer, 2005; LeBlanc, 2008). RFM is a substantial predisposing factor for endometritis, and is associated with an increase in the severity of uterine bacterial disease (metritis and endometritis).

### Metritis and endometritis

Unusually among the domestic species, bacterial contamination of the uterus at the time of calving is normal in cattle (Williams _et al._, 2008). A variety of defence mechanisms are responsible for clearing this

---

**Box 4.9.** Risk factors for retained fetal membranes.

---

- Abnormalities relating to myometrial contractions (either in terms of frequency or amplitude): uterine atony is important, and common causes for this include
  - clinical or subclinical hypocalcaemia; and
  - prolonged dystocia
- **Interference with the normal maturation of the placentome** (involving changes in collagen and alteration in binucleate cell numbers in the villi on the fetal side), resulting in failure of adequate separation of maternal and fetal tissues. Potential causes of this include
  - negative energy balance;
  - micronutrient deficiencies (e.g. vitamins E and A, selenium);
  - premature calving: spontaneous (e.g. twins) or induced;
  - prolonged gestation;
  - inflammatory conditions (e.g. some specific causes of abortion);
  - trauma/oedema; and
  - hyperaemia/necrosis of fetal villi/placentome.

---

contamination in the post-partum period in order to allow normal uterine involution. However, some level of uterine bacterial infection is still present in as many as 40% of animals at one week post-calving (Sheldon *et al.*, 2009). Failure of these clearance mechanisms leads to uterine bacterial disease, specifically metritis and endometritis. There has been significant confusion between these terms, and Sheldon *et al.* (2006) suggest that for clarity the terms puerperal metritis, clinical metritis and clinical endometritis are used (see Box 4.5 for definitions). Cows may experience one or more of these syndromes during the early post-partum period, with puerperal or clinical metritis commonly followed by clinical endometritis. However, many cases of clinical endometritis are not preceded by evident signs of uterine bacterial disease earlier in lactation. More recently it has also been recognized that a subclinical inflammatory state also exists, and that the lactational incidence rate of this may be as high as 30% (Sheldon *et al.*, 2009). This state may be associated with partial recovery of the endometrium after clinical metritis or endometritis, trauma or other non-microbial disease, or can be the direct result of failure of uterine bacterial clearance mechanisms where no clinical disease has been evident.

Cows experiencing uterine bacterial disease tend to have longer intervals from calving to first service or conception and lower pregnancy rates (Borsberry and Dobson, 1989; LeBlanc *et al.*, 2002), and as a result it is implicated as one of the major causes of financial loss due to reproduction in dairy herds.

Development of clinical and/or subclinical endometritis depends on the balance between host immunity and microbial pathogenicity. It is generally held that the bacteria responsible for this group of syndromes are ubiquitous in the environment, and traditionally much importance has been attached to calving pen hygiene for prevention of disease. However, several studies have failed to associate environmental hygiene with endometritis (Noakes *et al.*, 1991; Potter *et al.*, 2010), and this may play a negligible role. Instead, factors such as trauma to the reproductive tract during parturition, speed and extent of uterine involution and immune function may be more significant.

Several studies have evaluated risk factors for endometritis: Potter *et al.* (2010) reported significant associations between the likelihood of endometritis and the occurrence of a case of RFM in the same lactation, assisted calving, stillbirth, vulval angle, primiparity and a male calf. Similarly, Gautam (2010) found associations between probability of a case of endometritis and assisted calving, RFM and concurrent periparturient disease. Further workers have found additional associations between endometritis and delivery of twin calves

(LeBlanc *et al.*, 2002). An earlier study evaluating risk factors for clinical metritis (Bruun *et al.*, 2002) found similar associations (although in this study the effect of parity was different, with second-lactation cows at lower risk), supporting the view that these syndromes have a common aetiology (Sheldon, 2004). The role of energy balance in the development of uterine bacterial disease is controversial, and research evidence in this field is not comprehensive. Negative energy balance and clinical ketosis have been associated with increased incidence of disease (Butler and Smith, 1989; Hammon *et al.*, 2006), but other workers have failed to find such associations. There is a clear and plausible role for energy balance: a large body of research evidence suggests that cows in peri-parturient negative energy balance have impaired immune function (Hammon *et al.*, 2006), and this has also been demonstrated within the uterine environment (Zerbe *et al.*, 2000). Since the immune system plays a key role in clearance of bacterial contamination from the uterus post-calving (Sheldon *et al.*, 2009), it is likely that management of peri-parturient energy balance is important in prevention of this syndrome. Energy balance is also likely to be important in terms of timely return to cyclicity: oestrus represents a key opportunity for cure of bacterial disease (Sheldon and Dobson, 2004), and negative energy balance can delay first ovulation and return to normal cyclicity post-partum. It is also plausible that micronutrient nutrition (especially selenium and vitamins A and E) is important for the same reason, and parenteral administration of vitamin E has been associated with a lower risk of clinical metritis (Erskine *et al.*, 1997), although dietary supplementation is preferable (see Chapter 8).

### Anovulatory anoestrus and cystic ovarian disease

These conditions are related to disruption of normal post-partum return to ovarian cyclicity. In both conditions, follicular waves develop in response to follicle-stimulating hormone (FSH) stimulation, but in affected cows there is failure of the dominant follicle (DF) to ovulate. In anovulatory anoestrus, it is thought that there is insufficient luteinizing hormone (LH) release from the anterior pituitary (AP) to trigger ovulation, and that this results from perturbation of the hypothalamo-pituitary-ovarian axis (HPOA). This leads to regression and atresia of the DF, and development of a subsequent follicular wave. This process continues in a cyclical fashion until such time as the HPOA is sufficiently functional to stimulate ovulation of a DF. In cystic ovarian disease (COD), LH is sufficient to support the DF, but insufficient to cause ovulation. The DF therefore persists, and may continue to secrete high levels of oestrogen, become luteinized (forming a luteal cyst) or become functionally inactive.

Disruption of the HPOA leading to subnormal LH release is therefore the key element in the pathogenesis of both diseases. A number of potential causes for this disruption have been suggested, and many of these have also been associated with one or both diseases in epidemiological studies. Established risk factors for delayed ovarian cyclicity include dystocia, abnormal vaginal discharge, concurrent disease and severe negative energy balance (Opsomer *et al.*, 2000). Control of anoestrus therefore centres around managing peri-parturient energy balance and minimizing early-lactation diseases (see Chapter 8). Risk factors for COD are less clear, although several studies have found associations between disease and later-parity animals (Laporte *et al.*, 1994; Nelson *et al.*, 2010) and animals with higher milk production (Laporte *et al.*, 1994; Hooijer *et al.*, 2001). Therefore, nutrition and management in the peri-parturient period are again likely to be important (see Chapter 8).

### Abortion

Abortion is defined as the expulsion of a recognizable dead or non-viable fetus prior to the end of normal gestation (Cabell, 2007). A certain level of fetal loss is generally considered to be 'natural' or unavoidable, but investigation should be considered where the rate of abortion is above 3–5% of pregnancies. Abortion may be due to a wide range of infectious and non-infectious causes, many of which are sporadic in nature. Common causes of abortion are listed in Box 4.10.

A detailed description of monitoring and management of the infectious diseases is provided in Chapter 7. The key role of the herd health advisor is to monitor the rate of abortion, and ensure that appropriate diagnostic measures are implemented where rate exceeds the suggested level. Diagnosis involves submission of maternal blood, complete aborted fetus and placenta (as soon as possible) to an appropriate laboratory. Control measures will relate to the specific cause of an outbreak and are outlined briefly in Box 4.10.

## Conclusion

Reproductive performance is a major determinant of the efficient working and profitability of a dairy enterprise, and as such is a key focus for the practitioner of herd health. Monitoring of reproductive performance is a central, fundamental aspect of dairy herd health and is heavily reliant on good-quality data. Analysis of reproductive data provides an excellent insight into the areas where herd performance can be improved, and is useful in highlighting the impact of interventions carried out. There is significant scope for improved fertility in the vast majority of dairy herds, and this represents a large reservoir of untapped potential for the herd health advisor to unlock.

---

**Box 4.10.** Common causes of abortion in dairy cows.

**Non-infectious causes**

| | |
|---|---|
| Nutritional (including gross malnutrition and deficiencies in iodine, vitamin E and selenium) | Nutritional problems may be revealed by examination of aborted fetus (e.g. iodine deficiency), or may require sampling of the herd for diagnosis. A careful history will often be useful where toxic, physical or stress-related causes are involved. Genetic abnormalities may be implicated where a specific sire is involved. Control of such cases involves correcting or removing the underlying cause. |
| Toxic (a variety of toxic compounds, including mycotoxins) | |
| Physical (e.g. pyrexia, trauma, twin pregnancies) | |
| Stress | |
| Genetic abnormalities of the fetus | |

**Infectious causes**

| | |
|---|---|
| *Neospora caninum* | Mostly sporadic abortions at various stages of gestation (and stillbirths), although infected herds can suffer high incidence rates. Vertical transmission is effective, and other modes of infection possible (see Chapter 7 for details of control). |
| *Bacillus licheniformis* | Often sporadic late abortions. Infection and pathogenesis not well understood, but spoilt feedstuffs and silage run-off are thought to be important sources of infection. |
| *Arcanobacter pyogenes* | Again usually a sporadic cause of late abortions. Pathogenesis and epidemiology very poorly understood, and no specific measures are generally recommended for control. |
| Bovine viral diarrhoea (BVD) | Often associated with a low incidence rate of abortions in infected herds, although introduction of disease to a previously naïve herd can result in a large proportion of abortions (dependent on reproductive status). Diagnosis and control are covered in Chapter 7. |

*Continued*

| Box 4.10. Continued. | |
| --- | --- |
| *Salmonella* spp. | Affected cows are often (but not always) pyrexic and diarrhoeic. Control is very dependent on the clinical scenario: *Salmonella dublin* is endemic in many dairy herds and may cause sporadic abortions, but introduction of a species to which a herd is naïve can be associated with clusters of abortions. Control may involve vaccination. |
| *Leptospira hardjo* | Abortions (usually at >6 months) can be a feature of an infected herd, and clusters of abortions can result from introduction of disease to a naïve herd. See Chapter 7 for details of control. |
| Mycotic agents (e.g. *Aspergillus fumigatus*) | Usually sporadic abortions from mid-term onwards. Commoner in winter in UK herds. Spoiled feedstuffs (especially forages) are thought to be an important source of infection. |
| Infectious bovine rhinotracheitis (IBR) | Abortions (usually from mid-term onwards) can be a feature of an infected herd, and outbreaks can result from introduction of disease to a naïve herd. See Chapter 7. |
| *Campylobacter fetus venerealis* | See Box 4.8. |

# References and Further Reading

Arbel, R., Bigun, Y., Ezra, E., Sturman, H. and Hojman, D. (2001) The effect of extended calving intervals in high-yielding lactating cows on milk production and profitability. *Journal of Dairy Science* 84, 600–608.

Borsberry, S. and Dobson, H. (1989) Peri-parturient diseases and their effect on reproductive performance in five dairy herds. *Veterinary Record* 124, 217–219.

Breen, J.E., Hudson, C.D., Bradley, A.J. and Green, M.J. (2009) Monitoring dairy herd fertility performance in the modern production animal practice. *Cattle Practice* 17, 196–201.

Britt, J.H., Scott, R.G., Armstrong, J.D. and Whitacre, M.D. (1986) Determinants of estrous behavior in lactating Holstein cows. *Journal of Dairy Science* 69, 2195–2202.

Britt, J.S., Thomas, R.C., Speer, N.C. and Hall, M.B. (2003) Efficiency of converting nutrient dry matter to milk in Holstein herds. *Journal of Dairy Science* 86, 3796–3801.

Bruun, J., Ersbøll, A.K. and Alban, L. (2002) Risk factors for metritis in Danish dairy cows. *Preventive Veterinary Medicine* 54, 179–190.

Butler, W.R. (1998) Review: effect of protein nutrition on ovarian and uterine physiology in dairy cattle. *Journal of Dairy Science* 81, 2533–2539.

Butler, W.R. (2001) Nutritional effects on resumption of ovarian cyclicity and conception rate in post-partum dairy cows. *BSAS Occasional Publication* 133–146.

Butler, W.R. (2003) Energy balance relationships with follicular development, ovulation and fertility in post-partum dairy cows. *Livestock Production Science* 83, 211–218.

Butler, W.R. and Smith, R.D. (1989) Interrelationships between energy balance and post-partum reproductive function in dairy cattle. *Journal of Dairy Science* 72, 767–783.

Cabell, E. (2007) Bovine abortion: aetiology and investigations. *In Practice* 29, 455.

Cavalieri, J., Hepworth, G., Fitzpatrick, L.A., Shephard, R.W. and Macmillan, K.L. (2006) Manipulation and control of the estrous cycle in pasture-based dairy cows. *Theriogenology* 65, 45–64.

Collick, D., Ward, W. and Dobson, H. (1989) Associations between types of lameness and fertility. *Veterinary Record* 125, 103–106.

Compton, C.W.R. and McDougall, S. (2010) A longitudinal study of reproductive performance and management of 82 dairy herds in the Waikato region with differing policies on the routine use of induction of parturition. *New Zealand Veterinary Journal* 58, 175–183.

Cook, J. (2010) Measuring and monitoring reproductive performance in dairy herds. *In Practice* 32, 432–436.

De Rensis, F., Valentini, R., Gorrieri, F., Bottarelli, E. and Lopez-Gatius, F. (2008) Inducing ovulation with hCG improves the fertility of dairy cows during the warm season. *Theriogenology* 69, 1077–1082.

DeJarnette, J.M. (1999) Factors affecting the quality of frozen semen after thawing. In: *Proceedings of the Society of Theriogenology*, presented at the *Semen Cryopreservation and Artificial Insemination Symposium*, Nashville, TN, pp. 267–276.

DeJarnette, J.M., Marshall, C.E., Lenz, R.W., Monke, D.R., Ayars, W.H. and Sattler, C.G. (2004) Sustaining the fertility of artificially inseminated dairy cattle: The role of the artificial insemination industry. *Journal of Dairy Science* 87, E93–E104.

deVries, A. and Risco, C.A. (2005) Trends and seasonality of reproductive performance in Florida and Georgia dairy herds from 1976 to 2002. *Journal of Dairy Science* 88, 3155–3165.

Dhaliwal, G.S., Murray, R.D., Dobson, H., Montgomery, J. and Ellis, W.A. (1996) Reduced conception rates in dairy cattle associated with serological evidence of *Leptospira interrogans* serovar *hardjo* infection. *Veterinary Record* 139, 110.

Diskin, M. and Morris, D. (2008) Embryonic and early fetal losses in cattle and other ruminants. *Reproduction in Domestic Animals* 43, 260–267.

Doig, P.A., Ruhnke, H.L., Mackay, A.L. and Palmer, N.C. (1979) Bovine granular vulvitis associated with urea-plasma infection. *Canadian Veterinary Journal* 20, 89–94.

Dransfield, M.B.G., Nebel, R.L., Pearson, R.E. and Warnick, L.D. (1998) Timing of insemination for dairy cows identified in estrus by a radiotelemetric estrus detection system. *Journal of Dairy Science* 81, 1874–1882.

Eppink, E. (2005) A survey of bull breeding soundness evaluations in the south east of Scotland. *Cattle Practice* 13, 205–209.

Erskine, R.J., Bartlett, P.C., Herdt, T. and Gaston, P. (1997) Effects of parenteral administration of vitamin E on health of peri-parturient dairy cows. *Journal of the American Veterinary Medical Association* 211, 466–469.

Esslemont, R.J. (2003) The costs of poor fertility and what to do about reducing them. *Cattle Practice* 11, 237–250.

Esslemont, R.J. and Kossaibati, M. (2002) DAISY Research Report No. 5: The costs of poor fertility and disease in UK dairy herds - Trends in DAISY herds over 10 seasons. University of Reading, UK.

Evans, R.D., Wallace, M., Shalloo, L., Garrick, D.J. and Dillon, P. (2006) Financial implications of recent declines in reproduction and survival of Holstein-Friesian cows in spring-calving Irish dairy herds. *Agricultural Systems* 89, 165–183.

Fenwick, M.A., Fitzpatrick, R., Kenny, D.A., Diskin, M.G., Patton, J., Murphy, J.J. and Wathes, D.C. (2008) Interrelationships between negative energy balance (NEB) and IGF regulation in liver of lactating dairy cows. *Domestic Animal Endocrinology* 34, 31–44.

Ferguson, J.D. (2005) Nutrition and reproduction in dairy herds. *Veterinary Clinics of North America: Food Animal Practice* 21, 325–347.

Fetrow, J., McClary, D., Harman, R., Butcher, K., Weaver, L., Studer, E. *et al.* (1990) Calculating selected reproductive indices: Recommendations of the American Association of Bovine Practitioners. *Journal of Dairy Science* 73, 78–90.

Firk, R., Stamer, E., Junge, W. and Krieter, J. (2003) Improving oestrus detection by combination of activity measurements with information about previous oestrus cases. *Livestock Production Science* 82, 97–103.

Foote, R.H. (1975) Estrus detection and estrus detection aids. *Journal of Dairy Science* 58, 248–256.

Foulkes, J.A., Cookson, A.D. and Sauer, M.J. (1982) AI in cattle based on daily microtitre plate enzymeim-munoassay of progesterone in whole milk. *British Veterinary Journal* 138, 515–521.

Frazer, G.S. (2005) A rational basis for therapy in the sick post-partum cow. *Veterinary Clinics of North America: Food Animal Practice* 21, 523–568.

Garnsworthy, P.C., Sinclair, K.D. and Webb, R. (2008) Integration of physiological mechanisms that influence fertility in dairy cows. *Animal* 2, 1144–1152.

Gautam, G., Nakao, T., Koike, K., Long, S.T., Yusuf, M., Ranasinghe, R.M. *et al.* (2010) Spontaneous recovery or persistence of post-partum endometritis and risk factors for its persistence in Holstein cows. *Theriogenology* 73, 168–179.

Gilbert, R.O., Shin, S.T., Guard, C.L., Erb, H.N. and Frajblat, M. (2005) Prevalence of endometritis and its effects on reproductive performance of dairy cows. *Theriogenology* 64, 1879–1888.

Gomez, F., de Boer, H. and van Eerdenburg, F.J.C.M. (2003) Relationship between mild lameness and expres-sion of oestrus in dairy cattle. *Veterinary Record* 152, 403–404.

Gonzalez-Recio, O., Perez-Cabal, M.A. and Alenda, R. (2004) Economic value of female fertility and its rela-tionship with profit in Spanish dairy cattle. *Journal of Dairy Science* 87, 3053–3061.

Grove-White, D. (2004) Rumen healthcare in the dairy cow. *In Practice* 26, 88–95.

Hammon, D.S., Evjen, I.M., Dhiman, T.R., Goff, J.P. and Walters, J.L. (2006) Neutrophil function and energy status in Holstein cows with uterine health disorders. *Veterinary Immunology and Immunopathology* 113, 21–29.

Hawk, H.W. (1987) Transport and fate of spermatozoa after insemination of cattle. *Journal of Dairy Science* 70, 1487–1503.

Hertl, J.A., Grohn, Y.T., Leach, J.D.G., Bar, D., Bennett, G.J., Gonzalez, R.N. *et al.* (2010) Effects of clinical mastitis caused by gram-positive and gram-negative bacteria and other organisms on the probability of conception in New York State Holstein dairy cows. *Journal of Dairy Science* 93, 1551–1560.

Holman, A., Thompson, J., Routly, J.E., Cameron, J., Jones, D.N., Grove-White, D. *et al.* (2011) Comparison of oestrus detection methods in dairy cattle. *Veterinary Record* 169, 47–52.

Holt, L.C., Whittier, W.D., Gwazdauskas, F.C. and Vinson, W.E. (1989) Early post-partum reproductive profiles in Holstein cows with retained placenta and uterine discharges. *Journal of Dairy Science* 72, 533–539.

Hooijer, G.A., Lubbers, R.B.F., Ducro, B.J., van Arendonk, J.A.M., Kaal-Lansbergen, L.M.T.E. and van der Lende, T. (2001) Genetic parameters for cystic ovarian disease in Dutch Black and White Dairy Cattle. *Journal of Dairy Science* 84, 286–291.

Hudson, C., Breen, J., Bradley, A. and Green, M. (2010) Fertility in UK dairy herds: Preliminary findings of a large-scale study. *Cattle Practice* 18, 89–94.

Humblot, P. (2001) Use of pregnancy-specific proteins and progesterone assays to monitor pregnancy and determine the timing, frequencies and sources of embryonic mortality in ruminants. *Theriogenology* 56, 1417–1433.

Humblot, P., Freret, S. and Ponsart, C. (2009) Epidemiology of embryonic mortality in cattle; practical implications for AI and embryo production. In: CETA/ACTE AETA Joint Convention, Montreal, Canada, p. 17.

Hunter, R.H.F. and Greve, T. (1997) Could artificial insemination of cattle be more fruitful? Penalties associated with ageing eggs. *Reproduction in Domestic Animals* 32, 137–141.

Hurnik, J.F., King, G.J. and Robertson, H.A. (1975) Estrous and related behaviour in post-partum Holstein cows. *Applied Animal Ethology* 2, 55–68.

Kasimanickam, R., Duffield, T.F., Foster, R.A., Gartley, C.J., Leslie, K.E., Walton, J.S. *et al.* (2004) Endometrial cytology and ultrasonography for the detection of subclinical endometritis in post-partum dairy cows. *Theriogenology* 62, 9–23.

Knutson, R.J. and Allrich, R.D. (1988) Influence of nutrition on serum concentrations of progesterone, luteinizing hormone and estrous behavior in dairy heifers. *Journal of Animal Science* 66, 90–97.

Kreplin, C.M., Ruhnke, H.L., Miller, R.B. and Doig, P.A. (1987) The effect of intrauterine inoculation with *Ureaplasma diversum* on bovine fertility. *Canadian Journal of Veterinary Research* 51, 440–443.

Laporte, H., Hogeveen, H., Schukken, Y. and Noordhuizen, J.P.T. (1994) Cystic ovarian disease in Dutch dairy cattle, I. Incidence, risk factors and consequences. *Livestock Production Science* 38, 191–197.

LeBlanc, S. (2007) Economics of improving reproductive performance in dairy herds, in: Doepel, L. (ed.), Advances in Dairy Technology, Vol 19, Advances in Dairy Technology. University Alberta Dept Agr, Food & Nutr Sci, Edmonton, pp. 201–214.

LeBlanc, S.J. (2008) Post-partum uterine disease and dairy herd reproductive performance: A review. *The Veterinary Journal* 176, 102–114.

LeBlanc, S.J., Duffield, T.F., Leslie, K.E., Bateman, K.G., Keefe, G.P., Walton, J.S. *et al.* (2002) Defining and diagnosing post-partum clinical endometritis and its impact on reproductive performance in dairy cows. *Journal of Dairy Science* 85, 2223–2236.

Leroy, J.L.M.R., Vanholder, T., Mateusen, B., Christophe, A., Opsomer, G., de Kruif, A. *et al.* (2005) Non-esterified fatty acids in follicular fluid of dairy cows and their effect on developmental capacity of bovine oocytes in vitro. *Reproduction* 130, 485–495.

Loeffler, H.S. and Van Vliet, J.H. (1996) Detection of oestrus in dairy cows: a new approach to an old problem. *The Veterinary Quarterly* 18, 52.

Lopez, H., Satter, L.D. and Wiltbank, M.C. (2004) Relationship between level of milk production and estrous behavior of lactating dairy cows. *Animal Reproduction Science* 81, 209–223.

López-Gatius, F., Pabón, M. and Almería, S. (2004) *Neospora caninum* infection does not affect early pregnancy in dairy cattle. *Theriogenology* 62, 606–613.

López-Gatius, F., Santolaria, P. and Almería, S. (2005) *Neospora caninum* infection does not affect the fertility of dairy cows in herds with high incidence of *Neospora*-associated abortions. *Journal of Veterinary Medicine, Series B* 52, 51–53.

Lucy, M.C. (2001) Reproductive loss in high-producing dairy cattle: Where will it end? *Journal of Dairy Science* 84, 1277–1293.

Maatje, K., Loeffler, S.H. and Engel, B. (1997) Predicting optimal time of insemination in cows that show visual signs of estrus by estimating onset of estrus with pedometers. *Journal of Dairy Science* 80, 1098–1105.

Machado, V.S., Caixeta, L.S., McArt, J.A.A. and Bicalho, R.C. (2010) The effect of claw horn disruption lesions and body condition score at dry-off on survivability, reproductive performance, and milk production in the subsequent lactation. *Journal of Dairy Science* 93, 4071–4078.

Mawhinney, I. and Biggadike, H. (1998) A field study of the Intercept planned breeding routine for dairy cows involving GnRH and PGF2alpha. *Cattle Practice* 138, 515–521.

McDougall, S. (2001) Effects of peri-parturient diseases and conditions on the reproductive performance of New Zealand dairy cows. *New Zealand Veterinary Journal* 49, 60–67.

McGowan, M. (2004) Approach to conducting bull breeding soundness examinations. *In Practice* 26, 485.

McGowan, M.R., Kirkland, P.D., Rodwell, B.J., Kerr, D.R. and Carroll, C.L. (1993) A field investigation of the effects of bovine viral diarrhea virus infection around the time of insemination on the reproductive performance of cattle. *Theriogenology* 39, 443–449.

Mee, J.F. (2004) Temporal trends in reproductive performance in Irish dairy herds and associated risk factors. *Irish Veterinary Journal* 57, 158–166.

Melendez, P., Bartolome, J., Archbald, L.F. and Donovan, A. (2003) The association between lameness, ovarian cysts and fertility in lactating dairy cows. *Theriogenology* 59, 927–937.

Merkal, R.S., Larsen, A.B. and Booth, G.D. (1975) Analysis of the effect of inapparent bovine paratuberculosis. *American Journal of Veterinary Research* 36, 837–838.

Moore, A.S. and Spahr, S.L. (1991) Activity monitoring and an enzyme immunoassay for milk progesterone to aid in the detection of estrus. *Journal of Dairy Science* 74, 3857–3862.

Morton, J.M. (2003) The InCalf Project - identifying risk factors for reproductive performance in Australian dairy herds. *Cattle Practice* 11, 201–208.

National Milk Records plc (2009) Annual Production Report. Chippenham, UK.

Nebel, R.L. and Jobst, S.M. (1998) Evaluation of systematic breeding programs for lactating dairy cows: a review. *Journal of Dairy Science* 81, 1169–1174.

Nebel, R.L., Whittier, W.D., Cassell, B.G. and Britt, J.H. (1987) Comparison of on-farm and laboratory milk progesterone assays for identifying errors in detection of estrus and diagnosis of pregnancy. *Journal of Dairy Science* 70, 1471–1476.

Nebel, R.L., Walker, W.L., McGilliard, M.L., Allen, C.H. and Heckman, G.S. (1994) Timing of artificial insemination of dairy cows: Fixed-time once-daily versus morning and afternoon. *Journal of Dairy Science* 77, 3185–3191.

Nelson, S.T., Martin, A.D. and Osteras, O. (2010) Risk factors associated with cystic ovarian disease in Norwegian dairy cattle. *Acta Veterinaria Scandinavica* 52, 60–70.

Noakes, D., Wallace, L. and Smith, G. (1991) Bacterial flora of the uterus of cows after calving on two hygienically contrasting farms. *Veterinary Record* 128, 440–442.

Norman, H.D., Wright, J.R., Hubbard, S.M., Miller, R.H. and Hutchison, J.L. (2009) Reproductive status of Holstein and Jersey cows in the United States. *Journal of Dairy Science* 92, 3517–3528.

Opsomer, G., Gröhn, Y.T., Hertl, J., Coryn, M., Deluyker, H. and de Kruif, A. (2000) Risk factors for post partum ovarian dysfunction in high producing dairy cows in Belgium: A field study. *Theriogenology* 53, 841–857.

Paisley, L.G., Mickelsen, W.D. and Anderson, P.B. (1986) Mechanisms and therapy for retained fetal membranes and uterine infections of cows: A review. *Theriogenology* 25, 353–381.

Pennington, J.A., Albright, J.L., Diekman, M.A. and Callahan, C.J. (1985) Sexual activity of Holstein cows: Seasonal effects 1. *Journal of Dairy Science* 68, 3023–3030.

Penny, C. (2005) Practical semen collection and examination techniques for breeding soundness evaluation of bulls. *Cattle Practice* 13, 199–204.

Penny, C. (2009) The new BCVA bull pre-breeding examination certificate. *Cattle Practice* 17, 202–207.

Peralta, O.A., Pearson, R.E. and Nebel, R.L. (2005) Comparison of three estrus detection systems during summer in a large commercial dairy herd. *Animal Reproduction Science* 87, 59–72.

Peter, A.T. and Bosu, W.T.K. (1986) Post-partum ovarian activity in dairy cows: Correlation between behavioral estrus, pedometer measurements and ovulations. *Theriogenology* 26, 111–115.

Phillippo, M., Humphries, W.R., Atkinson, T., Henderson, G.D. and Garthwaite, P.H. (1987) The effect of dietary molybdenum and iron on copper status, puberty, fertility and oestrous cycles in cattle. *The Journal of Agricultural Science* 109, 321–336.

Phillips, N.J., Mcgowan, M.R., Johnston, S.D. and Mayer, D.G. (2004) Relationship between thirty post-thaw spermatozoal characteristics and the field fertility of 11 high-use Australian dairy AI sires. *Animal Reproduction Science* 81, 47–61.

Pinedo, P.J., Melendez, P., Villagomez-Cortes, J.A. and Risco, C.A. (2009) Effect of high somatic cell counts on reproductive performance of Chilean dairy cattle. *Journal of Dairy Science* 92, 1575–1580.

Platz, S., Ahrens, F., Bendel, J., Meyer, H.H.D. and Erhard, M.H. (2008) What happens with cow behavior when replacing concrete slatted floor by rubber coating: a case study. *Journal of Dairy Science* 91, 999–1004.

Potter, T.J., Guitian, J., Fishwick, J., Gordon, P.J. and Sheldon, I.M. (2010) Risk factors for clinical endometritis in post-partum dairy cattle. *Theriogenology* 74, 127–134.

Ravagnolo, O. and Misztal, I. (2002) Effect of heat stress on nonreturn rate in Holsteins: Fixed-model analyses. *Journal of Dairy Science* 85, 3101–3106.

Redden, K.D., Kennedy, A.D., Ingalls, J.R. and Gilson, T.L. (1993) Detection of estrus by radiotelemetric monitoring of vaginal and ear skin temperature and pedometer measurements of activity. *Journal of Dairy Science* 76, 713–721.

Refsdal, A.O. (2007) Reproductive performance of Norwegian cattle from 1985 to 2005: trends and seasonality. *Acta Veterinaria Scandinavica* 49, 7.

Roche, J.F. (2006) The effect of nutritional management of the dairy cow on reproductive efficiency. *Animal Reproduction Science* 96, 282–296.

Roelofs, J., Vaneerdenburg, F., Soede, N. and Kemp, B. (2005) Pedometer readings for estrous detection and as predictor for time of ovulation in dairy cattle. *Theriogenology* 64, 1690–1703.

Roelofs, J., López-Gatius, F., Hunter, R.H.F., van Eerdenburg, F.J.C.M. and Hanzen, C. (2010) When is a cow in estrus? Clinical and practical aspects. *Theriogenology* 74, 327–344.

Royal, M., Mann, G.E. and Flint, A.P.F. (2000) Strategies for reversing the trend towards subfertility in dairy cattle. *The Veterinary Journal* 160, 53–60.

Sangsritavong, S., Combs, D.K., Sartori, R., Armentano, L.E. and Wiltbank, M.C. (2002) High feed intake increases liver blood flow and metabolism of progesterone and estradiol-17 [beta] in dairy cattle. *Journal of Dairy Science* 85, 2831–2842.

Senger, P.L. (1994) The estrus detection problem: New concepts, technologies, and possibilities. *Journal of Dairy Science* 77, 2745–2753.

Sheldon, I.M. (2004) The post-partum uterus. *Veterinary Clinics of North America: Food Animal Practice* 20, 569–591.

Sheldon, I.M. and Dobson, H. (2003) Reproductive challenges facing the cattle industry at the beginning of the 21st century. *Reproduction Supplement* 61, 1–13.

Sheldon, I.M. and Dobson, H. (2004) Post-partum uterine health in cattle. *Animal Reproduction Science* 82/83, 295–306.

Sheldon, I.M., Lewis, G.S., LeBlanc, S. and Gilbert, R.O. (2006) Defining post-partum uterine disease in cattle. *Theriogenology* 65, 1516–1530.

Sheldon, I.M., Cronin, J., Goetze, L., Donofrio, G. and Schuberth, H.-J. (2009) Defining Post-partum uterine disease and the mechanisms of infection and immunity in the female reproductive tract in cattle. *Biology of Reproduction* 81, 1025–1032.

Sheldon, M. (1997) Bovine fertility – practical implications of the maternal recognition of pregnancy. *In Practice* 19, 546.

Statham, J.M.E. (2012) Fertility management of dairy cows. *Cattle Practice* 20, 48–56.

Stevenson, J.S. (2008) Progesterone, follicular, and estrual responses to progesterone-based estrus and ovulation synchronization protocols at five stages of the estrous cycle. *Journal of Dairy Science* 91, 4640–4650.

Sturman, H., Oltenacu, E.A.B. and Foote, R.H. (2000) Importance of inseminating only cows in estrus. *Theriogenology* 53, 1657–1667.

Trimberger, G.W. (1948) Breeding efficiency in dairy cattle from artificial insemination at various intervals before and after ovulation. *University of Nebraska Agriculture Experimental Station Research Bulletin* 153.

USDA (1961) Dairy statistics through 1960 (Statistical Bulletin No. 303). Economic Research Service, US Department of Agriculture, Washington, DC.

USDA (1998) Milk cow numbers and yield. Economic Research Service, US Department of Agriculture, Washington, DC.

van der Burgt, G., Clark, W. and Knight, R. (2007) Cattle fertility problems and *Histophilus somni*. *Veterinary Record* 160, 600.

Van Vliet, J.H. and Van Eerdenburg, F.J.C.M. (1996) Sexual activities and oestrus detection in lactating Holstein cows. *Applied Animal Behaviour Science* 50, 57–69.

Van Vliet, R. and Van Eerdenburg, F. (2006) Estrus detection in dairy cattle: how to beat the bull? *Vlaams Diergeneeskundig Tijdschrift* 75, 61.

Vanroose, G., Nauwynck, H., Van Soom, A., Vanopdenbosch, E. and de Kruif, A. (1997) Susceptibility of zona-intact and zona-free in vitro-produced bovine embryos at different stages of development to infection with bovine herpesvirus-1. *Theriogenology* 47, 1389–1402.

Vanroose, G., Nauwynck, H., Van Soom, A., Vanopdenbosch, E. and de Kruif, A. (1998) Replication of cytopathic and noncytopathic bovine viral diarrhea virus in zona-free and zona-intact in vitro-produced bovine embryos and the effect on embryo quality. *Biology of Reproduction* 58, 857–866.

Veerkamp, R.F., Koenen, E.P.C. and De Jong, G. (2001) Genetic correlations among body condition score, yield, and fertility in first-parity cows estimated by random regression models. *Journal of Dairy Science* 84, 2327–2335.

Villa-Godoy, A., Hughes, T.L., Emery, R.S., Chapin, L.T. and Fogwell, R.L. (1988) Association between energy balance and luteal function in lactating dairy cows. *Journal of Dairy Science* 71, 1063–1072.

Walker, S.L., Smith, R.F., Jones, D.N., Routly, J.E. and Dobson, H. (2008a) Chronic stress, hormone profiles and estrus intensity in dairy cattle. *Hormones and Behavior* 53, 493–501.

Walker, S.L., Smith, R.F., Routly, J.E., Jones, D.N., Morris, M.J. and Dobson, H. (2008b) Lameness, activity time-budgets, and estrus expression in dairy cattle. *Journal of Dairy Science* 91, 4552–4559.

Wall, E. and Coffey, M. (2005) Improving dairy cattle fertility through genetic selection. *Cattle Practice* 13, 19–22.

Wapenaar, W., Green, M., Huxley, J., Reader, J., Biggs, A., Burnell, M. *et al.* (2008) Measuring and comparing reproductive performance in dairy herds: strengths and weaknesses of frequently used parameters. *Cattle Practice* 14, 36–41.

Washburn, S.P., Silvia, W.J., Brown, C.H., McDaniel, B.T. and McAllister, A.J. (2002) Trends in reproductive performance in Southeastern Holstein and Jersey DHI herds. *Journal of Dairy Science* 85, 244–251.

Wathes, D.C., Fenwick, M., Cheng, Z., Bourne, N., Llewellyn, S., Morris, D.G. *et al.* (2007) Influence of negative energy balance on cyclicity and fertility in the high producing dairy cow. *Theriogenology* 68, S232–S241.

Weaver, L.D., Daley, C.A. and Borelli, C.L. (1989) Effect on pregnancy rate of nonestrus insemination in previously inseminated dairy cows. *Theriogenology* 32, 603–606.

Whitaker, D.A. (1998) Are links between blood urea and fertility in dairy cattle a diversion from reality? *Cattle Practice* 6, 399–403.

Whitlow, L.W. and Hagler, W.M. (1999) An association of mycotoxins with production, health and reproduction in dairy cattle and guidelines for prevention and treatment. In: *Biotechnology in the Feed Industry, Proceedings of Alltech's 15th Annual Symposium* (eds TP Lyons and KA Jacques), Nottingham University Press, UK, p. 401.

Wilde, D. (2005) Mycotoxins - are they a threat to the UK dairy industry? *Cattle Practice* 13, 131–133.

Williams, E.J., Herath, S., England, G.C.W., Dobson, H., Bryant, C.E. and Sheldon, I.M. (2008) Effect of *Escherichia coli* infection of the bovine uterus from the whole animal to the cell. *Animal* 2, 1153–1157.

Wilson, D.J., Grohn, Y.T., Bennett, G.J., González, R.N., Schukken, Y.H. and Spatz, J. (2008) Milk production change following clinical mastitis and reproductive performance compared among J5 vaccinated and control dairy cattle. *Journal of Dairy Science* 91, 3869–3879.

Xu, Z.Z., McKnight, D.J., Vishwanath, R., Pitt, C.J. and Burton, L.J. (1998) Estrus detection using radiotelemetry or visual observation and tail painting for dairy cows on pasture. *Journal of Dairy Science* 81, 2890–2896.

Yoshida, C., Yusuf, M. and Nakao, T. (2009) Duration of estrus induced after GnRH-PGF$_{2\alpha}$ protocol in the dairy heifer. *Animal Science Journal* 80, 649–654.

Zerbe, H., Schneider, N., Leibold, W., Wensing, T., Kruip, T.A.M. and Schuberth, H.J. (2000) Altered functional and immunophenotypical properties of neutrophilic granulocytes in post-partum cows associated with fatty liver. *Theriogenology* 54, 771–786.

# 5 Control of Mastitis and Enhancement of Milk Quality

**Andrew Bradley,**[1,2] **Herman Barkema,**[3] **Andrew Biggs,**[4]
**Martin Green**[2] **and Theo Lam**[5]

[1]*Quality Milk Management Services Ltd, Cedar Barn, Easton Hill, Easton, Wells BA5
IDU, UK;* [2]*School of Veterinary Medicine and Science, University of Nottingham,
Sutton Bonington Campus, Leicestershire LE12 5RD, UK;* [3]*Department of Production
Animal Health, Faculty of Veterinary Medicine, University of Calgary, Calgary, AB,
Canada;* [4]*Vale Veterinary Group, The Laurels, Tiverton, Devon EX16 4LF, UK;* [5]*Dutch
Udder Health Centre UGCN at GD Animal Health Service and Department of
Farm Animal Health, and Department of Farm Animal Health, Faculty of Veterinary
Medicine, Utrecht University, The Netherlands*

## Introduction

Mastitis is one of the most common and costly diseases of dairy cattle and therefore one of the most important in dairy herd health. The aims of this chapter are to give the herd health professional an insight into udder health management in the modern dairy herd and to equip him or her with the necessary background to pursue the latest approaches to control.

From a mammary gland perspective a healthy herd will have a low bulk milk somatic cell count (BMSCC), a low incidence of clinical mastitis, a low proportion of teats with teat end lesions and low numbers of cows culled for udder health reasons. Cows will have four functional quarters and produce milk that is wholesome and of required constituent value. Whilst this is a worthy aim, it is not always attained in modern productions systems where compromise too often rules the day.

## An international perspective on mastitis and milk production

Reducing numbers of producers, increasing herd size and yield – industrialization of milk production. In 2005, the average herd size globally was only 2.4 cows and 12–14% of the world's population were to some extent directly dependent on dairy farming (http://www.fao.org/docrep/012/i1522e/i1522e02.pdf). In contrast, in the UK the 20,000 producers represent less than 0.001% of the population with an average herd size of 98 cows (http://www.dairyco.net/datum.aspx, http://www.usda.gov/wps/portal/usda/usdahome). In the developed world, milk production in the early 21st century has been defined by a relentless decline in producer numbers, an increasing herd size (see Fig. 5.1) and increasing individual animal output (see Fig. 5.2). The lack of inflationary increases in farm income from milk production relative to other commodities such as

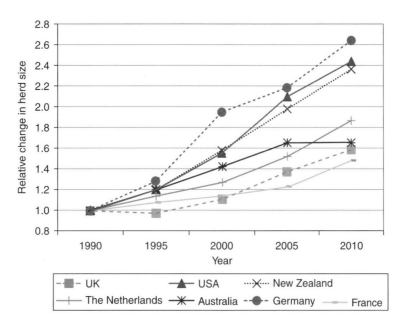

**Fig. 5.1.** Change in average herd size (relative to 1990) in exemplar of developed dairy-producing countries.

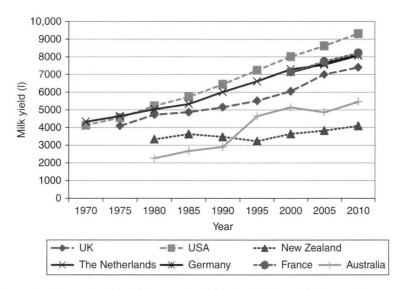

**Fig. 5.2.** Approximate annual milk yield in exemplar of developed dairy-producing countries.

feed, energy (diesel and electricity) and fertilizer has driven a requirement for greater efficiency. The changes in social acceptance of
long working hours and the introduction of
technical input in terms of improved cow
genetics (greater potential for milk produc-

tion), nutrition (realization of that potential)
and technology in terms of mechanization of
feed production, milking process and disease
monitoring have all contributed to both
increased productivity and efficiency. In the
developed world, the latter half of the 20th

century and early 21st century saw average herd sizes increase from tens of cows to hundreds, with some of the largest herds now being counted in the thousands or tens of thousands.

Increasing herd size, to capitalize on 'economies of scale', seems inevitable to maintain farm income and at the farm level there has been, and continues to be, an erosion of skill as experienced labour is lost. These are significant challenges in the pursuit of 'quality milk' production which make the herd health approach, as described in Chapter 1, essential in the modern dairy herd.

### Polarization in the industry: differing approaches to milk production

In understanding the approach to mastitis control and production of quality milk, there are two areas in particular, nutrition and milk harvesting, where technology has had an impact and has resulted in polarization of the approach to milk production. These polarizations are seen worldwide and are discussed below.

Nutrition of the dairy cow can be very complex, particularly when trying to optimize output in high-yielding Holstein-Friesian cows. In this situation, significant labour and financial inputs are required to support the high level of production per cow. Often cows in such systems are housed year round to ensure control and consistency of their diet (high input – high output production). In areas of the world where forage can be grown and preserved in abundance, cows with lower yield potential (often Channel Island or cross-bred cows) are fed on a simpler, less expensive and less labour-intensive, pasture-based diet (low input – low output production). Cows in these systems may not be housed at all, or for only a few months of the year compared with the 6 months or more seen in intensive production systems.

Milk harvesting has seen a technological revolution in terms of mechanical efficiency and technical ability. A car produced in the 1950s is very different from a car produced today, and similarly the milking parlour

of today has many more high-tech systems to monitor and modify its function as well as in-line, high-tech, solutions to aid the detection of abnormal milk and mastitis. Much of this sensor technology is still undergoing development and evaluation in terms of sensitivity and specificity of mastitis detection, as well as cost–benefit ratios, but it is likely to become more common as accuracy improves and costs come down. Adoption of this technology will also be influenced by the philosophy of the unit with high input – high-output systems more likely to be the early adopters.

Even the high-tech approach to milk harvesting has two directions of development, namely high-capacity parlours with a high throughput of cows per person per hour and automatic milking systems (AMS) where manual labour is replaced by a robot. To achieve high throughput in a parlour, labour needs to be used efficiently alongside automation (most commonly, automatic cluster removal (ACR) and possibly automatic application of post-milking teat disinfection (PMTD)). Despite this automation, which helps facilitate high throughput in these parlours, there is often only a few seconds available for teat preparation, which presents challenges for milk quality control. In single- or multiple-stall AMS the robot performs the manual tasks and the cows present themselves to be milked, hence the alternative name of voluntary milking system (VMS). Single-stall AMS as opposed to multiple-stall AMS systems have the potential disadvantage of a breakdown, leaving the farm without a functioning robot. A recent development in AMS is a multi-robot rotary parlour that can give flexibility of milking but may require batches of cows to be delivered to the parlour. Future developments will almost certainly see improvements in the ability of robots and further automation in conventional parlours, and these innovations will bring challenges in their own right.

### Clinical and subclinical mastitis

Mastitis can be classified as 'clinical' when inflammatory changes to the mammary gland or milk are visually apparent, or 'sub-clinical' when disease is present but the inflammatory changes cannot be detected visually. In most developed countries, the incidence of clinical and subclinical mastitis has decreased over the last few decades. For example, in the UK it is estimated that between the late 1960s and the early 1980s average clinical mastitis rates fell from in excess of 150 cases to around 40 cases per 100 cows per year (Bradley and Green, 2000). By the early 2000s the rate was 50–60 cases per 100 cows (Bradley *et al* 2007a). These changes in rate were accompanied by a significant change in the aetiology of mastitis, with a shift away from the classic contagious mastitis pathogens to those defined as environmental.

In a similar time frame, the UK BMSCC fell from around 600,000 to around 200,000 cells/ml. The most dramatic fall was in the mid-1990s, when EU directive 92/46 EEC (EU 1992a) made it unlawful for milk to leave a farm for human consumption when the geometric mean of 3 months' BMSCC was >400,000 cells/ml. This was coupled with the advent of milk buyers applying significant price penalties (often 25% of milk price) to encourage farmers to either improve their milk quality or leave the industry.

Whilst directives such as that implemented by the EU have not been universally adopted worldwide, the declining incidence, prevalence and shifting patterns described in the UK are common to the dairy industries of other developed countries around the world. Examples of the changing incidence and prevalence of bovine mastitis in parts of the developed world are outlined in Table 5.1.

*Milk hygiene*

EU directive 92/46 EEC (EU, 1992a) set a hygiene standard of 100,000 cells/ml total bacterial count (TBC), measured by agar plate count, for milk leaving a farm for human consumption. Payment penalties were again applied to encourage compliance. TBC – or, more accurately – total viable count (TVC) is costly and time consuming to perform and has been largely replaced by Bactoscan, a much more rapid and simple measurement with which it correlates well (http://www.food.gov.uk/multimedia/pdfs/mb_009_feb2001.pdf).

Within the EU the limits of 400,000 somatic cells/ml and 100,000 bacterial cells/ml are used as standards for intra- and extra-community trade. While similar levels have

**Table 5.1.** Examples of the change in incidence and prevalence of bovine mastitis in an exemplar of countries with a developed dairy industry.

| | 1980s | | Early 2000s | |
|---|---|---|---|---|
| | Incidence of clinical mastitis (cases/100 cows/year) | Bulk milk SCC ($\times 10^3$/ml) | Incidence of clinical mastitis (cases/100 cows/year) | Bulk milk SCC ($\times 10^3$/ml) |
| Canada | – | – | 23[c] | 230[c] |
| New Zealand | – | 350[a] | 19[d] | 232[e] |
| Norway | 19[a] | 248[a] | 19[f] | 114[f] |
| The Netherlands | 20–25[a] | 350[a] | 34[g] | 220[h] |
| USA | 48[a] | 500[a] | – | 224[i] |
| UK | 40[b] | 376[a] | 50–60[j] | 192[k] |

SCC, somatic cell count. [a] Booth (1996); [b] Wilesmith *et al.* (1986); [c] Sargeant *et al.* (1998; reports incidence of first cases of CM: Olde Riekerink *et al.* (2008), http://www.dairyinfo.gc.ca/index_e.php?s1=dff-fcil&s2=farm-ferme&s3=ssbc-clbt); [d] Petrovski *et al.* (2009); [e] NZ Dairy Statistics, http://www.lic.co.nz/pdf/DAIRY%20STATISTICS%2010-11-WEB.pdf; [f] Østerås and Sølverød (2009); [g] Sol (2002); [h] van den Borne *et al.* (2011); [i] USDA, http://www.aphis.usda.gov/animal_health/nahms/dairy/downloads/dairy_monitoring/BTSCC_2010infosheet.pdf; [j] Bradley *et al.* (2007a); [k] DairyCo Datum, http://www.dairyco.org.uk/datum/milk-supply/composition-and-hygiene/gb-milk-hygiene.aspx been adopted and implemented in other parts of the world, these limits act as barriers to trade for countries not able to demonstrate that their industry is producing to these standards. The figures used around the world for upper BMSCC limits for milk sold for human consumption vary, although both New Zealand and Australia use the 400,000 cells/ml upper limit, while all Canadian provinces will move to the same cut-off in the summer of 2012. The USA uses an upper limit of 750,000 cells/ml. However, it is important to add that while some countries have higher regulatory limits this does not necessarily reflect the milk quality situation within that country, with the majority of herds in the USA having similar BMSCCs to herds in the EU (see Table 5.1).

### The economics of bovine mastitis

Mastitis and suboptimal milk quality are considered to be the most costly production disease in dairying, and have been estimated to account for 38% of all the direct costs associated with such diseases (Kossaibati and Esslemont, 1997). The cost to the UK dairy industry alone is estimated to be in excess of £200 million annually, while worldwide costs are estimated in the region of US$35 billion.

The economic impact of mastitis can be viewed at world, national, herd or individual cow level and encompasses both treatment and preventive measures aimed at clinical and subclinical disease. Effectively, expenditure can be split into (i) investment in preventive measures and monitoring and (ii) costs due to suboptimal production, early culling and clinical disease. It is often considered that some preventive measures have a relatively high return on investment whilst others do not (Huijps et al., 2010) and could perhaps be best viewed as a form of 'insurance'. However, the cost–benefit of different control methods in different farm circumstances has been the subject of little research and remains relatively poorly understood. Clearly, treatment of cases of mastitis that have a good chance of success will be better value for

money than attempting to treat cases where success is very unlikely, and factors that influence this success rate are described later.

Mastitis costs can broadly be split into direct and indirect costs. Direct costs are those that are closely related to the mastitis or its treatment, whereas indirect costs are those incurred as a result of, or subsequent to, the mastitis. The costs associated with clinical mastitis are generally easier to calculate than those with subclinical mastitis, with the direct costs being the most simple to quantify. In addition, there are also significant costs to the industry of ongoing preventive measures.

The costs of preventive management measures are usually attributed equally to all cows in a herd, since the benefits are assumed to be equally shared. In terms of treatment costs, the effects of a successful treatment of a single infected quarter are not restricted to the cow under treatment; the removal of an infected quarter from a herd, by successful treatment (or culling), reduces the chance of spread within the herd and thus benefits the herd as a whole. Such benefits will vary between herds, depending on the likelihood of transmission of infection from infected to uninfected cows.

The costs of clinical and subclinical mastitis vary widely between herds. For example, the average cost of a case of clinical mastitis has been estimated to be between £100 and £2000 per case depending on the severity, the stage of lactation when disease occurs and farm circumstances (such as milk price). Therefore, when evaluating the cost of mastitis on a dairy unit, it is essential to estimate costs using herd-specific values, rather than average figures. The costs associated with mastitis can be estimated as shown below.

#### Clinical mastitis costs

The direct and indirect costs associated with clinical mastitis are shown in Box 5.1.

#### Subclinical mastitis costs

Subclinical mastitis costs are difficult to estimate, but again can be divided into direct and indirect costs in a similar way to

---

**Box 5.1.** Direct and indirect costs of mastitis.

| Direct costs | Indirect costs |
|---|---|
| Treatment costs | Reduction in cow yield following case |
| Labour costs | Recurrent clinical case in later lactation |
| Veterinary surgeon's (veterinarian's) time (if required) | Culling |
|  | Transmission to uninfected cow(s) |
| Reduced milk sales from discarded milk during treatment and withholding period | |
| Mortality | |

---

those outlined above for clinical mastitis. Direct costs attributable to increased BMSCC are perhaps the most obvious cost to farmers, and these take the form of payment penalties or lost bonuses. Different payment penalties in pence per litre (ppl) are levied on individual farms, but are often triggered by a BMSCC >200,000 or >250,000 cells/ml. These penalties are generally banded, becoming more severe with increasing BMSCC, and typically represent between <1% and 5% of milk value depending on the milk contract and BMSCC level. The indirect costs of subclinical mastitis are difficult for producers to appreciate, but a reasonable estimate is that herd yield decreases approximately 2.5% for every 100,000 cells/ml that the BMSCC increases over a threshold of 200,000 cells/ml. While losses associated with subclinical mastitis will vary hugely, for a UK herd, for example, on a typical milk supply contract and with a BMSCC of 250,000 cells/ml and an average yield of 8500l, subclinical mastitis costs could be expected to be in the range of £30–50 per cow per year.

### Additional indirect costs

In addition to the costs outlined above, there are further indirect herd costs associated with mastitis that are difficult to estimate:

- spread to other cows, resulting in increased clinical and subclinical mastitis;
- increase in preventive management and monitoring costs enforced due to increased disease prevalence (see later);

- loss of genetic potential from the herd due to forced culling; and
- further financial penalties from:
  - potential effect on BMSCC once milk returned to the bulk tank;
  - potential effect on bacterial count in milk/Bactoscan; and
  - potential to cause an antibiotic milk failure having significant economic impact.

### Preventive management costs

As well as the costs associated with the occurrence of disease, it is also necessary to consider the cost of routine preventive measures. Examples, though not an exhaustive list, of typical preventive management costs are:

- labour: time involved in:
  - maintaining general hygiene of cow accommodation;
  - good milking routine;
  - monthly routine milk recording;
  - maintaining accurate clinical and drying-off records;
  - evaluating action lists from analysis and interpretation of SCC and clinical records; and
  - segregation of cows.
- consumables:
  - teat preparation material (paper/medicated towels/milking gloves, etc.);
  - teat dip/spray (pre- and post-milking);
  - dairy chemicals for cleaning parlour (and cluster disinfection);
  - antibiotic dry cow tubes or teat sealants; and

○   somatic cell counting and bacterio-
    logical monitoring.

Clearly, many of the preventive management costs outlined above have benefits
with respect to other aspects of disease control, cow comfort and cow welfare, and thus
such costs should not solely be attributed to
mastitis control.

## Welfare implications of bovine mastitis

The Farm Animal Welfare Council (FAWC),
an independent advisory body established
by the UK Government in 1979, stated that
'The welfare of an animal includes its physical and mental state and we consider that
good animal welfare implies both fitness
and a sense of well-being'. They have provided a framework to define ideal states that
are applicable to all animal production systems, termed the 'Five Freedoms'. The third
freedom states 'Freedom from pain, injury
or disease'.

There is no question that clinical mastitis can be a painful condition and, in very
severe cases, cows will appear sick and dis-
tressed. Research has shown that even in
relatively mild cases cows show a reduced
threshold for pain, indicating that pain can
be a significant consequence for a cow suffering from even a mild case of clinical mastitis (Kemp et al., 2008). For this reason, the
use of anti-inflammatory drugs such as non-
steroidal anti-inflammatory drugs (NSAIDs)
is an important part of the veterinary
armoury in mastitis treatment.

The influence of husbandry and management on mastitis incidence, and the predominant types of pathogens present in a
herd, have a part to play in the welfare of
the cows in that herd. It is worth considering the relative welfare implications in two
contrasting herds with different patterns of
disease: a herd with a high BMSCC (~350,000
cells/ml) but an acceptable clinical mastitis
rate (20 cases/100 cows/year) compared
with a herd with a low BMSCC (<100,000
cells/ml) but a high clinical mastitis rate
(80 cases/100 cows/year). Which herd has
the most significant welfare concerns? What

approaches are appropriate for each herd?
While we may not completely understand
the impact that mastitis has on cow welfare,
it is clear that reducing the incidence and
prevalence of mastitis in dairy herds will
result in an important welfare improvement. However, we should be mindful that
the change in aetiology of mastitis that may
occur following implementation of mastitis
control measures could have an adverse
effect on a small proportion of cows – for
instance, an increase in severe coliform
mastitis following control of contagious
pathogens. This balance is discussed more
fully in later sections.

## The public health implications
## and perception of bovine milk

### Bacterial risks: pasteurization

Milk has the potential to harbour a range of
pathogens harmful to human health. These
can be the result of (i) an intra-mammary
infection with a mastitis pathogen resulting
in clinical or subclinical mastitis; (ii) asymptomatic, non-significant intra-mammary
infection with a potential human pathogen
such as Campylobacter spp.; or (iii) contamination of the milk after or during harvesting from the cow. Pasteurization reduces
the overall viable bacterial load in milk,
diminishing the chance of harmful bacteria
being present and increasing the shelf life of
milk and milk products. Consumption of
dairy products from unpasteurized sources
carries significant risks from a number of
pathogens, including but not limited to
Salmonella spp. and Listeria spp.

### Adverse effects of mastitis on milk quality

Mastitis has a variety of effects on the constituents of milk, many of which have implications for the food industry. Cows identified
with clinical mastitis have their milk discarded during the clinical episode and for a
period afterwards, i.e. within the antibiotic
withhold time. However, changes in milk
quality associated with subclinical mastitis
can have significant effects on both the

keeping quality (i.e. the shelf life) and yield of milk products such as cheese. More specifically, somatic cells that are present in increased numbers in milk during an infection are involved in the conversion of plasminogen to plasmin. Plasmin, a proteolytic enzyme produced by the cow, can break down casein and decrease cheese yield.

### Medicines residues

Developed dairy nations have in place strict rules and regulations to prevent contamination of the food chain by veterinary medicinal products. All medicines licensed for use in dairy cattle have a milk withhold period to ensure that residues are below the maximum residue limit (MRL) when the milk from treated cows is offered for human consumption.

Antibiotics are of special concern because of their potential effect on human bacterial populations in terms of antibiotic resistance, as well as their potential to elicit allergic reactions in humans. Many of the antibiotics used in the treatment of mastitis are similar to therapeutic antibiotics used in human medicine, giving rise to concerns regarding the development and amplification of antibiotic resistance. While there is much debate about antibiotic resistance in human pathogens being influenced by use in animals, there is a need for constant appraisal, vigilance and responsible use of antibiotics in animals.

Certain antibiotics reserved for use in critical life-threatening conditions in human patients shine a spotlight on their use in veterinary medicine, and the veterinary clinician needs to be aware of these concerns and question whether it can be justified to use these types of drugs in a routine and widespread manner. There exists the precedent of the removal of chloramphenicol for veterinary use in food-producing animals, to safeguard its use in diarrhoeic patients, particularly children in Africa with cholera. There are two other antibiotic classes where there are major areas of concern: the fluoroquinolones and 3rd- and 4th-generation cephalosporins. Concerns regarding fluoroquinolone use are enhanced because the resistance mechanism can confer resistance across all members of the groups quinolones and fluoroquinolones. Third- and fourth-generation cephalosporin concerns surround the emergence of extended spectrum beta lactamase (ESBL) resistance. Some countries and farms use these drugs routinely as part of their protocols for various infectious diseases, including mastitis; however, without responsible and prudent use the risk will remain that these drugs may be withdrawn from use in food-producing animals.

One area of particular concern that will receive increased attention is the disposal of waste milk. Waste milk often contains antibiotic residues and is commonly fed to calves. This practice raises considerable worry over transmission of disease and encouraging of antibiotic resistance. A principle that should perhaps be followed is that 'if it isn't good enough for humans it isn't good enough for calves'.

### On-farm avoidance of antibiotic residues

Test kits such as DelvotestSP-NT (DSM Food Specialties, Heerlen, The Netherlands), BetaStar (Neogen Corporation, Lansing, MN) or Snap (IDEXX, Westbrook, ME) are commercially available and are used by milk buyers to detect antimicrobials in milk, and by producers to test milk when they feel there may be a risk of an antibiotic violation. This could be in the case of a suspicion of cow identity recording error or if a dry cow calves unexpectedly early.

DelvotestSP-NT is an 'inhibitory substance' test as opposed to the BetaStar and Snap, which are immunological tests specific for beta lactam antibiotics. Furthermore the various kits have different thresholds of detection and these thresholds are, in some instances, well below the MRL. These differences in sensitivity and specificity can often lead to apparent discrepancies in results between on-farm tests (often conducted using the rapid immunological kits) and the tests conducted by the milk buyer to fulfil their regulatory commitments. Also worthy of mention is the fact that it is possible for false-positive reactions to inhibitor tests to occur as a result of high levels of natural inhibitors such as lactoferrin, and high fat levels can also interfere with the tests.

## Underlying Principles of Disease

### Anatomy and physiology

Although the complete anatomy and physiology of the mammary gland is beyond the scope of this chapter, it is worth reviewing pertinent facts as they relate to host susceptibility. The mammary gland is a mucosal surface and is essentially a highly specialized apocrine sweat gland. The gland in cattle is split into four anatomically separate quarters which function as discrete units. The teat comprises the teat cistern, which opens via the streak canal and the teat orifice. The streak canal is lined with stratified squamous epithelium and is held closed by a smooth muscle sphincter. The teat cistern joins the gland cistern, which is connected via a 'branching tree' of intralobular and secretory ducts to the secretory alveoli, which are the functional units of milk production. While the teat and gland cistern serve as milk reservoirs, in cattle the majority of milk is stored within the secretory tissue of the gland prior to initiation of the 'milk let-down reflex'. The secretory alveolus is an epithelial-lined sac surrounded by smooth muscle. In the lactating animal, milk is continually synthesized within the epithelial cells and secreted into the alveolar lumen.

Physiologically, the function of the reproductively active adult mammary gland can be split into the lactating and non-lactating phases, commonly known as the lactation cycle. The non-lactating phase (the dry period) can be further subdivided into three distinct phases. First is involution, which follows the cessation of milking and is the period during which the gland returns to a 'quiescent' (though still metabolically active) state after a lactation. Second is the steady state, which is characterized by the involuted gland, the length of which is determined by the time until the next calving. Third is colostrogenesis or transition,

when the gland 'gears up' for the next lactation. This cycle is critically important in terms of mastitis epidemiology since it results in dramatic fluctuations in gland susceptibility to infection, as will be outlined later.

### Host immune defence

The host defence against pathogens invading the mammary gland can be divided into the innate and acquired immune systems, and may be further subdivided into anatomical, soluble and cellular components (Sordillo et al., 1997). These are outlined below.

The primary anatomical defence of the mammary gland is the teat sphincter that is supplemented by keratin within the streak canal, which, as well as providing a physical barrier to the ingress of microorganisms, also forms a chemical barrier in the form of esterified and non-esterified fatty acids. Compromise in the integrity of this barrier, either through teat end damage, extreme hyperkeratosis or depletion/inadequate production of keratin, will result in an increase in susceptibility to infection (Neijenhuis et al., 2001).

The soluble components of the immune defence in the bovine mammary gland are diverse and not fully understood. Perhaps the most studied and best understood component is lactoferrin. This iron-binding protein helps protect the gland by depleting free iron and therefore inhibiting bacterial growth, as well as being immunomodulatory to some leukocytes. It is particularly important in the non-lactating gland, as its effectiveness is relatively reduced by the higher levels of citrate present in the lactating gland. The soluble arm of the acquired immune system comprises the immunoglobulins, but the role of this secondary arm of the immune defence in the bovine mammary gland is not fully understood. Despite significant research efforts into developing mastitis vaccines, this is likely to remain a problematic area given the diversity of aetiological agents and the fact that mastitis is primarily a reflection of the

host's natural response to invading pathogens rather than a direct effect of the pathogens themselves.

The cellular arm of the mammary gland
defence comprises both innate and acquired
components. The 'sentinel' cells within the
uninfected gland are primarily macrophages, though neutrophils and lymphocytes will also be present. The immune
response following ingress of pathogens
will result in non-specific recruitment of
large numbers of neutrophils following
release of chemotactic factors by resident
macrophages. This recruitment phase takes
4–6 h, a time period that can be crucial in
the early stages of some mastitis cases, particularly those caused by Gram-negative
organisms.

Leukocytes and small numbers of epithelial cells also present in milk are collectively known as 'somatic cells', literally
'cells of the body'. The number of these cells
in milk, the somatic cell count (SCC), is routinely measured both in bulk milk and individual cows, and is used as a proxy for
intra-mammary infection. Due to their easy
availability and the low cost of the test, SCC
measurements provide a useful tool for
monitoring and diagnosing patterns of

disease within a herd, as will be outlined
later in this chapter.

*The interaction between phases of the
lactation cycle and the immune defence*

It is crucial to understand the interaction
between the immune system and the lactation cycle because of the impact this has on
cow susceptibility to infection and therefore, inevitably, on the epidemiology of
mastitis. The fluctuation in mammary gland
susceptibility to intra-mammary infection
(IMI) is illustrated in Fig. 5.3.

The variation in susceptibility can be
explained by changes in the physiological
and immunological function of the lactating cow. There are two peaks in the risk of
new infection in the lactating cycle, one
during involution and another centred
around the time of calving. The peak during
involution is, at least in part, explained by
(i) the cessation of milking and therefore of
the regular 'flushing' of the streak canal,
coupled with an increase in intra-mammary
pressure that compromises the streak canal;
(ii) the cessation of post-dipping; (iii) the
fact that it takes some time (up to 28 days)
for lactoferrin concentrations to rise in the

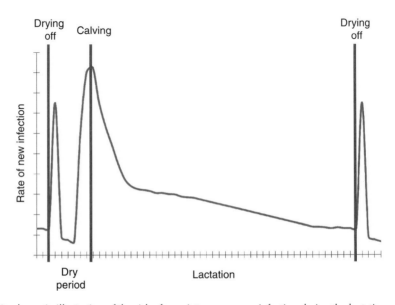

**Fig. 5.3.** A schematic illustration of the risk of new intra-mammary infection during the lactation cycle.

dry gland; and (iv) the inhibitory effect of fat and casein levels from milk remnants on leukocyte function. It is also worthy of note that the peak in new infection risk, after drying off, is considerably higher in cows not receiving any form of dry cow therapy. The peak of new infection at the end of the dry period is also driven by a variety of factors, many of these being similar to those seen in involution as the gland reverts to the lactating state. However, in addition there are direct inhibitory effects of colostrum on the function of white blood cells, as well as the impending era of negative energy balance associated with the freshly calved cow and the negative impact this also has on neutrophil function. In contrast, the fully involuted mammary gland is relatively resistant to colonization by pathogens by virtue of high levels of lactoferrin, a relatively higher SCC and, importantly, an environment more conducive to leukocyte function.

One area not yet discussed, though much studied and of great importance, is the keratin plug. This physical and chemical barrier is a key component of the natural defence in the non-lactating mammary gland and is slow to develop even in those cows most competent at forming the seal. In reality, the modern, high-yielding dairy cow is poor at forming this natural defence (for reasons not yet fully understood) and a significant number of cows fail to form a functional keratin plug throughout the dry period (Dingwell et al., 2004), while in heifers a large percentage of the teats are open weeks before first calving (Krömker and Friedrich, 2009). It is this lack of ability that has led to the relatively recent interest in both internal and external sealants and the additional protection they can confer in the non-lactating period.

### Somatic cells and their role in the host defence

There has been much debate in recent years as to whether there is a critical lower number of somatic cells in milk that afford an effective immune defence. As a proxy for intra-mammary infection, there is little doubt that as SCCs rise there is an increased risk of disease being present. However, as a part of the normal immune defence there must be an optimum number of cells in milk and below that threshold one would expect an increase in the risk of new intra-mammary infection.

The relationship between clinical mastitis and SCC is both controversial and complex, which is reflected in the peer-reviewed literature. However, research in recent years has improved our understanding of the relationship between the number (concentration) of somatic cells in milk and the subsequent susceptibility of that gland to clinical mastitis. As long ago as the 1960s, experimental evidence demonstrated that elevated SCCs in a quarter could protect against coliform infection (Schalm et al., 1964). More recent experimental studies have demonstrated a negative association between SCC and severity of experimentally induced infections (Shuster et al., 1996; van Werven, 1999), clearly demonstrating the risk associated with an 'inadequate' number of somatic cells in milk.

A number of field studies have also examined the association between SCC and clinical mastitis, though this is a difficult area of research as the diagnosis of clinical mastitis is subjective and double-blinded studies are difficult to conduct. In a field study in the UK on cows with toxic mastitis, it was found that cases were more likely to occur in herds with a lower BMSCC in that month than control herds (Green et al., 1996). Since this early work there have been a number of additional field studies, both in the UK and overseas, that have examined the relationship between SCC and clinical mastitis. Barkema et al. (1998) found no difference in the incidence of clinical mastitis in low (<150,000), medium (150,000–250,000) and high (250,000–400,000cells/ml) cell count herds, though systemic signs of illness associated with mastitis were more common in the low-cell count (<150,000 cells/ml) herds. Tadich et al. (1998) also reported low BMSCC as being a risk factor for severe clinical mastitis. Suriyasathaporn et al. (2000) also found that low SCC was associated with an increased risk of clinical mastitis. More recently, studies at both the quarter and herd level have indicated that low numbers of somatic cells in milk are associated with an increase in clinical disease. Peeler *et al.* (2003) and Green *et al.* (2004) both demonstrated that quarters with a low and high number of somatic cells were at increased risk of clinical mastitis. These findings have led to the description of a 'j-shaped' distribution of risk of clinical mastitis associated with SCC. This distribution of risk is illustrated in Fig. 5.4, and could be equally applied to SCCs at the quarter, cow and herd level; Beaudeau *et al.* (2002) investigated the risk of clinical mastitis in herds with a high proportion of cows with low SCC, and concluded that such herds were at increased risk of clinical disease.

While the arguments laid out above are of interest, they are not yet useful in predicting the outcome for an individual cow. However, if these findings are applied at the herd level in terms of the proportion of cows falling within different risk categories, they give the practitioner a useful insight into the relative risks facing cows in different types of herd. The proportions of cows falling within each of the risk categories, as defined by Beaudeau *et al.* (2002) in herds

of differing BMSCC, are outlined in Table 5.2, based on data from 427,244 individual cow recordings on 3865 test days in 52 herds, spread throughout England and Wales. This table illustrates the potential impact of different cell count bands on the distribution of cows in the different 'risk' groups. While clearly reducing BMSCC has the positive benefit of significantly reducing the number of cows in the high cell count at-risk category, it is likely to have the effect of increasing the number of cows susceptible to severe disease.

While this increase in risk is not a problem per se, it does mean that as mastitis overall is controlled and BMSCC falls it becomes even more important to ensure optimal environmental management to ameliorate the increased risk experienced by low-SCC cows. This is perhaps best illustrated by considering the absolute number of cases of clinical mastitis occurring on these farms in each of the categories of cows, as illustrated in Fig. 5.5. While all other things being equal, a low-BMSCC herd may not necessarily experience an overall increase in clinical cases, a significant proportion of cases is likely occur in low-SCC cows resulting in a more severe disease.

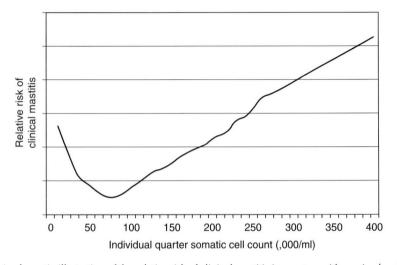

**Fig. 5.4.** A schematic illustration of the relative risk of clinical mastitis in quarters with varying levels of somatic cell count.

**Table 5.2.** Proportion of milking cows falling within different cell count (and risk) categories according to bulk milk somatic cell count, based on 427,244 cow recordings and using the risk categories proposed by Beaudeau *et al.* (2002).

| Bulk milk somatic cell count (,000 cells/ml) | Proportion of cows (%) falling within each cell count band and 'risk' categories proposed by Beaudeau *et al.* (2002) | | |
| --- | --- | --- | --- |
| | >250 | >49 and <251 | <50 |
| | At increased risk of clinical mastitis | At least risk of clinical mastitis | At increased risk of severe clinical mastitis |
| >200 | 26.07 | 48.87 | 25.06 |
| 151–200 | 17.69 | 46.76 | 35.55 |
| 101–150 | 12.56 | 42.30 | 45.14 |
| 51–100 | 7.37 | 35.96 | 56.67 |
| <50 | 3.59 | 21.34 | 75.06 |

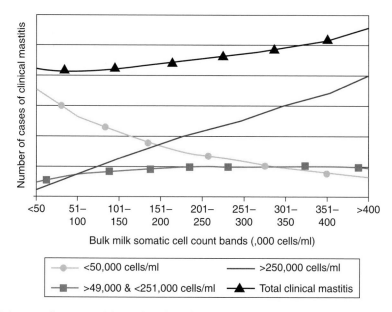

**Fig. 5.5.** Schematic illustration of the predicted number of cases of clinical mastitis in cows in different cell count groups as herd bulk milk somatic cell count increases (lines represent the number of cases occurring in cows in different somatic cell count categories).

### Genetic susceptibility of the host

Resistance to clinical mastitis and SCCs are heritable and offer opportunities, albeit small, to improve udder health. How these relate to udder health management is covered later in this chapter, along with sire selection in Appendix 2.

### Pathogens and their behaviour

While in excess of 150 different organisms have been implicated in bovine mastitis, the majority of cases are caused by a relatively small number of species. Historically bovine mastitis pathogens have been classified as either contagious or environmental, as illustrated for the key pathogens in Table 5.3.

Contagious mastitis pathogens are characterized by their adaptation to the mammary gland and their proclivity to cause persistent intra-mammary infection, and therefore to be spread from cow to cow during the milking process. *Streptococcus agalactiae* is probably the best example of a contagious pathogen; it is unable to survive for protracted lengths of time outside the mammary gland, causes only mild clinical signs and is easily transmitted from cow to cow. Other examples of contagious pathogens include *Staphylococcus aureus*, and arguably *Streptococcus dysgalactiae* (although this organism also has a significant environmental reservoir). *Staphylococcus aureus* is probably the commonest classic contagious pathogen in dairy herds today and is also probably the most troublesome to cure, often resulting in chronic subclinical infection and the need to cull the affected cow. Although the exact epidemiology of *Mycoplasma* spp. has not been fully elucidated, it can also be considered as primarily contagious since the main mode of spread is from cow to cow during the milking process.

In contrast, environmental mastitis pathogens are considered opportunistic invaders from an environmental reservoir. Cow-to-cow spread is not the major mode of spread and, although reported, persistent infection is probably relatively rare when compared with the contagious mastitis pathogens. However, in herds where the classical contagious mastitis pathogens are under control, environmental pathogens can be a significant cause of recurrent clinical disease (Bradley and Green, 2001a). The main environmental mastitis pathogens are the Enterobacteriacae (in particular *Escherichia coli*) and *Streptococcus uberis*, and the non-lactating period has been demonstrated to be of particular importance in their epidemiology (Smith *et al.*, 1985; Bradley and Green, 2000). Coliform organisms have classically been associated with severe mastitis resulting in systemic signs as a result of endotoxin release. However, though more likely to cause systemic disease than Gram-positive pathogens, the vast majority of coliform mastitis (>90%) does not result in peracute clinical disease (Bradley and Green, 2001a).

It is important to note that while the characteristics of contagious and environmental behaviour are useful indicators of the best way to approach mastitis control on an individual unit, we cannot adequately evaluate this simply from identification of a particular species of bacteria. Recent research has demonstrated clear variation in the ability of different strains of the same species to behave quite differently; for instance, some strains of *S. uberis* are thought to be far more capable of causing persistent infection and chronic intra-mammary infection than others that behave in a more classically environmental manner (Zadoks *et al.*, 2003). Similarly, some strains of *E. coli* have been demonstrated to persist intracellularly in mammary epithelial cells (Passey *et al.*, 2008), causing recurrent episodes of clinical disease (Bradley and Green, 2001a), while some strains of *S. aureus* have been shown to behave in a more environmental manner (Sommerhäusera *et al.*, 2003).

When one considers pathogens in this light, the approach to control will inevitably

**Table 5.3.** Summary of the key bovine mastitis pathogens and their historical classification simply as contagious or environmental.

| Contagious pathogens | Environmental pathogens |
| --- | --- |
| *Streptococcus agalactiae* | *Escherichia coli* |
| *Streptococcus dysgalactiae* | *Streptococcus uberis* |
| *Staphylococcus aureus* | *Klebsiella* spp. |
| *Mycoplasma* spp. | Other Enterobacteriaceae |
| *Corynebacterium* spp. | |
| Coagulase-negative Staphylococci | |

have to be tailored to the individual herd and the apparent behaviour of the predominant species and strains of pathogen present at that time. The ability to spread will be a feature of both opportunity and ability, with ability being influenced by the infectious dose and the duration/persistence of intramammary infection. Opportunity for contagious spread will improve with increased duration of infection, increased shedding and a minimal infectious dose. In contrast, environmental behaviour as a minimum demands a robust ability to survive in the environment and possibly an ability to cause infection at a relatively low dose – being shed in large numbers is not a prerequisite as the main reservoir of infection is the environment. This is currently an area of intensive research and it is likely that, in the near future, research into bacterial genetics and host–pathogen interactions will allow us to use genetic methods to differentiate bacterial strains of a mastitis pathogen, in terms of the mode of transmission and infection.

Key characteristics of different strains of the same mastitis pathogen are illustrated in Fig. 5.6. Using this classification, *S. agalactiae* is perhaps the ultimate contagious pathogen: bovine strains would appear to be confined to that niche since these are unable to survive for long in the environment, are shed in large numbers and intramammary infections are of long duration, thereby maximizing the opportunity to spread to a new host. In contrast, environmental strains of *S. uberis* will cause infections of only short duration and therefore, despite being shed in large numbers, will have a limited ability to be transmitted to a new host via a route such as the milking machine; however, should a strain acquire the ability to persist it will be able to transmit with relative ease. Finally, if one considers *E. coli*, while flourishing in the environment most infections are of short duration and, despite a low infectious dose spread between cows is uncommon. If persistence occurs (and with some strains it evidently can) the potential for spread is limited by the fact that the organism is generally shed in relatively low numbers.

### Major versus minor pathogens

Historically, as well as classifying pathogens by epidemiological behaviour, organisms

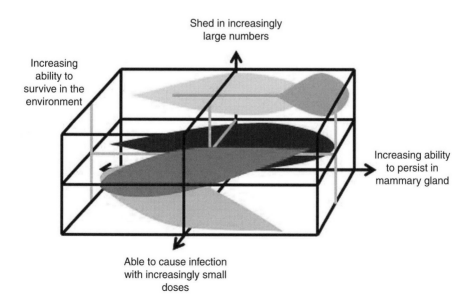

**Fig. 5.6.** Schematic illustration of the relationship between the ability of mastitis pathogens to survive in the host or environment, to be shed in large numbers and to carry a relatively large or small infectious dose.

have also been classified as 'major' or 'minor' pathogens. The minor pathogens have been characterized due to their proclivity to engender only a mild immune response and rarely clinical signs of disease. *Corynebacterium* spp. and the group of organisms classified as the coagulase-negative *Staphylococcus* spp. (CNS) have most commonly been considered the minor pathogens. Whilst this is a useful categorization, the groupings may be a little simplistic as some strains of *S. aureus* are coagulase negative and, by simple interpretation, could be classed as minor pathogens which they are clearly not. Moreover, these groups of pathogens are very diverse, encompassing a wide range of different species and it seems very likely that there will be important within- and between-species differences in pathogenicity. The minor pathogens are commonly associated with streak canal colonization and are common commensals of teat skin, so it is not unsurprising that they are also often isolated in milk samples. The role of the minor pathogens as significant causes of intra-mammary infection and clinical mastitis is hotly debated. While in some countries the CNS spp. are associated with clinical disease (most notably Scandinavia and Israel) in other countries their role is equivocal – their prevalence is similar in low and high SCC quarters and, when found, are typically attributed to raising the SCC by only a few tens of thousands of cells/ml. In contrast, Piepers *et al.* (2011) found that heifers infected with CNS spp. in early lactation outproduced their non-infected herd mates. The reason for this is unclear, but there is emerging evidence suggesting that a persistent CNS infection may have a protective effect against IMI caused by some of the major pathogens (De Vliegher *et al.*, 2004; Piepers *et al.*, 2011), although the effect may very well be species-specific.

*Corynebacterium* spp. are probably even more benign, being associated with an even smaller rise in SCC than the CNS spp., and while they may be the most prevalent organism on most farms, even in low-SCC herds, they are not thought to play any significant role in BMSCC. Whilst most coryneforms of bovine mammary origin are considered to be *Corynebacterium bovis*, in

reality there are many other species isolated from the bovine gland and these may have varying significance. Perhaps the most notable feature of *Corynebacterium* spp. is that they are keratolytic meaning they can break down keratin; their persistence in the streak canal has been associated with delay in formation of the keratin plug after drying off, which may (or may not) have implications for the subsequent acquisition of intra-mammary infection.

The importance of the minor pathogens in susceptibility to infection with a major mastitis pathogen is a poorly understood area, with a number of papers presenting conflicting findings (Huxley *et al.*, 2003). The rationale behind a role for minor pathogens is that they may reduce the likelihood of super-infection with a major pathogen, either directly through competitive exclusion or indirectly through elevation of SCC. This concept, along with the observation that herds in which contagious pathogens are well controlled may experience an increase in environmental mastitis, supports the theory that the mammary gland provides an ecological niche and that when a species adapted to filling that niche (e.g. *S. agalactiae* or *C. bovis*) is removed, then a true opportunist has the opportunity to move in and temporarily (or perhaps more permanently) occupy that niche.

As a summary to this section, we conclude that is it too simplistic to consider the bovine mammary gland as an aseptic environment. The udder, as a mucosal surface with direct communication to the external environment, will have been challenged by microorganisms for millions of years and while some organisms have become pathogens and uniquely adapted to fill this ecological niche, others may have adopted a more benign commensal-type role. While one would reasonably expect the depths of the mammary gland to be 'sterile', it is reasonable to expect a 'normal flora' to be present at the periphery of the gland (i.e. the teat and streak canal). An important challenge lies in understanding the role of these organisms, their impact on measures of udder health and therefore the definition of a healthy mammary gland. The future of control (see later) probably lies in maintaining a healthy balance rather than trying to 'blitz' the udder with antibiotics. It would seem unusual if the mammary gland were the only mucosal surface meant to be sterile; this is an area that has received significant attention in recent years, and the concept of a mammary microbiome is likely to be an area of productive research in the future.

## Mastitis Diagnostics

It is important that milk, as a food product, undergoes diagnostic and quality testing at all stages of production from the cow to the cup. Veterinarians have an interest in milk quality throughout this process and in particular the production of high-quality, clean, nutritionally wholesome milk up to the point where it leaves the farm. On the farm, milk quality can be adversely affected by the management of mastitic cows, hygiene and nutrition. Milk can also be adversely affected by conditions after it has left the farm. Although these factors are outside the scope of this book, they include storage temperature and hygiene. Milk is susceptible to contamination, an issue that can affect large volumes of stored milk such as bulk tanks on farms or silos at a milk-processing factory. Examination of milk is commonly performed as an element of a diagnostic or monitoring process. This can be as part of day-to-day quality management, a diagnostic investigation or routine quality control incorporated into a herd health programme.

### Detection or diagnosis

Current cow-side mastitis tests commonly used on the farm are effectively detection rather than diagnosis. In contrast, tests such as bacteriological culture or polymerase chain reaction (PCR), where milk is often transported to a laboratory, are diagnostic to the point of implicating a causal pathogen. Both diagnosis and detection can be performed at the herd (most commonly bulk tank milk),

cow (composite, co-mingled sample from all four quarters) or quarter level.

## Mastitis detection

Inspection of milk for abnormality (most commonly achieved by fore-stripping prior to milking) is a legal requirement in many countries around the world. At its simplest mastitis detection starts with visual observation. Consequently, the role of the milker is central to both identification and control of bovine mastitis. Detection rates, and therefore sensitivity and specificity, will vary depending on the milker's method of observation (e.g. whether fore-stripping is performed), the criteria for a positive mastitis diagnosis (degree of milk changes) and the conditions during observation (such as light levels and demeanour and workload of the operator). These differences will inevitably impact the absolute rates of disease recorded both within and between farms over time and need to be considered when analysing any recorded data.

In addition to visual observation a widely used, cheap and simple supplement that also allows detection of subclinically affected quarters is the California milk test (CMT). The CMT can be used to identify affected quarters in cows identified in routine recording, to confirm mastitis in cows showing only subtle visual changes, or to assess therapy success by estimating SCC of clinically recovered cows.

While technological advances bring new tools and techniques to the market place, visual observation and the measurement of SCC remain the mainstays of mastitis detection in the majority of dairy herds. However, additional testing modalities are gaining momentum in the market despite some significant shortfalls. Examples of these technologies and estimates of their performance are outlined in Table 5.4.

The benefits of timely on-farm, cow-side, real-time detection, such as that facilitated by fore-stripping or in-line conductivity, will be a balance of the inputs (time, cost and compliance) and benefit (potential or

**Table 5.4.** Outline of examples of mastitis detection modalities and approximate sensitivities and specificities (where known).

| Test | Estimated sensitivity (%) | Estimated specificity (%) | Time to result | Location |
|---|---|---|---|---|
| Milk or cow inspection | 80 | 100 | Seconds | Cow side |
| SCC (DHI testing) | 75 | 75 | Minutes | Lab |
| SCC (on-farm testing)[a] | ≤75 | ≤75 | Minutes | On farm |
| CMT[b] | 75 | 75 | Seconds | Cow side |
| Conductivity (hand held) | 80 | – | Seconds | Cow side |
| Conductivity (AMS) | – | – | Seconds | Cow side |
| Milk temperature | 50 | 70 | Seconds | Cow side |
| Yield: manual assessment | 20–40 | Low | Seconds | Cow side |
| NAGase | 70–100 | 95 | Minutes | Lab |
| Milk colour using real-time digital camera technology | – | – | Seconds | Cow side |
| Acute phase proteins (e.g. MAA) | – | – | Minutes | Lab |
| LDH | – | – | Minutes | Lab |
| ATP | – | – | Minutes | Lab |
| 'Electronic tongue': using an array of chemical sensors and computer data algorithm processing | – | – | Seconds | Cow side |

SCC, somatic cell count; DHI, dairy herd improvement; CMT, California milk test; AMS, automatic milking systems; NAGase, N-acetyl-beta-D-glucoaminidase; MAA, milk amyloid A; LDH, lactate dehydrogenase; ATP, adenosine triphosphate.
[a] Will vary according to methodology used. [b] When undertaken by trained operator and referring to detection of a high somatic cell count (after J.E. Hillerton, National Mastitis Council Annual Meeting Proceedings, 2000).

perceived) of outputs (mastitis detection). While early detection of mastitis has potential benefits in cow welfare, treatment success and milk quality, the accuracy (sensitivity and specificity on that farm) of early detection must be balanced against the risks of false-positives, available time, cost, effort and the likely compliance of performing the test.

### Somatic cell counting

Automated SCC determination using composite (co-mingled) milk from all four quarters to give an individual cow SCC (ICSCC) has become a cornerstone of mastitis management in many systems. These data are regularly collected (most commonly monthly) as part of a dairy herd improvement (DHI) scheme and, as well as offering individual cow information to facilitate treatment and culling decisions, the information is increasingly used to monitor herd performance and diagnose patterns of disease on the farm.

It is important when interpreting SCCs to remember that they are a measure of the inflammatory response and a proxy for infection status. Although intra-mammary infection is primarily responsible for elevating SCC it also impacted, to a lesser extent, by other factors; it varies during the day, over the lactation cycle and with yield as well as with other factors. In addition, as BMSCCs rise, mainly affected by the prevalence of high-cell count cows, SCCs of individual animals within the herd also tend to rise, regardless of their infection status (i.e. very low-SCC cows also tend to experience a rise in their SCC); this may be a result of increased challenge, as the prevalence within the herd increases. In late lactation, SCCs tend to rise as yield decreases. Within a few days after calving, SCCs also tend to be higher; this increase is the result of an increased SCC in all four quarters and may be increased by transient infections (particularly with coagulase-negative staphylococci). In quarter samples collected between milkings, SCC is not a reliable indicator of intra-mammary infection status. To be enable optimal interpretation of SCC tests, whether by laboratory, portable SCC devices or CMT, milk samples should be taken immediately before milking (Olde Riekerink *et al.*, 2007a).

Despite their limitations, ICSCCs are very useful for indicating infected and uninfected cows. Importantly, the threshold used to define infection will be influenced by the purpose of the test. For instance, if the aim is to identify 'infected cows' for the purposes of sampling for bacteriology, then a relatively high (e.g. 400,000 cells/ml) threshold is appropriate as this will increase the specificity of the test. In contrast, if the aim is to identify uninfected cows for purchase, a lower threshold should be used (e.g. 100,000 cells/ml) to increase sensitivity. Thus, as with any test, varying the threshold will result in changes in both sensitivity and specificity: increased thresholds resulting in increased specificity and reduced sensitivity and decreased thresholds resulting in increased sensitivity and reduced specificity. Furthermore, as outlined earlier, the sensitivity and specificity of a given threshold will also vary depending on the herd BMSCC. Because of the factors influencing sensitivity and specificity, individual cow management decisions should always be made on the basis of at least three SCC recordings as repeated measurements of SCC will add to the confidence of correctly defining a cow's infection status.

While varying the threshold is legitimate when making management decisions, when used for monitoring purposes a policy of selecting a fixed SCC threshold is essential. For this purpose, using a 200,000 cells/ml threshold effectively provides a good balance between sensitivity and specificity (both being around 75–80%), and is thus commonly used (Dohoo and Leslie, 1991).

## Mastitis diagnosis

Since individual farm treatment and control programmes vary depending on the predominant mastitis pathogens, as well as the patterns of disease, accurate and timely microbial pathogen identification is essential. However, mastitis diagnostics will become more useful when pathogen behaviour can be differentiated as well as bacterial species. As with many diagnostic procedures there is often a compromise between cost, speed and accuracy, which has led to a diversity of approaches to diagnosis varying from the quick, but rather crude, on-farm culture systems (e.g. Petri-film, Tri-plate) through to laboratory-based culture. While laboratory-based culture remains the 'gold standard', it has significant disadvantages including the need for experience and technical expertise, the time and resources required and the shortcomings of some biochemical typing methods.

The advent of new molecular technologies, some of which have already been commercialized, offers alternatives to conventional bacteriology. Some aspects of these new technologies confer clear advantages, whilst others fall short of current methods. The most notable of these new technologies commercially available are real-time PCR, which is a diagnostic tool in its own right, and MALDI-TOF-MS (matrix-assisted laser desorption ionization time-of-flight mass spectrometry), which offers a rapid and alternative method to conventional biochemical typing when combined with standard culture. The relative advantages and disadvantages of these methodologies are outlined in Table 5.5. Other new techniques on the cusp of commercialization that are worthy of mention are the detection of volatile bacterial metabolites and the use of array technology, both of which are likely to become available in the near future.

While the techniques outlined above are primarily focused on identification of pathogens at the species level, there is increasing interest in subspecies level or strain typing. The interest in this field stems from a need to better understand the epidemiology of mastitis outbreaks on individual farms, as the line between contagious and environmental behaviour of pathogens has become blurred. Different techniques are applicable to different species and for different purposes; this typing can be undertaken using either phenotypic or genotypic variation and, with respect to phenotypic

**Table 5.5.** A comparison of commercially available mastitis diagnostic techniques.

| | Conventional bacteriology | Bacteriology with MALDI-TOF-MS-assisted pathogen ID | RT-PCR |
|---|---|---|---|
| Number of pathogens identified | >150[a] | >150[a] | 11 |
| Sensitivity testing | Unlimited | Unlimited | Penicillin resistance |
| Detection of non-viable microorganisms | – | – | + |
| Detection in preserved samples | – | – | + |
| Interpretation | Well understood | Well understood | Problematic |
| Easy identification of contaminated samples | + | + | – |
| Speed (h) | 24–72 | 24 | 4–6 |
| Subspecies typing | – | + | – |
| Sensitivity (CFU/ml) | 10[b] | 10[b] | 100[c] |
| Cost | Low | Low | Moderate |

MALDI-TOF-MS, matrix-assisted laser desorption ionization time-of-flight mass spectrometry. [a] *Mycoplasma* spp. detected only with the use of specialist agar and prolonged incubation. [b] Viable bacteria only and assuming use of selective media and increased volume of secretion plated. [c] Viable and non-viable, assuming 2 ml of secretion used and copy number of 5 for gene of interest in bacterium detected.

variation, can vary from the crudest such as differences in colony morphology and anti-biograms through to the much more sophisticated MALDI-TOF-MS. Options for genotyping also vary with regard to discriminatory ability; examples include random amplified polymorphic DNA (RAPD), pulse field gel electrophoresis (PGFE), amplified fragment length polymorphism (AFLP) and multi-locus sequence typing (MLST).

### Selecting a diagnostic technique

With an increased number of choices for mastitis diagnostics, the practitioner will need to be able to select the most appropriate approach for the task in hand. For the foreseeable future there is likely to be a compromise between speed and accuracy.

#### *Bacteriological culture*

This can be performed at the herd (bulk milk), cow or quarter level. Bulk tank bacteriology has a role to play in investigation of issues surrounding elevation in TVC, and can also be a useful technique when screening

a herd for contagious pathogens such as *S. agalactiae* or *S. aureus*. However, the practitioner must be aware of the shortfalls of this approach, particularly its poor sensitivity (~75 and 60%, respectively, for the pathogens above) and the need for repeated culture. Furthermore, isolation in the case of *S. aureus* is not necessarily diagnostic of intra-mammary infection, indicating that specificity is not 100% and that repeated measures are needed (Jayarao *et al.*, 2004). The use of bulk tank analysis to draw conclusions about environmental pathogens is difficult if not impossible, as any such organisms isolated may have been derived from non-specific contamination from cow skin, bedding, manure or water, although they may provide an indicator of farm hygiene.

Cow (composite) samples have been recommended as a way of screening for contagious pathogens, and could form part of a biosecurity programme, but the findings need to be interpreted with caution as intermittent shedding can be an issue and this will also be compounded by the decreased sensitivity resulting from dilution of any pathogens from infected quarter(s). This technique will probably work well for *S. agalactiae* (Dinsmore *et al.*, 1991) and *Mycoplasma* spp. (Biddle *et al.*, 2003); however, approximately 40% of quarters infected with *S. aureus* will not be cultured from composite milk samples (Lam *et al.*, 1996a). Additionally, for *Mycoplasma* spp., samples should not be frozen because freezing and thawing is harmful to this pathogen (Biddle *et al.*, 2004).

Individual quarter bacteriology is undoubtedly the most useful and representative way to collect data on intra-mammary infection dynamics within a herd, and need not be prohibitively expensive. It is arguably best applied proactively through the pre-treatment sampling and frozen storage of all clinical cases. This allows culture of a proportion of samples on a rolling basis and targeting of sampling towards problem cows. Additionally, samples can be collected from problem quarters of cows identified by using ICSCCs supplemented with CMT. It is possible using this technique to build up a picture of, and monitor, mastitis aetiology on a unit and use this for the basis of prescription of intra-mammary antibiotic treatments.

### PCR diagnostics

While bacterial culture has been used for decades for mastitis diagnosis, PCR and real-time PCR are more recent developments. Commercially available kits based on the detection of 16s DNA gene sequences allow both the detection of live and dead bacteria as well as detecting the *blaZ* gene that confers resistance to beta lactam antibiotics. PCR-based techniques have the advantage of speed, but interpretation remains difficult, particularly if sampling technique is suboptimal. PCR is particularly useful where the pathogen of interest is rarely found in the environment (e.g. *S. agalactiae*) or if the screen is for a human pathogen when the source of contamination is immaterial.

### Factors influencing diagnostic accuracy

Accurate diagnosis goes beyond purely identifying potential mastitis pathogens in a milk sample. Interpretation of results such that insignificant or contaminant microbes can be distinguished from causal ones is essential. The quality of the sample delivered to the laboratory determines the diagnostic usefulness and is influenced by the conditions at collection, during storage and transport.

The first step to acquiring meaningful diagnostic samples is an adequate aseptic collection technique, which requires diligence and training and is often overlooked. Standard operating procedures (SOPs) and materials necessary for collection need to be readily available on the farm if consistent samples are to be collected. If collecting and freezing samples, the use of a cryopreservant such as glycerol can prove useful in protecting the species (Gram-negative organisms) most susceptible to freezing. A SOP for the collection of an aseptic milk sample is given in Box 5.2.

As well as poor sampling technique, there are a number of other factors that affect diagnostic accuracy. The timing of sampling can be important: pre-milking samples generally give higher detection rates than post-milking sampling (Sears *et al.*, 1991) and the use of repeated sampling will increase diagnostic accuracy. Repeated sampling, for instance, will improve sensitivity for intermittently shed pathogens as long as a single isolation remains the criterion for defining an IMI. However, if criteria such as isolation on more than one occasion are applied this will increase specificity, but at the expense of sensitivity. If the time between repeated samples is increased, agreement between those samples will decrease and results will become biased towards organisms causing persistent infection (possibly resulting in the loss of useful diagnostic information).

Another factor that is often overlooked is the limitations of many of the approaches to organism identification in the practice or professional laboratory. It is not safe to extrapolate findings from a pathogen in one host species to another. Colony morphology and growth on selective agar are not adequate criteria for identification, and many biochemical tests developed for identification of organisms isolated in human medicine have poor diagnostic accuracy in bovine mastitis.

138 A. Bradley *et al.*

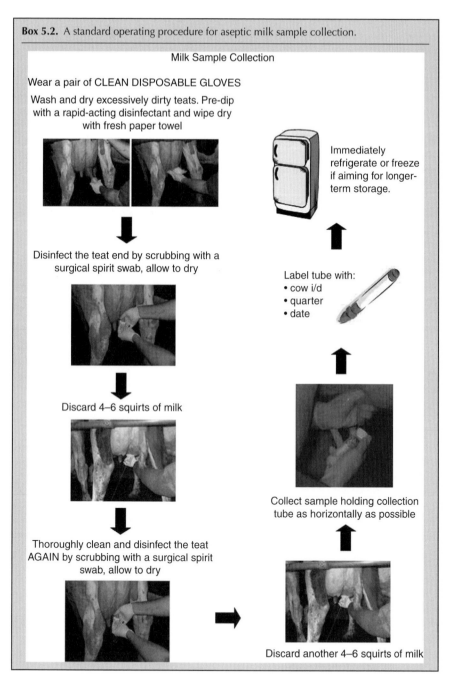

Box 5.2. A standard operating procedure for aseptic milk sample collection.

Milk Sample Collection

Wear a pair of CLEAN DISPOSABLE GLOVES

Wash and dry excessively dirty teats. Pre-dip with a rapid-acting disinfectant and wipe dry with fresh paper towel

Disinfect the teat end by scrubbing with a surgical spirit swab, allow to dry

Discard 4–6 squirts of milk

Thoroughly clean and disinfect the teat AGAIN by scrubbing with a surgical spirit swab, allow to dry

Discard another 4–6 squirts of milk

Collect sample holding collection tube as horizontally as possible

Label tube with:
• cow i/d
• quarter
• date

Immediately refrigerate or freeze if aiming for longer-term storage.

While this is a potential minefield for the practitioner, the simple questions 'Does this result make sense?' and 'Does it fit with what I'm seeing on farm?' are often sufficient filters to pick up diagnostic inaccuracies in the laboratory.

In short, the herd health practitioner cannot afford to divest all responsibility for testing modalities and interpretation to the laboratory, and they need to be aware of the approaches used, the pros and cons of these different approaches and should tailor the requests they require to best suit the aim of the diagnostic procedure they are undertaking. Equally, the findings need to be interpreted in a herd context: the identification of a single quarter infected with *S. aureus* does not necessarily make this the most significant pathogen on the farm. The value of any diagnostic or detection system should not be judged just by its technical ability or characteristics but by whether it can facilitate faster and more effective intervention on the farm.

## Monitoring and Analysis of Mastitis Data

An essential aspect of herd health is to monitor mastitis in a way that *allows identification of the main herd problems and improves use of control strategies*. While the presence of mastitis pathogens can be monitored through bacteriology or similar tests, analysis of clinical mastitis or cell count records provides the best picture of the overall farm situation. The aim of this section is to focus on the analysis of SCC and clinical mastitis data collated through a DHI process or on the farm. While clinical mastitis data are free and relatively easy to collate (given a computer), these are a subjective measure, place an additional onus on the producer and do not provide a useful way of monitoring subclinical infection. In contrast, SCC data can be easily collated via a DHI recording service with little input from the producer, but have the disadvantages of additional cost and a bias towards monitoring Gram-positive pathogens (and within that grouping pathogens most able to cause prolonged infection). Another disadvantage is that with the increased use of in-line measurements (in AMS systems and otherwise) in some countries the number of herds participating in SCC measurement in DHI systems is decreasing. A monitoring system should encompass both SCC and clinical mastitis data, because relying exclusively on one method is likely to lead to both erroneous conclusions and a bias in any control approach. Monitoring and analysis can be carried out at the herd, cow or quarter level

and, while each have their relative advantages and disadvantages, a combination of all three is important in putting in place an effective monitoring system for a herd health programme.

The aim of any analytical and monitoring approach should be to inform farm treatment and control plans. Historically these have often been based on the predominant bacteria identified on that farm in the knowledge that different mastitis pathogens have different modes of transmission. As described earlier, it is recognized that most pathogens have the potential to behave in both a contagious and environmental manner, but there are no direct genetic or phenotypic markers for contagious or environmental behaviour. Molecular diagnostic and typing techniques such as PGFE, RAPD and MALDI-TOF-MS will become more generally available and will increasingly be used to distinguish between clonal (single-strain) and non-clonal (multiple-strain) disease outbreaks. When multiple strains are identified in a mastitis outbreak, opportunistic infections originating from the environment are most likely, whereas if a single predominant strain is identified it can be inferred that contagious spread is likely to be occurring (or possibly multiple cows are becoming infected from an environmental point source).

The availability of detailed individual cow clinical mastitis and SCC data on many farms has increased the use of computer analysis and interpretation of these data such that inferred behaviour and the origin of intra-mammary infections are increasingly becoming an important part of data analysis. Such an analysis underpins an individual farm mastitis control plan. Using pattern recognition and integrating both clinical mastitis and SCC data, it is possible to infer whether new intra-mammary infections are likely to be derived from the dry period or from lactation. This differentiation, coupled with an analysis of herd prevalence, disease persistence and recurrence, also allows an insight into whether pathogen behaviour appears primarily environmental or contagious. The approach to 'categorization' of herds has been adopted as a cornerstone of the DairyCo Mastitis Control Plan in the UK (www.mastitiscontrolplan.co.uk), where herds are defined as experiencing either contagious or environmental patterns of disease that are either predominantly of dry period or lactating period origin. This approach has been tested and validated under field conditions (Green *et al.*, 2007a) and offers one method of targeting and implementing mastitis control measures.

## Monitoring and interpreting somatic cell count data

Analysis of regular milk recording (DHI) data is the cornerstone of SCC monitoring. This is best achieved using regular monthly recording, though less regular recording regimes can still reveal useful data and have been described in the literature (Bradley *et al.*, 2002, 2007b; Bradley and Green, 2004). Individual cow SCCs are used to identify cows as either infected or uninfected, with new infections being defined as cows moving from below to above a given cell count threshold. Chronically infected cows are defined by their persistence above a given threshold. The widely adopted threshold for detection of infection is 200,000 cells/ml, although the use of a higher threshold in early lactation and a lower threshold in primaparous animals may be appropriate (a threshold of 150,000 or 250,000 cells/ml will work, but different target figures to evaluate SCC changes may be required).

Computers allow a herd-based approach to analysis of these SCC data (based on the accumulation of probabilities from many individual cows) that better reflects the true biological situation, including allowing cows to move through different infection statuses from uninfected to infected, to chronically infected or back to uninfected through intervening periods of uncertainty. Even though every cow will not be correctly categorized using SCC, when these analyses are conducted on a herd basis a sufficient number of cows are correctly classified to provide an accurate herd picture. An impor-

tant and crucial aspect of any approach to analysing SCC data is to deal with 'missing data' – this can only be sensibly achieved with access to reliable clinical mastitis data, thereby allowing an 'intelligent' interpretation of the implication of 'absent' cows (cows absent from a milk recording). Cows absent with clinical mastitis should be attributed a high SCC reading. Integrating clinical data and allowing for absent cows when analysing DHI data increases the confidence and adds credibility to the calculated SCC indices, because the analysis is more likely to reflect the true temporal distribution of mastitis in the herd. Currently this approach to SCC monitoring is available in the TotalVet Software (QMMS and SUM-IT computer systems) in the UK and in the Dairy Data WareHouse (UniformAgri) in other parts of the world, and is used in this chapter to illustrate the principles of monitoring using SCC and clinical mastitis data. Other software packages and approaches are available in local markets and will vary in their approach to analysis, use of thresholds and interpretation, although the basic principles of analysis remain the same. The results obtained when using different software will differ slightly, and the herd health practitioner needs to be aware of these differences and vary their interpretation accordingly.

### BMSCC

The bulk milk SCC, as calculated from individual cow recordings, provides a useful first oversight of the infection prevalence in a herd. It circumvents on-farm manipulation of the bulk tank, though it may still be an underestimate if significant numbers of cows are not sampled at a given recording. As a rule of thumb, for every 100,000 cells/ml increase in bulk milk SCC there will be an 8–10% increase in the proportion of cows infected in the herd (Lievaart *et al.*, 2009). At the extremes, herds with a high BMSCC are generally more likely to be experiencing contagious patterns of disease, and low-BMSCC herds environmental patterns of disease. However, in herds with an intermediate level of BMSCC it is impossible to predict the underlying patterns of disease. As the BMSCC becomes lower, individual cow SCCs become relatively less useful as a tool for understanding mastitis patterns and the practitioner becomes increasingly reliant on clinical mastitis data (see later).

### ICSCC

Individual cow SCCs provide an invaluable tool for tracking and tracing infection within a herd. The use of a threshold of 200,000 cells/ml is commonly used to define and monitor key infection parameters within the herd. Some key indices with suggested targets are outlined in the sections below and summarized in Table 5.6.

LACTATION NEW INFECTION RATE.    This provides a measure of the proportion of cows acquiring a new intra-mammary infection between consecutive milk recording (DHI) tests, based on movement in SCC from below to above 200,000 cells/ml. This proportion can be plotted over time to allow the user to visualize patterns and trends, as illustrated in Fig. 5.7. When interpreting SCCs it is important to bear in mind aspects of the normal physiology of the bovine mammary gland that may be influencing the analysis,

such as the potential effect of yield and stage of lactation, and therefore to always examine the animals that are included in the analysis before drawing firm conclusions.

PROPORTION OF THE HERD INFECTED AND CHRONICALLY INFECTED.    These are defined, respectively, as the proportion of cows currently infected (above the threshold) and the proportion of those persistently infected (e.g. above the threshold for two of the previous three consecutive tests) at a particular time point. The relationship between these two parameters can provide a useful insight into disease dynamics, as illustrated in Fig. 5.8. When the rolling proportions of the herd chronically infected and above 200,000 cells/ml are both rising but converging, this is suggestive of a situation involving pathogens that are more likely to cause persistent infection and less likely to cure (i.e. contagious pathogens); when both are rising but diverging it suggests that cell counts may be being driven by pathogens less likely to cause persistent infection and more likely to cure (i.e. environmental pathogens).

DRY PERIOD INFECTION RATES.    Using the data from the first monthly milk recording in a lactation ($\leq 30$ days in milk), it is possible to

**Table 5.6.** Mastitis monitoring indices with sample UK target ranges.

| Index | Target level | Mean[a] | Best 25th percentile[a] |
|---|---|---|---|
| SCC indices | | | |
| Lactation new infection rate (%) | <5.0–7.0 | 10.0 | 7.6 |
| % herd > 200,000 cells/ml | <15.0 | 24.1 | 18.5 |
| % herd chronically infected | <5.0 | 15.9 | 11.5 |
| Fresh calver infection rate (%) | <10.0 | 22.3 | 17.0 |
| Dry period new infection rate (%) | <10.0 | 18.9 | 13.6 |
| Dry period cure rate (%) | >85.0 | 72.5 | 79.5 |
| Clinical mastitis indices | | | |
| Incidence rate of clinical mastitis (per 100 cow years) | <25 | 76.4 | 42 |
| Incidence rate of cows affected (per 100 cow years) | <20 | 38.4 | 27 |
| Apparent clinical mastitis cure rate (%) (All cases) | >40 | 31.4 | 39 |
| Apparent clinical mastitis cure rate (%) (Index cases) | >50 | 40.9 | 50 |
| Apparent subclinical mastitis cure rate (%) | >35 | – | – |
| Putative dry period origin cases (cows in 12) | <1 | 1.3 | 0.7 |
| Putative lactating period origin cases (cows in 12) | <2 | 3.12 | 2.16 |

SCC, somatic cell count. [a] Based on data collated from 653 UK dairy herds participating in a mastitis control programme.

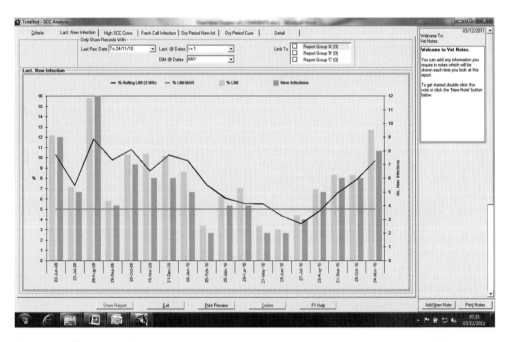

**Fig. 5.7.** An illustration of lactation new infection rate over time, showing seasonal variation in infection rate typical of a herd experiencing environmental patterns of disease (TotalVet©). The light grey bars represent the percentage of animals at each recording (of those eligible) that experience a lactation new infection (i.e. they were previously defined as 'uninfected' and their somatic cell count rose from below to above 200,000 cells/ml). The dark grey bars indicate the number of animals experiencing a lactation new infection. The upper line provides a 3-recording rolling average rate. The lower line represents an acceptable rate.

gain an insight into the likely origin of intra-mammary infection and the importance of the dry period in mastitis epidemiology on an individual unit. The proportion of cows with an SCC >200,000 at the 1st DHI test (fresh calver infection rate) is a useful measure of cows calving with an infection, as illustrated in Fig. 5.9. It is important to divide those cows infected into either *new* intra-mammary infections acquired during the dry period (proportion of cows with last DHI test in the previous lactation <200,000 that have a 1st DHI test in this lactation >200,000) and *failure of existing infections to cure* (proportion of cows with last DHI test in the previous lactation >200,000 that have a 1st DHI test in this lactation >200,000). Failure to cure is often expressed more intuitively as the proportion that do cure (dry period cure rate). Another important facet of interpretation of SCC data in early lactation is to consider the normal physiological ele-

vation in SCC in very early lactation; this scenario is the justification for utilizing a higher threshold at this time (Sargeant *et al.*, 2001).

When interpreting dry period outcomes, it is important to understand the relationship between apparent dry period cure and new infection rates. As new infection rates increase, apparent cure rates will tend to decrease. The underlying basis of this relationship is illustrated in Fig. 5.10 and is as a result of reinfection of previously high-SCC quarters that had cured earlier during the dry period. It is important to factor this effect into the interpretation of dry period data, particularly in herds with poor apparent cure rates, because otherwise an erroneous conclusion may be drawn about the efficacy of the current dry cow therapy. Therefore, herds that have a high dry period new infection rate are also likely to have a low dry period cure rate, but, to improve the herd mastitis

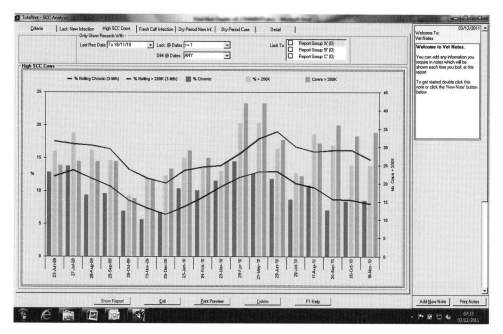

**Fig. 5.8.** An illustration of the interaction between the percentage of cows infected and chronically infected, typically seen in a herd with an environmental pattern of disease (TotalVet©). The light grey bars represent the percentage of the milking herd with an elevated somatic cell count (SCC); the medium grey bars indicate the number of animals with an elevated SCC; the dark grey bars show the percentage of the milking herd defined as chronically infected. The upper horizontal line provides a 3-recording rolling average proportion of the herd 'infected' and the lower horizontal line the 3-recording rolling average proportion of the herd chronically 'infected'.

situation, it is the new infections that should be addressed initially rather than cure rates (see section 'Control of Mastitis').

The importance of interpretation and integration of clinical mastitis data to account for 'missing' data is probably best highlighted when considering dry period infection rates. This is because of the higher incidence of clinical mastitis in early lactation.

THE NET TRANSMISSION INDEX (NTI).    This offers a simple way to assess monthly SCC records and to give an assessment of the transmission dynamics within a herd (Bradley and Green, 2004). It provides a single figure that is easy to understand and monitor, is an overview

for the veterinarian and farmer but should be viewed as an initial indicator of infection issues. It is a simple ratio, as shown below (see equation at bottom of page);

The ratio gives an approximation of the ratio of 'new infections' to 'cures', and can be used to assess both lactation and dry period performance. A ratio of <1 suggests new infections <cures and that there is a reducing prevalence of infection; a ratio of >1 suggests new infections >cures and that there is an increasing prevalence of infection. This indicates a potential problem and that action is needed, starting with further analysis of SCCs and mastitis records. A ratio of 1 suggests that new infections and cures are equal and that there is no net

$$NTI = \frac{\text{number of cows with SCC increasing from below to above threshold}}{\text{number of cows with SCC decreasing from above to below threshold}}$$

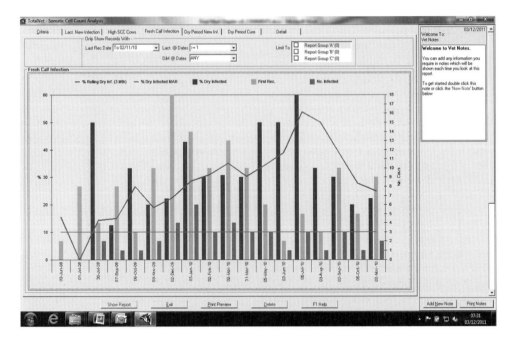

**Fig. 5.9.** An illustration of the 'fresh calver infection rate' over time (TotalVet©). The dark grey bars represent the percentage of cows, within 30 days of calving with a somatic cell count >200,000 cells/ml; the light grey and medium grey bars illustrate the number of cows at the first recording (and <30 days in milk) and the number defined as 'infected', respectively; the upper line illustrates the rolling 3-recording rate and the lower horizontal line represents the acceptable rate.

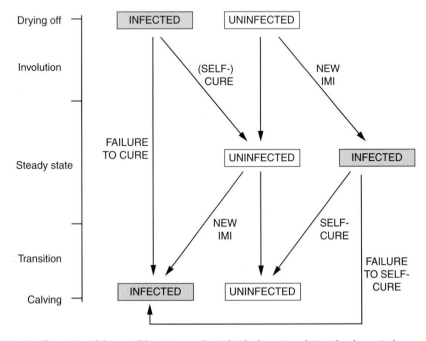

**Fig. 5.10.** An illustration of the possible outcomes for individual quarters during the dry period.

increase in the prevalence of infection occurring in the herd.

The SCC indices outlined above inform the practitioner of the epidemiology of mastitis on a unit. For example, a poor dry period cure rate, coupled with a rising prevalence of infection and a rapidly rising prevalence of chronic cows with a lack of seasonality in rates of new infection, is suggestive of a contagious pattern of disease. In contrast, seasonality, a low ratio of chronic to infected cows and a high dry period new IMI rate tend to indicate an environmental pattern of disease.

While all of the analysis up to this point undoubtedly provides a useful insight into mastitis control, it provides only a one-dimensional approach to the issue of mastitis control. The other and equally important aspect of monitoring mastitis for the herd health advisor is to evaluate patterns of clinical mastitis.

### Monitoring and interpreting clinical mastitis data

Clinical mastitis data are of particular use in herds with bulk milk SCCs <200,000 cells/ml when analysis of and reliance on cell count data alone can lead to a false 'sense of security'. As a minimum the date, cow and quarter affected should be recorded for all clinical cases of mastitis on a farm and ideally this should be supplemented with severity and treatment data. However, it has to be noted that the quality of clinical mastitis data needs continuous attention – only a limited number of farmers have the capacity and motivation to collect these data in a reliable way. If, however, complete data are available, they are very valuable.

Conventional approaches to clinical mastitis analysis have focused on basic quarter and cow rates and incidences, as well as a number of ratios such as the case–cow case ratio. While the absolute rates are important and the ratios/recurrence rates can give some indication of the likely aetiology of mastitis on a unit, they do not assist the practitioner in the 'targeting' of interventions and have become increasingly less useful as the dis-

tinctive behaviour of classical contagious and environmental pathogens has become less clear. As a result of these inadequacies, an alternative approach to analysing clinical mastitis that assists the practitioner in tracing the apparent origins (as lactation or the dry period) and defining patterns of mastitis on the farm has been developed (Bradley et al., 2008). This approach has been utilized in a recently published mastitis intervention study and has been shown to be a useful tool in targeting mastitis interventions (Green et al., 2007a).

The central precept of this approach to clinical mastitis analysis is to categorize clinical mastitis by putative origin based on the temporal occurrence during the lactation cycle, with cases in early lactation attributed to the dry period (Bradley et al., 2008). Once an index case (i.e. the first case in lactation) has been identified, subsequent cases are then 'linked' to the index case and recurrences attributed accordingly. Using this approach it is possible to define target rates and recurrences and to plot herd performance in terms of overall, putative lactation and putative dry period rates.

#### Incidence rates of clinical mastitis

For the purposes of calculating a base level of clinical mastitis on a unit and for benchmarking, the overall rate of clinical mastitis needs to be calculated. This is often expressed as a number of cases/100 cows/year. While it is difficult to define targets for these parameters applicable to all herds, the following ranges are achievable in the UK: 25–35 cases/100 cows/year, 20–25 cows affected (one or more cases)/100 cows/year. Local conditions and management systems in other countries may make different targets applicable.

#### Apparent clinical and subclinical mastitis cure rates

Once basic clinical mastitis data have been captured in herds undertaking DHI testing, it is possible to calculate apparent cure rates for cases of clinical mastitis (and, if recorded, subclinical mastitis). This is done by tracking individual cow performance after a recorded incidence of disease and monitoring both SCCs and clinical mastitis for predefined periods of time within the same lactation. A number of definitions can be used, but one proposal has been to define a cure as being no recurrence of clinical mastitis and either two or three consecutive cow SCCs <100,000 or <200,000 cells/ml, respectively (Bradley *et al.*, 2008).

### Analysing mastitis cases by their putative origin

As outlined earlier, a first case of clinical mastitis in lactation can be attributed as being of either dry- or lactating-period origin, recurrences within a lactation cycle thereafter being linked to this index case. A simple plot of these cases over time can be enlightening to both the practitioner and farmer alike in understanding the relative importance of the dry and lactating periods

within a herd, as illustrated in Fig. 5.11. A putative dry-period origin can be attributed to cases occurring within a defined period of calving; generally cases occurring in the first 30 days of lactation are accepted as likely to be of dry-period origin. In this instance, a recommended target level is that fewer than 1 in 12 cows should develop clinical mastitis in the first 30 days of lactation (Bradley *et al.*, 2008). In contrast, a putative lactating-period origin can be attributed to index cases of mastitis occurring after the first 30 days of lactation. In this instance a target is that fewer than 2 in 12 cows should develop clinical mastitis in the remainder of lactation, giving an overall rate of fewer than 3 in 12 cows affected in a lactation cycle (Bradley *et al.*, 2008).

Using this approach it is possible to calculate apparent rates on a monthly, quarterly and annual basis and this allows for identification of seasonal patterns, giving an insight into the relative importance

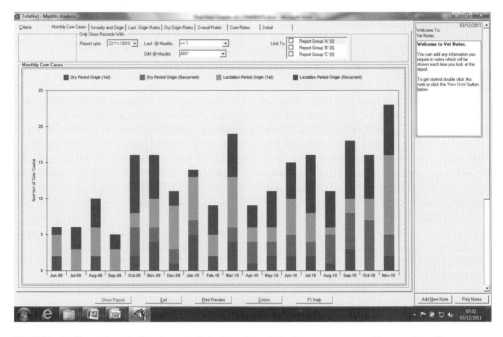

**Fig. 5.11.** An illustration of a bar chart of clinical mastitis; clinical cases are grouped by month and by apparent origin (TotalVet©). The bars represent the actual number of clinical mastitis cases per month; dark shading indicates index cases of apparent dry period origin (occurring in the 1st 30 days of lactation); medium shading indicates recurrent cases in quarters first affected in the 1st 30 days (within a lactation cycle); light shading indicates index cases of apparent lactating period origin (occurring after the 1st 30 days of lactation); very dark shading indicates recurrent cases in quarters first affected after the 1st 30 days (within a lactation cycle).

of the dry and lactating periods and clinical mastitis recurrence.

## Summary of monitoring

A comprehensive mastitis monitoring programme should take into account both herd and individual cow level parameters, encompass both clinical and SCC data and should generate analyses that are useful and meaningful to the farmer while allowing an insight into the epidemiological patterns of disease on the farm. The indices used should also facilitate tracking and measurement of outcomes. It is crucial that monitoring tools enable the farmer and herd health advisor to develop a better understanding of clinical and subclinical mastitis on a dairy unit and therefore give specific direction towards areas where control can be improved. In Box 5.3 we provide examples of areas where further subdivisions of data will give even more detailed analyses, and add to the understanding of herd mastitis patterns.

While monitoring of mastitis provides the practitioner with an opportunity to track and trace intra-mammary infection in a herd, it is necessary to define the point ('alarm' level) at which intervention is necessary. These 'alarm' levels are often measured at the highest level (e.g. BMSCC or overall rate of clinical mastitis), and practitioners should be aware that these highest-level measures are blunt tools and are often slow to respond to changes in individual animal infection rates. As a rule, new infection rates are more informative and an earlier indicator of emerging issues than measures of prevalence. It is crucial that 'targets' are influenced by farm-specific goals that will vary according to farmer aspirations, the size of the herd, calving patterns and milk supply contracts.

## Control of Mastitis

### Principles of control

The overriding aims when attempting to control mastitis in dairy herds are to reduce the prevalence of infection (i.e. reduce the number and duration of existing infections) and to minimize the incidence of new infections. Both aspects are crucial, and while reducing current prevalence will result in short-term gains and could in itself impart a downward influence on new infection rates, reducing the incidence of new infections is essential for success in the medium to long term. If the control of new infections is not achieved, there will be a continual battle to reduce prevalence and this is usually very costly. Therefore, preventing new infections must be the major focus of a mastitis herd health programme.

It is often useful to consider reducing the incidence and prevalence of intra-mammary infections as two separate components of mastitis control. It should be acknowledged that cure of existing infections is usually very difficult (except in the relatively uncommon circumstance of *S. agalactiae* infection) and that culling or management of chronically infected cows to prevent transmission is an important element of control. Indeed, evidence indicates that the best chance to cure chronic infections is during the dry period and thus careful management of these cows until drying off is essential (see section on 'Contagious mastitis control').

When addressing the control of new intra-mammary infections, a critical consideration is to determine when the new infections occur and this should be apparent from the monitoring being conducted (see earlier section). In particular, we need to establish whether the main infection pressure is during the dry period or during lactation and whether transmission is occurring mainly from cow to cow or from environment to cow. This is an area in which mastitis control has progressed in the last decade, with generic farm plans (such as the five-point plan (Dodd *et al.*, 1969) and ten-point plan (NMC, 2011)) being enhanced by individually tailored, detailed control plans that depend upon herd-specific patterns of infection. Improvements in the understanding of the epidemiology and monitoring of dairy cow mastitis have enabled this improvement. An overview of an approach to monitoring and improving udder health

---

**Box 5.3.** Examples of interpretation of data to improve the understanding of mastitis within a herd.

**Interpreting Mastitis Data – Useful Indicators**

- The incidence of *repeat cases*: investigate the potential effect of a small number of cows on the overall clinical incidence rate. The example below shows a positively skewed distribution of incidence, with 21 of the 195 cows affected in a 2-year period (11%) recorded with 4 or more incidences of clinical disease contributing 119 of the total of 392 incidences (30%).

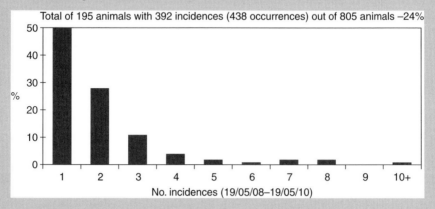

- The current *cure rate* of the 1st clinical mastitis case in lactation: cure rates <30% (as judged by no recurrence of clinical disease and either two consecutive cow somatic cell counts <100,000 or three < 200,000 cells/ml) may indicate issues surrounding rapid identification and treatment of cases, inadequate treatment duration, a high re-infection pressure or persistence of major pathogens.
- The effect of *seasonality* in clinical and/or sub-clinical mastitis patterns highlights likely variation in environmental infection pressure. In the example below, the rate of new infection in lactation (as measured by cows moving above the 200,000 cells/ml threshold between test-days) is increased in summer months and around turnout, indicating likely pasture-acquired infection.

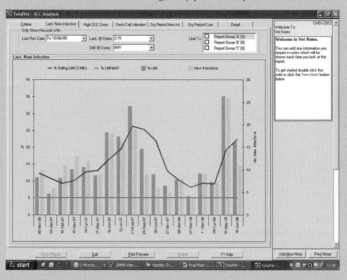

- Any effect of *parity* in the data patterns: for example restricting the dry period cure rate in routine somatic cell count analysis to cows in the 4th lactation and above to investigate if older cows are responsible for a fall in herd apparent dry period cure rate. Similarly, the incidence rate of clinical mastitis in the 1st 30 days of lactation may be heavily influenced by parity 1 animals already infected at calving.

*Continued*

**Box 5.3.** Continued.

- The effect of *'legacy'* cows on the herd infection prevalence: apparently high prevalence (i.e. increased sub-clinical disease) herds may be heavily influenced by carry-over of infection from previous lactations. In the example below, >50% of the infected, high SCC cows during winter 2010 were carrying that infection from earlier lactations. This generally reflects poor mastitis control in an historical context rather than the current time period.

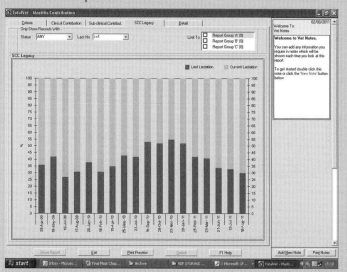

- The effect of individual *cows* on the calculated herd average test-day somatic cell count. In the example below, cow 114 contributes nearly 20% of the herd average SCC.

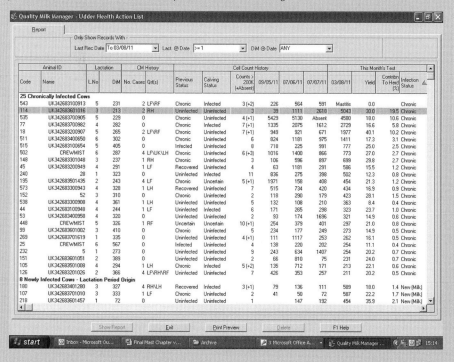

is outlined in Fig. 5.12, further details of which are covered later in this section.

Another recent change has been recognition that mastitis control extends beyond the technical aspects of reducing the incidence and prevalence of infection. Understanding farmer motivations and improving communications between advisors and herdspersons are now understood to be crucial to enhance uptake of control measures (Jansen *et al.*, 2010; Lam *et al.*, 2011; Valeeva *et al.*, 2007). In fact this can be a major barrier when it comes to

mastitis control and has to be addressed in order to successfully implement any mastitis scheme. This is discussed in detail in Chapter 2.

### Action and reaction

When attempting to control mastitis, it should be recognized that the disease is complex, involving both major and minor intra-mammary pathogens and an interaction

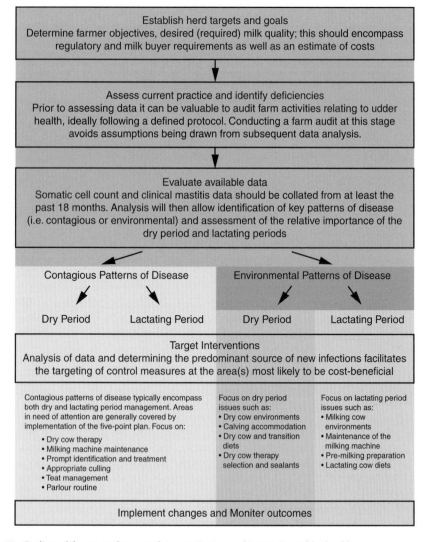

**Fig. 5.12.** Outline of the general approach to monitoring and improving udder health.

between host defence mechanisms and pathogen virulence. This means that any control programme requires close monitoring and should be viewed as a continuous, dynamic process because the alteration of one component may have an impact on another. Some of the complexities of mastitis are not fully understood, such as the potential protective effects of minor pathogens such as *C. bovis* and CNS spp. against major pathogen infection, or the interaction between host immunity and increased risk of severe clinical mastitis. However, these complexities demonstrate the importance of the principles of herd health established in Chapter 1, because monitoring outcomes and readjusting control measures is essential when certain elements of disease pathogenesis are uncertain. Moreover, a consequence of control of contagious mastitis pathogens in a herd may be an increase in environmental mastitis, in both relative and absolute terms. Examples of this phenomenon have been reported in the literature, demonstrating an increase in coliform mastitis in herds utilizing post-milking teat disinfection and in cows receiving antibiotic dry cow therapy (Bradley *et al.*, 2010).

### National control schemes

National schemes, programmes and campaigns have been used for mastitis control in dairy cows for many years. An early example in the 1960s was the five-point plan in which a basic set of measures was proposed that were considered to have a beneficial effect on clinical and subclinical mastitis. At this time, control plans were relatively straightforward because, with mastitis incidence and prevalence at very high levels and contagious pathogens being responsible for the majority of mastitis that occurred, the scope for improvement, using relatively simple measures, was huge. Since then, levels of production have escalated, cow genetics have altered radically and systems have changed dramatically, and

thus the management of mastitis has become much more challenging. In general, environmental pathogens have become increasingly important and the prevention of environmental infections is often more complicated than reducing the transmission of contagious pathogens: environmental management often requires more detailed, close-to-farm evaluations and farm-specific advice.

Implementing mastitis control on a national basis requires knowledge, motivation, widespread participation, excellent communication, financial backing, industry and political cooperation and probably most of all a dogged determination. Some examples of successful schemes that have been set up include Countdown Downunder (Australia), the SAMM Plan (now Smart SAMM, New Zealand), the Dutch Udder Health Program and the Norwegian Mastitis Control Program. More recently a scheme has been launched in the UK led by a collaboration of the National Dairy Levy Board (DairyCo) and a team of researchers and veterinary surgeons. These various schemes, while sharing the same objective of improving mastitis and milk quality, have taken quite different approaches to implementation: from generic education at one end of the scale to focused delivery of farm-specific management plans at the other. Ultimately, all large-scale approaches try to reach a variety of farmers with different outlooks and lifestyles (as discussed in Chapter 2), in an attempt to have a wide-ranging impact on mastitis control.

### Contagious mastitis control

Contagious mastitis pathogens are characterized by their ability and proclivity to persist within the host and by their transmission from host to host rather than from the environment to host. Prior to domestication of dairy cows, transmission by this route would have been slow, relying for instance on cross-suckling or flies, and therefore would have necessitated essentially lifelong colonization of the host mammary gland. However, domestication and subsequently the advent of modern dairying and the use of the milking machine would have suddenly made transmission much easier and ultimately, one could argue, have opened this mode of transmission to pathogens capable of only shorter durations of persistence. While the classic contagious pathogens such as *S. agalactiae* and *S. aureus* were the target of initial mastitis control programmes (e.g. the five-point plan), the principles of control of this type of mastitis remain similar and include prevention of contagious spread of organisms previously considered 'environmental'.

There are two main components to the control of contagious mastitis. The first is to reduce the prevalence of infected quarters within the herd to a minimum; this effectively reduces the challenge to other cows. The second is to put in place measures that minimize the risk of new intra-mammary infections, and this means primarily preventing spread from cow to cow (both within the herd and from outside).

### Reducing the prevalence of infection

The prevalence of infected quarters within a herd can be reduced in several ways, each with their advantages and disadvantages. Important economic decisions have to be made when deciding between strategies, although in some areas the lack of solid evidence from independent research means that empirical decisions sometimes have to be made. Reducing the herd prevalence of infection can be achieved through a combination of treatment, culling and drying off infected cows (or quarters). These are described below.

### Treatment

A prolonged description of different treatment protocols and their pros and cons is not within the remit of this book, and there are many publications on which the practitioner can draw to inform his or her decisions. Importantly, as an overriding principle the first approach should always be to use licensed regimes; should these fail then other approaches such as extending treatment duration and combining systemic and intra-mammary antibiotics can be considered. However, this should always be undertaken incorporating the principles of responsible antibiotic use and consideration of the likely cost–benefit. When non-licensed treatment regimes are considered and implemented, the monitoring of treatment outcomes is essential. It is imperative that if treatment regimes are used outside data-sheet recommendations, that diligence is shown with milk withdrawal periods; exact recommendations will vary from country to country, but best practice must dictate always to test milk from each treated cow for antibiotic residues prior to consignment of milk to the bulk tank.

When embarking on treatment regimes, one should also consider the factors likely to affect treatment outcome. As well as factors associated with the organism, research has identified various other factors important in determining the likelihood of treatment success. More than one quarter of a cow affected, increasing parity, a beta lactamase-producing strain of *S. aureus*, delay in the initiation of treatment, increasingly high and increasingly chronic SCC, clinical signs of abscessation/fibrosis within the mammary gland, severe teat lesions, other health problems, as well as an increasing prevalence of infection in the herd, have all been associated with a poorer chance of cure (Barkema *et al.*, 2006).

While there is a great deal of interest and debate around treatment in lactation and huge amounts of time and resources are focused in this direction, the reality is that cure rates in the dry period are consistently and substantially better than those achieved in lactation; as such, the dry period should be the time of choice for treatment of sub-clinical mastitis (with the exception of *S. agalactiae*). There has also been considerable debate around supplementing intra-mammary dry cow therapy with systemic antibiotics; however, there is both a dearth of peer-reviewed research evidence to support this approach and it is rarely likely to be cost effective given the high cure rates already achieved in the dry period with conventional approaches (Newton *et al.*, 2008; Bradley *et al.*, 2010, 2011).

### Culling

Culling a chronically infected cow offers a quick and easy way to reduce both herd prevalence and the risk of subsequent spread of infection. However, it comes at a significant cost. The decision to cull is complex and depends on the herd prevalence of infection, the ability within the herd to prevent the spread of infection, other pressures on culling and economic factors such as the influence that culling might have on SCC penalty/bonus payments. It is important to remember that culling alone will not provide a permanent answer to a high-SCC problem – too often a policy of culling is all that is implemented in a herd; in the absence of the institution of appropriate measures to control the spread of infection, the end result is likely to be just more culls at a substantial financial cost.

### Drying off or culling a quarter

In some herds drying off a quarter can prove to be a useful procedure, particularly when there is limited scope for culling cows and lactation-based treatment is deemed ineffective. At its simplest, chronically infected quarters are identified and milking of the quarter is suspended for the remainder of that lactation; antibiotic dry cow therapy is then administered in this quarter when other quarters are treated at drying off. More complex approaches involving 'simulation of a dry period' in individual quarters have been described (Newton *et al.*, 2006), but only small-scale studies have been conducted. Use of an escharotic agent (e.g. povidineiodine or chlorhexidine) to destroy secretory tissue in the offending quarter has been suggested, but this is a welfare concern and should be avoided. Simple cessation of milking in a quarter for part of the lactation essentially gives that quarter a prolonged 'dry period' and often gives cure rates of over 50%, although if advocating this technique the practitioner should be aware that it should be avoided when clinical signs persist, and that adverse effects such as abcessation may occur in some cases.

### Controlling the spread of infection

Control of the spread of infection between cows is based mostly on aspects of the milking routine and a correctly functioning milking machine. The aim is to prevent infected milk from one quarter reaching the teat of another cow either via the milking equipment or the milker. In most instances, attention to set-up and practices in the parlour is effective in minimizing contagious spread. Minimizing the risk of introducing fresh infection into the herd either from maiden heifers or bought-in stock is also essential (Barkema *et al.*, 2009).

### Segregation

Often overlooked, possibly because it is unpopular with owners and herdspersons, is the practice of segregation of infected cows. As with many infectious diseases, this is an effective way to prevent spread. Segregation can vary in its application – from attempts to effectively segregate cows using chemical and physical barriers in the milking apparatus (liner shields, cluster back-flushing and disinfection), to milking infected cows separately (after uninfected cows), to physically separating cows during both milking and in their accommodation. Infected quarters can also be segregated within cows by techniques such as quarter milking, or the use of clusters that segregate quarters during the milking process (e.g. IQ cluster, Gea Farm Technologies). While 'back-flushing' systems offer an attractive alternative to segregation, primarily as less effort is involved, there is, as yet, a lack of field study evidence of the efficacy of this technique in preventing the spread of intra-mammary infection; there is little doubt that these systems result in a reduction in bacterial numbers in the liner, but it remains unclear whether there is an associated reduction in intra-mammary infection.

Once one accepts that segregation is useful in controlling the spread of contagious pathogens, then implementation is key.

The exact approach will inevitably vary from farm to farm and according to the number of infected cows. In herds with a very high prevalence of infection it may be appropriate to consider segregation of the 'clean' cows rather than the 'infected' animals. The exact approach needs to be pragmatic and should take into account the capabilities of the farmer and available facilities; for instance, if segregating and milking problem cows last it may be appropriate to create a group that is equivalent in size to the number of available units in the parlour and then institute a policy of full washing and disinfection of the milking plant after every milking. If attempting to establish a 'clean' group, the priority is to correctly identify the uninfected cows, and a low threshold is therefore justified (e.g. <100,000 cells/ml), thereby minimizing the risk of including infected cows. If establishing a 'dirty' group, then the priority is to identify infected cows and thereby reduce the challenge to the pool of animals currently uninfected. It is obviously not practical in this case to have such a low threshold, and a policy of segregating cows with a SCC >400,000 cells/ml is likely to be adequate to make a significant impact on the challenge to other cows in the herd if other aspects of infection control are implemented.

### Minimizing spread in the parlour

MILKING ROUTINE. A clean, methodical approach to milking is essential to minimize the risk of spread in the parlour and should ideally encompass a regime summarized by 'Strip, Dip, Dry and Apply'. The milking routine should maximize mammary stimulation and optimize timing in order to promote adequate milk let-down (grossly contaminated teats and udders should be washed first). This approach and order is advocated for the reasons outlined below.

1. Strip by removing foremilk to detect clinically affected quarters, to flush pathogens from the streak canal and to discard the milk likely to have the highest SCC.
2. Dip using a product with a rapid kill time to kill pathogens present on the teat or deposited there during fore-milking (some authors advocate dip before strip, as this

facilitates fore-milking, but this runs the risk of exacerbating the spread of contagious pathogens if these are transferred between teats in the fore-milking process).
3. Dry with a single-use (paper) towel to ensure clusters are applied to dry teats, thereby minimizing the risk of liner slip.
4. Attach the cluster (ideally within 60–90 s of initial tactile stimulation, although delay is perhaps less detrimental than previously thought).

(NB: application of pre-milking disinfectants is not allowed in some jurisdictions).

In addition there should be no common towels or rags used between teats, and clean, disposable, regularly disinfected gloves should be used for milking. As outlined earlier, segregation of infected cows should be employed, ideally by milking the high-SCC and clinically affected cows last.

After a cow is milked, post-milking teat disinfection (PMTD) should be applied and is widely regarded as one of the most important elements for controlling contagious mastitis. PMTD reduces new infections by killing bacteria that are deposited on the teat during the milking process. Another important role is to preserve healthy teat condition and thereby maintain natural teat defences. Formulation of dips is beyond the scope of this book (see http://www.nmconline.org/docs/Teatbibl.pdf for further information), but as well as using an efficacious product, teat coverage is also important in ensuring effectiveness. Correct storage and handling of dips is vital. Dipping with a teat cup gives more reliable coverage than spraying, although if carefully and thoroughly used both methods can work. Around 10–12 ml of disinfectant/cow/milking is recommended when dipping, whereas at least 15 ml is recommended when spraying. Automated spraying and application methods can be less effective than conventional dipping, and they are prone to mechanical failure; if used, their operation should be regularly evaluated. Although PMTD is essential in the prevention of contagious mastitis, it can result in an increase in clinical coliform mastitis cases (Lam *et al.*, 1997).

### The milking plant

The milking plant can facilitate transmission of pathogens by acting as a vector to transfer bacteria between quarters and cows, and by causing teat damage that predisposes cows to subsequent infection. A clean, well-maintained machine with appropriate milk flow characteristics is a prerequisite for minimizing pathogen spread. Daily and weekly cleaning and maintenance should be carried out by the herdsperson according to the manufacturer's recommendations. A full machine test should be performed six-monthly, by an independent machine expert. Common faults associated with milking machine function are given in Box 5.4. While the herd health advisor will not necessarily be an expert on milking machine function, it is important to understand the importance of the milking machine in mastitis and milk quality. A key role for the herd health practitioner is to be able to work with an appropriate milking plant specialist, put machine issues within the context of a herd mastitis problem and arrive at the best decisions for mastitis

---

**Box 5.4.** Common factors associated with poor milking machine function that may impact on mammary gland health.

- Excessive operating vacuum: the level of vacuum at which the machine operates will depend on the design of the parlour (a 'high-milk line' installation will require a higher level of system vacuum (45.0–48.0 kPa) to draw milk up the long milk tubes than a 'low-milk line' installation (40.0–44.0 kPa). Excessive system vacuum (or insufficient stability, see below) may cause increased vacuum at the teat end and tissue damage, commonly manifesting as cyanosis and oedema (acute) and/or hyperkeratosis of the teat orifice (chronic).
- Overmilking: automatic cluster removal (ACR) systems should be set at milk flow rates that allow some milk to remain in the udder and the cow not to be 'over-milked' (it is commonly recommended that a milk flow rate falling below 400 ml/min should trigger the ACR to remove the cluster (Billon et al., 2007)). Removal of the cluster at very low milk flow rates (<200 ml/min), manual removal of the cluster without prior vacuum shut-off or machine stripping (excessive manual application of the milking machine, usually when applying extra downward pressure on the clawpiece) may all cause tissue damage and an increased risk of mastitis.
- Poor vacuum stability: any blockage or improper function of the regulator may cause inappropriate volumes of air to 'bleed' into the system to counteract the extraction of air via the vacuum pumps, potentially causing fluctuations in vacuum at the teat end. This may be detected audibly as 'liner slip'. Liner slip may also be caused by suboptimal cluster position beneath the cow (e.g. caused by very long milk tubes). Liner slipping can result in air being forced up the teat canal and contamination of the quarter with milk from other (potentially infected) quarters. The installation of liner shields can reduce this, in addition to correcting vacuum instability issues.
- Insufficient vacuum reserve: the vacuum pump(s) are not able to generate sufficient extra air to compensate for the air admitted when clusters are attached. There should be sufficient air extraction capacity to cope with one or more units allowing air into the system (e.g. when one unit is being placed on to a cow and another is kicked off during milking by another cow) and maintain system vacuum within 2.0 kPa of the norm. A vacuum distribution vessel (a large hollow vessel, typically 200 l or more in volume) is sometimes added to the system to improve vacuum stability during milking.
- Inadequate pulsation: the massage phase may be insufficient to allow blood circulation in the teat if the milking 'b' phase (i.e. when air is drawn out of the shell causing the liner to open) is more than 60% of the total pulsation cycle.
- Inadequate shell liner replacement: liners are the interface between the teat and the milking machine and, if not replaced as frequently as recommended by the manufacturer (usually every 2500 milkings or six-monthly for many rubber liners), will rapidly degrade and harbour bacterial pathogens. For example, a 200-cow herd, milked twice daily through a 20-unit, 20-stall herringbone parlour will need to replace all liners every 125 days. The use of silicone liners provides a longer liner life.

management. While automated milking systems present different challenges with respect to mastitis management, in general the principles of mastitis control remain the same. For example, correct pre-milking teat preparation is a vital component of mastitis control whether that is undertaken by a human or a robot – the methods of ensuring an adequate routine are different, but the principle of clean teats remains.

### Environmental sources of traditionally contagious pathogens

While environmental sources of infection with apparent contagious pathogens are rare, they need to be considered. The relative importance of the environment will vary with pathogens. Environmental sources of *S. agalactiae*, by virtue of its inability to survive outside the host for more than a couple of weeks, do not need considering beyond the acute stages of an outbreak and management. In contrast, research suggests that some strains of *S. aureus* tend to have more of an 'environmental' behaviour than others (Sommerhäusera *et al.*, 2003), thereby necessitating more general control measures; environmental sources of this pathogen should be considered when more traditional approaches based on the five-point plan yield disappointing results. Finally, and perhaps obviously, when dealing with apparent 'contagious' behaviour of a more environmental pathogen (e.g. *S. uberis*), environmental control measures will need to be implemented at the same time.

### Biosecurity

Biosecurity plays a crucial role in the control of any infectious disease and is discussed in more detail later. However, in relation to contagious mastitis, maintaining a low prevalence of infection means minimizing the risk of introducing infected heifers or cows (whether bought-in or home-bred) to the milking herd (Barkema *et al.*, 2009). An individual plan should be drawn up for each farm based on current infection status and acceptability of risk; this area will be expanded later in the chapter.

### Vaccination

To increase host resistance, vaccination has generally proved a valuable tool for preventing infectious disease. For mastitis, however, the added value of vaccination so far has been limited. One reason for this is that mastitis can be caused by many different bacterial species and subspecies. In spite of promising data on antibody titres and enhancement of phagocytosis following injection of *S. aureus* antigen conjugates in microspheres (O'Brien *et al.*, 2000), no convincing data are yet available on vaccines being effective in preventing intra-mammary infection with *S. aureus* or other Gram-positive bacteria.

## Environmental mastitis control

Intra-mammary infections originating from pathogens in the environment are described as 'environmental mastitis'. For many years environmental mastitis was considered to be of an acute nature: a cow was infected, became acutely ill, died or survived and the infection was removed. In the 1990s it was shown that typical environmental bacteria such as *E. coli* can also lead to chronic infections (Lam *et al.*, 1996b; Döpfer *et al.*, 1999). It has also been identified that environmental infections can originate in the dry period and result in clinical mastitis in early lactation (Bradley and Green, 2000).

The occurrence of environmental mastitis can be thought of as a balance between infection pressure (being exposed to the pathogen) and the capability of the cow to prevent pathogen invasion or infection. To control mastitis, management measures need to be taken to reduce infection pressure and increase cow resistance. Some management factors (such as breeding and vaccination) specifically influence host resistance, while others (such as cubicle hygiene) are focused on infection pressure. Many factors, however, influence both: feeding regimen, for instance, will influence host resistance, and, through manure consistency, will also have an impact on infection pressure. In terms of environmental mastitis control it is important to identify areas in which cow resistance and infection pressure can be improved, and these are discussed below.

*Breeding*

Selection for resistance to mastitis can have an important impact on clinical mastitis incidence. It does not solve immediate problems, but should be a component of mastitis control in the long term. Selection can be carried out to a limited extent by culling problem cows and raising offspring of healthier cows. More reliable improvements can be made through bull selection (see Appendix 2). The effect of breeding is slow and it also takes many years to correct mistakes made. Selection of the best bulls can lead to a decrease in the percentage of cows affected by clinical mastitis of up to 10–20% per generation (de Haas *et al.*, 2008).

To be able to select for resistance to clinical mastitis, large volumes of reliable data have to be available. Scandinavian countries have made use of data on clinical mastitis for genetic evaluations – in Norway, for instance, analyses have been performed using records of several millions of cows and thousands of bulls since 1978 (Heringstad *et al.*, 2003). In Sweden, all veterinary treatments have been recorded since 1985, being available for estimation of breeding values (Andersson-Eklund and Danell, 1993). The Norwegians have shown that it is possible to select against clinical mastitis and substantially decrease clinical mastitis incidence. If mastitis data are ignored in a breeding programme, and selection is based only on milk production, this will lead to an increase in clinical mastitis incidence (Heringstad *et al.*, 2003).

Most countries, however, do not have these data available. Recent work in the Netherlands showed that test-day records of SCCs, including analysis of peak patterns, can be used as an indicator for susceptibility to clinical mastitis, with an accuracy only slightly inferior to using direct information on clinical mastitis alone (Windig *et al.*, 2010). In the Netherlands a breeding

index for udder health based on this work commenced in 2009. This new index improved the accuracy of the previous index (based on average SCC, udder height, fore udder attachment, teat length and speed of milking) from 0.7 to 0.9 (de Haas *et al.*, 2008).

*Vaccination*

In North America vaccination against *E. coli* mastitis has been used for approximately 20 years. Vaccines using the J5 core antigen are applied twice – at drying off and 3–4 weeks before calving (Wilson *et al.*, 2007). In the 1990s large decreases in the incidence of clinical mastitis were described (Hogan *et al.*, 1992), whereas more recent reports describe a reduction in severity of clinical signs of clinical *E. coli* mastitis, with less culling and death, but not with a decrease in incidence (Wilson *et al.*, 2007). In several countries worldwide researchers are working on the development of mastitis vaccines, and new products are scheduled to appear. Although this research may lead to new products that do have a value in preventing new intra-mammary infections or the consequences of these infections, vaccines are not likely to be a panacea for mastitis prevention.

*Heat stress*

While in tropical countries the effect of heat stress is very well known and accounted for, its effect may be underestimated in countries with a more moderate climate. Both intra-mammary infection and clinical mastitis have a clear species-specific seasonal pattern (Olde Riekerink *et al.*, 2007b); as a result, BMSCC is often highest in the summer months. Heat stress leads to production losses following reduced feed intake and to effects on glucose and lipid homeostasis (Wheelock *et al.*, 2010), with a consequent negative energy balance and impaired host resistance. A recent study (do Amaral *et al.*, 2011) indicated that heat stress during the dry period may also lead to altered immune function in the peri-parturient period and subsequent lactation, and thus it is not surprising that heat stress is a risk factor for mastitis.

Reduced dry matter intake during lactation can be a direct effect of high ambient temperature alone, but can also be a consequence of impaired claw health. In a study by Cook *et al.* (2007), a temperature–humidity index of 68 resulted in the behaviour of dairy cows changing that led to decreased lying times and increased time standing in alleys and cubicles (see Table 5.7). This altered behaviour was associated with a significantly worse locomotion score. Based on these findings, it is wise to consider cooling strategies such as the use of shade, increased ventilation (fans) and

water sprays at environmental temperatures above around 21°C.

### Cow comfort

While comfort itself may be important in terms of affecting the cow's well-being, the specific positioning of a cow, particularly in a cubicle, can be important in terms of reducing infection pressure on the teat. The dimensions and design of cubicle housing are discussed in detail in Chapter 6. Here, we concentrate on cow comfort and housing design with a focus on mastitis. A checklist for aspects of cubicle design related to prevention of environmental mastitis is provided in Box 5.5.

### Other diseases

Any disease that reduces food intake has the potential to increase the risk of mastitis through negative energy balance (see Chapter 8). Lameness is a major cause for reduced feeding time and thus feed intake, as are peri-parturient diseases such as (sub-clinical) hypocalcaemia. Other diseases can also have an effect on mastitis by impairing immune function, as has been described for Blue Tongue (Santman-Berends *et al.*, 2011) and bovine viral diarrhoea (BVD) infection (Berends *et al.*, 2008). Furthermore, mastitis is not independent of other diseases –

**Table 5.7.** The effect of heat stress on behaviour of dairy cows (after Cook *et al.*, 2007).

| Temperature–humidity index[a] | 56.2 | 73.8 |
|---|---|---|
| Time lying (hr) | 10.9 | 7.9 |
| Time standing in stall (hr) | 3.4 | 4.3 |
| Time standing up in alley (hr) | 2.6 | 4.5 |
| Time drinking (hr) | 0.3 | 0.5 |
| Time feeding (hr) | 4.6 | 5.2 |
| Time milking (hr) | 2.2 | 2.3 |

[a] The temperature humidity index (THI) is a method for taking into account the combined effects of temperature and humidity and is calculated using the following equation: THI = (dry bulb temperature, °C) + (0.36 × dew point temperature, °C) + 41.2.

---

**Box 5.5.** Aspects of cubicle design important in the prevention of environmental mastitis (see Chapter 6 for more details on cubicle design).

- There should be >5–10% more cubicles than cows, for each group of milking animals.
- The design of the cubicles should be such that >90% of cows lying in cubicles are positioned correctly and that cows do not defaecate on the cubicle surface.
- The design of the cubicles should minimize the risk of injury to the udder and teats.
- The majority of cows should defaecate into the passageway when lying down; in order to achieve this there should be (i) a brisket board (positioned approximately 75% of the cubicle length from the rear but adjustable so that position can be changed to suit the individual herd); (ii) a neck rail (positioned just above withers height) that prevents cows from walking too far forward into the cubicle prior to lying down; and (iii) partitions to prevent cows from lying at an angle.
- There should be a slope in the cubicles (1 in 20 fall from front to back) to aid drainage of liquid from the bed and prevent build-up of pathogens around the udder.
- The kerb height should be sufficiently high to prevent slurry from splashing on to the back of the cubicles when scraping out.
- Adequate loafing area (>2–3m²/cow) and feed space (see chapter 8) should be provided to reduce competition and to reduce stocking density and subsequent soiling of the udder. Ideally there should be sufficient space for all cows to feed simultaneously.

mastitic cows, for instance, have poorer fertility (Heringstad and Larsgard, 2010). Optimizing general health in a dairy herd undoubtedly has a favourable effect on mastitis and milk quality.

### Nutrition

Feeding is crucial in host resistance, particularly in the dry and transition periods. This is discussed in detail in Chapter 8, and although we wish to highlight the importance of the role of nutrition in mastitis control, we shall not repeat the details here.

It is worth noting that some vitamins and minerals play a role in mastitis control. The importance of adequate supplementation with vitamin E and selenium (Se) is acknowledged (see Chapter 8 for further details); cows fed adequate vitamin E and Se have been shown to have reduced incidence rates of clinical mastitis (Weiss et al., 1990) and a lower prevalence of intra-mammary infection at calving (Ceballos-Marquez et al., 2010). Recently, however, it has been found that overdosing with vitamin E during the dry period can lead to adverse effects on the incidence of clinical mastitis (Bouwstra et al., 2010) and it is advisable to check the vitamin E status of a herd before supplementing with vitamin E.

Although some older studies claim an effect of vitamin A on the severity of mastitis (Chew et al., 1982), the literature is not conclusive. In experimental infections a protective effect has been described for copper and vitamin C levels in milk on the severity of clinical mastitis (Scarletti et al., 2003; Weiss et al., 2004), but conclusive evidence for use in the field is lacking.

### Milking machine and teat scoring

As described earlier, milking machines and milking routines are very important for mammary gland health and this applies to some extent to environmental mastitis. Teat preparation and pre-milking hygiene are of particular importance to reduce the risk of environmental infections, elements described in the earlier section on milking routines.

Scoring teat end condition gives a good impression of the functionality of the milking machine and milking routines (Neijenhuis et al., 2001). Teats should be scored just after removal of the milking cluster. If more than 10% of cows have pronounced teat rings or oedema, milking machine or milking routines require further attention. Teat ends should be scored approximately three-monthly (Hulsen and Lam, 2008). While much attention is placed on teat end hyperkeratosis, a large longitudinal study in the UK found an association only between severe teat end hyperkeratosis and clinical mastitis or new intra-mammary infection; in fact, mild teat end hyperkeratosis was found to be protective (Neijenhuis et al., 2001; Breen et al., 2009a, b). Thus the relationship between teat lesions and risk of mastitis is not clear-cut and further research is needed.

### The non-lactating period

The non-lactating period warrants mention in its own right when considering environmental mastitis control. Research has clearly demonstrated the importance of the dry period in mastitis epidemiology and, more recently, the central role it can play in environmental mastitis. UK studies around the turn of the century demonstrated that in excess of 50% of mastitis caused by the classic environmental mastitis pathogens occurring in the first 100 days of lactation could be as a result of infections acquired during the dry period (Bradley and Green, 2000). Subsequent studies demonstrated that use of antibiotic dry cow therapy with an extended spectrum of activity against Gram-negative pathogens could reduce the incidence of clinical coliform mastitis in the subsequent lactation (Bradley and Green, 2001b). More recently, non-antibiotic approaches such as internal teat sealants have been shown to result in a dramatic reduction in environmental mastitis in the subsequent lactation (Huxley et al., 2002; Sanford et al., 2006; Newton et al., 2008; Bradley et al., 2010). The most recent research in this area has also suggested that overzealous use of antibiotics may result in an increase in the incidence of coliform mastitis (Bradley *et al.*, 2010) – an interesting concept when tackling clinical environmental mastitis issues in very low-BMSCC herds where there is scope to reduce antibiotic dry cow therapy use. As in many areas of mastitis control and herd health, this is another example of where the practitioner may need to 'balance the risks' and modify/adjust interventions according to the herd priorities; reducing antibiotic dry cow therapy use may lower the risk of coliform mastitis in early lactation, but will be coupled with an increased risk of persistence of Gram-positive and contagious mastitis pathogens and a subsequent rise in BMSCC (Bradley *et al.*, 2010).

### Managing the environment to reduce infection pressure

Specifically for environmental mastitis, housing hygiene is very important throughout the lactation cycle – the environment is potentially an enormous source of infections. As a measure of general hygiene, a hygiene scoring system based on leg and udder scores has been described by Schreiner and Ruegg (2003), using a four-point scale ranging from 1 (very clean) to 4 (very dirty). It was reported that dirtier cows have a higher SCC and that more major pathogens are cultured from milk samples of dirtier cows. Hygiene scoring is a useful way to visualize the infection pressure from the environment – dirty cows indicate that environmental management needs to be improved in order to prevent problems. A recent study in the UK reported that cows with very dirty udders (udder hygiene score of 4) were significantly more likely to acquire a clinical case of mastitis in the next month (Breen *et al.*, 2009a). This is also the case at the herd level: Barkema *et al.* (1999) found that less hygienic herds (described as 'quick and dirty' had a higher BMSCC compared with 'clean and accurate' herds).

Assessing and making improvements to the environment is a critical aspect of environmental mastitis control. A checklist of important elements of environmental management, to minimize infection pressure, is provided in Box 5.6.

### Managing the milk-harvesting process

The aim of a milk-harvesting process is to extract milk from the cow, in a timely and efficient manner, while minimizing risk to udder health or contamination of the end product. The aim of this section is to look at the production of quality milk and how this can be monitored, assessed and managed.

As outlined earlier, producers have to maintain milk quality within strict criteria to maximize returns and retain their right to supply milk for human consumption. From an SCC perspective this involves control of mastitis within the herd, and this has been described in earlier sections. However, from a bacteriological perspective, managing milk quality can equally be a challenge.

When one considers the bacteriological quality of milk there are only a limited number of potential sources/breakdowns in the process that can result in a problem, and these can be conveniently split into four categories: (i) the udder; (ii) the environment; (iii) the result of poor plant cleaning; and (iv) the result of failure of refrigeration, which are reviewed below. It should be stressed that, on occasion, a thorough investigation will be required to identify the source of bacterial contamination.

### Intra-mammary sources of contamination

In certain circumstances the mammary gland can contribute significant numbers of bacteria to the bulk supply. Most notably and almost exclusively this relates to the *Streptococcus* spp., as these are generally the only species that are shed in sufficient numbers from infected glands to influence the bulk supply. Classically this phenomenon has been attributed to *S. agalactiae*, though in recent years it has also been increasingly associated with *S. uberis*, which is commonly associated with wide fluctuations in bacterial count. This area is easily monitored and investigated using the direct plating of bulk milk on to both selective and non-selective media and specific counts if necessary (though often gross plate assessment can be a sufficient indicator

**Box 5.6.** Important elements of environmental management for the prevention of environmental mastitis.

Bedding management
- Any material (particularly organic materials) used for bedding cows should be stored under cover to keep it dry and clean.
- Cubicle systems
  - Dung and soiled/wet bedding should be removed from cubicle beds at least twice daily and clean bedding material applied to the cubicles at least daily.
  - Sufficient bedding should be used to ensure that cows remain clean.
  - Drying agents (e.g. hydrated lime) and disinfectants may be used but their efficacy is uncertain. The aim should be to achieve a dry, clean bed.
  - The use of inorganic bedding materials, such as sand and ash, is excellent in reducing bacterial numbers in the environment, and thus decreasing infection pressure. If sand is used, it needs to be free of organic matter and significant quantities of clay (unwashed river sand is often unsuitable). While an excellent bedding material, sand has significant disadvantages, most notably that it can make pre-milking teat preparation more arduous, causes significant wear to mechanical equipment and can have a significant impact on soil pH over time when spread on pasture.
- Yard systems
  - Stocking density should be controlled when cows are kept on straw or sand yards; a bedded area of 1.25 m²/1000 l milk/cow (annual milk yield) is recommended (Green et al., 2007b).
  - Straw usage should be sufficient to keep cows clean (generally >300 kg/cow/month). It should be un-chopped, and spread evenly over the bedded area.
  - New, clean and dry straw or sand should be laid in milking and dry cow yards at least once daily, and more frequently if mastitis problems persist.
  - Straw yard systems should ideally be completely cleaned out and re-bedded at least every month; sand yard systems should be completely cleaned out and re-bedded at least every 6 months.

Slurry management and scraping routine
- All passageways, loafing areas and feed areas used for cows should be scraped out at least twice daily.
- If automatic scraping systems are used these should be run sufficiently often that passageways are kept clean and slurry does not overflow the sides of the scrapers.
- Sufficient drainage must be present so that pooling of liquid in passageways and feed areas is minimized.

Ventilation
- Check that cows do not show a preference for particular areas of the building and that there is good ventilation in all areas.
- Evaluate the central ridge air outlet requirements for the house to maximize the 'stack' effect; an open ridge >200 mm wide is usually required along the length of the building (allowing an outlet area ~0.10–0.15 m² per adult cow).
- The air inlet area should be 2–4 times the outlet area (i.e. increases with milk yield); avoid walls with no inlet at all. NB: excessive air inlet at cow level can lead to draughts and wind chill.
- Keep all inlets and outlets clean and free from obstruction.
- Where building design or ventilation are poor, consider forced (mechanical) ventilation to ensure adequate control of temperature and humidity.
- Check moisture management (e.g. leakage from drinking systems, gutters and downpipes and roof leaks) and ensure that water is directed away from the building.

Pasture management
- Cows should not remain on the same pasture/lying area for more than 2 weeks and cattle should not be returned to the same area for grazing for at least 4 weeks after use; in general, a policy of 'graze for 2 weeks and rest for 4 weeks' is recommended to reduce intra-mammary infections (Green et al., 2007b).
- If grazing management, grass growth rates and access to grazing are not conducive to a system optimal for udder health, then ensure that cows are fenced away from grossly contaminated areas.
- A stocking rate of not greater than 100 cows per acre per day in a 2-week period is recommended (e.g. 50 cows on 1 acre for 2 days).

*Continued*

**Box 5.6.** Continued.

- Sufficient drainage must be present to avoid flooding and significant poaching (trampling) of areas used to graze cattle: if this occurs, cattle should be moved to a different paddock.
- Tracks, gateways and areas around feed and water troughs should be actively managed to avoid excessive poaching, for example by using bark or wood chippings and/or routes and access points rotated to allow recovery of the ground.

Good fly control is essential for cows through the summer period, and sheltered areas associated with increased fly densities should be avoided.

given the sheer numbers of organisms that may be involved).

*Environmental sources of contamination*

The environment can be a significant source of contamination of the bulk supply, most commonly as a result of poor pre-milking teat preparation. This is often initially identified by direct plating revealing a diverse and heavy growth of a wide range of organisms. In addition, an elevated number of coliforms and psychrotrophic organisms has been associated with poor test preparation. Resolution of such issues is straightforward and requires improvements in the milk routine. However, this is often an area that needs to be managed with some sensitivity and often receives resistance because of the impact it can have on milking times.

*Plant cleanliness*

Inadequate plant cleaning most commonly, though not exclusively, manifests as a rise in bacterial numbers caused by thermoduric organisms. This may reflect a general issue (wash temperatures too low or insufficient volumes used) or a more focused issue driven by a nidus of contamination somewhere within the plant. In these instances review of plant cleaning is the first step, and the engagement of an experienced plant engineer may be necessary.

*Failure of refrigeration*

This usually manifests as a rise in the numbers of psychrotrophic bacteria and is likely to be a more significant issue in farms with less frequent milk collection (i.e. not daily).

Psychrotrophic bacteria are ubiquitous in the environment (and hence their use also as a measure of teat preparation and general milking cleanliness) and can grow successfully at low temperatures. Any compromise in milk refrigeration (even by a few degrees) will tend to manifest first as a rise in psychrotrophic count. Review of the efficiency of bulk tank cleaning and milk cooling is indicated.

As well as the examples outlined above, other more unusual causes of poor bulk milk bacterial quality do arise. These can encompass issues such as leaking pate coolers and contaminated water supplies. However, it is important to rule out the common causes of bacterial contamination initially before extending the search to other areas.

**Biosecurity**

Biosecurity is a key aspect of mastitis control on dairy farms and deserves particular attention. Biosecurity is important both from the perspective of preventing introduction of previously eradicated pathogens (e.g. *S. agalactiae*) or preventing introduction of new strains of existing pathogens, and from the perspective of preventing introduction of other pathogens that may have an indirectly deleterious impact on udder health (e.g. BVD) (see Barkema *et al.*, 2009 for an overview). For this reason it is crucial that all units should have a biosecurity plan that takes into account udder health risks and general disease risks (this is discussed further in Chapter 7).

Maintaining a closed herd is the ideal scenario and dramatically reduces the risk of introduction of pathogens affecting mammary gland health directly or indirectly. However, if animals are purchased, their mastitis history should be evaluated. Simple bulk tank screening and implementation of SCC thresholds for purchased animals can dramatically reduce the risk. When implementing an SCC threshold for biosecurity reasons it is important to remember the reason for the threshold – in this case to exclude infection – and for this reason a threshold to maximize sensitivity is key and therefore a lower SCC cut-off should be selected. While all herds should have an udder health biosecurity policy (even if contagious mastitis is already an issue), inevitably the stringency of any policy will reflect the current herd udder health status. Important details are outlined in Box 5.7. An optimal policy would encompass purchasing animals only from low-SCC herds (ideally, BMSCC <150,000 cells/ml) with the last three individual cow SCCs <100,000 cells/ml and a negative CMT, but this is difficult to achieve. Great caution should be exercised when purchasing animals without records, though this is inevitable when

purchasing heifers – in this instance a history of mastitis in the herd and previous heifer performance should be sought.

Transmission of infections by and to humans and non-bovine animals can occur, and these risks should also be considered; for example, relief-milkers should ideally have farm-specific clothing and equipment and while restricting them to just one farm is perhaps unrealistic, it might be wise at least to be aware of the disease status in other herds in which they operate. In addition, an area often overlooked is the level of personal hygiene prior to commencing the milking process; the mentality of being involved in a food-harvesting process should be engendered and encouraged in all milking personnel.

### The role of the heifer in mastitis control

There is little doubt that heifers entering the milking herd can be a significant source of intra-mammary infection, harbouring both contagious and environmental mastitis

---

**Box 5.7.** Key elements of a mastitis biosecurity protocol.

Maintain a closed herd if possible, otherwise:

Criteria for herds from which animals are purchased
- The herd should have had a rolling geometric mean BMSCC < 200,000 cells/ml for at least one year.
- The herd should have had individual at least bi-monthly cow SCC records for the previous six months.
- Information on pathogens present on the farm must be available for the herd, which must not have had any history of *S. agalactiae* or *Mycoplasma* spp. infection in the previous two years, and absence of these pathogens should be confirmed by serial bulk tank culture or PCR.
- The herd should be free of, or vaccinated against, BVD.
- The herd should not contain cows with severe teat lesions.

Criteria for animals purchased
- Although heifers can become infected before they calve for the first time, they are generally at less risk than older cows of carrying mastitis pathogens and thus represent a lower biosecurity risk in terms of mammary health.
- If older cows are purchased, they should be purchased with only complete lactation SCC records.
- Ideally, a cow should never have had a SCC of >200,000 cells/ml over her lifetime, and should preferably never have exceeded a SCC of 100,000 cells/ml during her lifetime.
- Failing this, a cow should have at least the three most recent SCCs in the current lactation <100,000 cells/ml.
- If purchased in the immediate post-calving period, the cow should meet the criteria defined above and have been treated with a dry cow therapy product at the previous drying off.
- Udder, teats and milk should be examined for signs of abnormalities and the cow should have been CMT negative for three consecutive days if purchased in early lactation.

pathogens. A number of studies have investigated intra-mammary infection in heifers and identified risk factors for contagious mastitis such as ineffective fly control, contact with lactating cows and a high BMSCC, whereas inadequate mineral supplementation and poor hygiene have been linked to environmental mastitis (Pieper *et al.*, 2011). Interestingly, teat apex colonization with CNS was associated with a reduced risk of infection by a major pathogen (Pieper *et al.*, 2011). However, this study concluded that heifer and quarter characteristics were more important than management in determining infection status at first calving (Pieper *et al.*, 2011). A number of intervention studies have investigated both antibiotic and non-antibiotic approaches to minimizing intra-mammary infection in nulliparous heifers; amongst others, these studies have suggested that post-milking teat dipping prior to calving (Lopez-Benavides *et al.*, 2009), the use of an internal teat sealant (Parker *et al.*, 2008) and intra-mammary antibiotic treatment (Sampimon *et al.*, 2009) may aid in reducing the prevalence of intra-mammary infection post-calving.

## Conclusions

Mastitis has, and will, remain a significant cause of loss to the modern dairy industry and will continue to be an area that will need significant input from herd health professionals. Due to its complex aetiology, it is likely that the disease will alter as we learn new approaches to control and implement new measures.

Arguably we have already seen the influence that our control measures have, not only on incidence and aetiology but also unintentionally on the behaviour of pathogens as ecological niches are freed of their historical occupants. The continued polarization of production techniques in the industry will present its own challenges. Increasing yields and the pressures on intensive systems will create one set of challenges while decreasing labour input, and the more 'hands-off' approach of extensive, low-output systems another.

In this chapter we have stressed the importance of monitoring mastitis in the dairy herd and the use of mastitis data to direct control strategies. We emphasize again that, since mastitis is a set of complex and dynamic infection processes, the herd health cycle (described in Chapter 1) of 'monitor – re-evaluate – make management changes – monitor' is *crucial* if mastitis control at herd level is to be achieved. Hopefully we have provided information in this chapter that will go some way to providing the herd health advisor with an insight into the flexible approach to mastitis management that will become essential when conducting herd health in the modern dairy herd.

## References and Further Reading

Andersson-Eklund, L. and Danell, B. (1993) Association of breeding values for disease traits and genetic markers in dairy cattle estimated with a mixed model. *Journal of Dairy Science* 76, 3785–3791.

Barkema, H.W., Schukken, Y.H., Lam, T.J., Beiboer, M.L., Wilmink, H., Benedictus, G. *et al.* (1998) Incidence of clinical mastitis in dairy herds grouped in three categories by bulk milk somatic cell counts. *Journal of Dairy Science* 81, 411–419.

Barkema, H.W., van der Ploeg, J.D., Schukken, Y.H., Lam, T.J.G.M., Benedictus, G. and Brand, A. (1999) Management style and its association with bulk milk somatic cell count and incidence rate of clinical mastitis. *Journal of Dairy Science* 82, 1655–1663.

Barkema, H.W., Schukken, Y.H. and Zadoks, R.N. (2006) Invited review: The role of cow, pathogen, and treatment regimen in the therapeutic success of bovine *Staphylococcus aureus* mastitis. *Journal of Dairy Science* 89, 1877–1895.

Barkema, H.W., Green, M.J., Bradley, A.J. and Zadoks, R.N. (2009) Invited review: The role of contagious disease in udder health. *Journal of Dairy Science* 92, 4717–4729.

Beaudeau, F., Fourichon, C., Seegers, H. and Bareille, N. (2002) Risk of clinical mastitis in dairy herds with a high proportion of low individual milk somatic-cell counts. *Preventive Veterinary Medicine* 53, 43–54.

Berends, I.M., Swart, W.A., Frankena, K., Muskens, J., Lam, T.J. and Gvan Schaik, G. (2008) The effect of becoming BVDV-free on fertility and udder health in Dutch dairy herds. *Preventive Veterinary Medicine* 84, 48–60.

Biddle, M.K., Fox, L.K. and Hancock, D.D. (2003) Patterns of *Mycoplasma* shedding in the milk of dairy cows with intra-mammary *Mycoplasma* infection. *Journal of the American Veterinary Medical Association* 223, 1163–1166.

Biddle, M.K., Fox, L.K., Hancock, D.D., Gaskins, C.T. and Evans, M.A. (2004) Effects of storage time and thawing methods on the recovery of *Mycoplasma* species in milk samples from cows with intra-mammary infections. *Journal of Dairy Science* 87, 933–936.

Billon, P., Pledel, D. and Gaudin, V. (2007). Effects of increasing the milk flow detachment level when using ACR's on milking and milk quality. In: *Proceedings of the Annual Meeting of the National Mastitis Council*, pp. 222–223.

Booth, J.M. (1996) Is bovine mastitis being reduced? In: *Proceedings of XIX World Buiatrics Congress*, Edinburgh, pp. 292–295.

Bouwstra, R.J., Nielen, M., Stegeman, J.A., Dobbelaar, P., Newbold, J.R., Jansen E.H.J. *et al.* (2010) Vitamin E supplementation during the dry period in dairy cattle. Part I: Adverse effect on incidence of mastitis postpartum in a double-blind randomized field trial. *Journal of Dairy Science* 93, 5684–5695.

Bradley, A.J. (2002) Bovine mastitis - an evolving disease. *The Veterinary Journal* 164, 1116–1128.

Bradley, A.J. and Green, M.J. (2000) A study of the incidence and significance of intra-mammary enterobacterial infections acquired during the dry period. *Journal of Dairy Science* 83, 1957–1965.

Bradley, A.J. and Green, M.J. (2001a) Adaptation of *Escherichia coli* to the bovine mammary gland. *Journal of Clinical Microbiology* 39, 1845–1849.

Bradley, A.J. and Green, M.J. (2001b) A randomized, temporally matched trial of the efficacy of dry cow therapy in the control of clinical coliform mastitis. *Journal of Dairy Science* 84, 1632–1639.

Bradley, A.J. and Green, M.J. (2004) Use and interpretation of somatic cell counts in the dairy cow. *In Practice* 27, 310–315.

Bradley, A.J., Green, M.J. and Huxley, J.N. (2002) Making better use of milk samples: monitoring and investigating herd mastitis. *Cattle Practice* 10, 105–112.

Bradley, A.J., Leach, K.A., Breen, J.E., Green, L.E. and Green, M.J. (2007a) A survey of the incidence rate and aetiology of mastitis on dairy farms in England and Wales. *Veterinary Record* 160, 253–258.

Bradley, A.J., Breen, J.E. and Green, M.J. (2007b) Mastitis pattern analysis – a fresh look at the analysis of bovine mastitis: Part 1 – somatic cell count data. *UK Vet* 12, 1–5.

Bradley, A.J., Breen, J.E. and Green, M.J. (2008) Mastitis pattern analysis – a fresh look at the analysis of bovine mastitis: Part 2 – clinical mastitis data. *UK Vet* 13, 1–5.

Bradley, A.J., Breen, J.E., Payne, B., Williams, P. and Green, M.J. (2010) The use of a Cephalonium-containing dry cow therapy and an internal teat sealant, both alone and in combination. *Journal of Dairy Science* 93, 1566–1577.

Bradley, A.J., Breen, J.E., Payne, B. and Green, M.J. (2011) A comparison of broad-spectrum and narrow-spectrum dry cow therapy used alone and in combination with a teat sealant. *Journal of Dairy Science* 94, 692–704.

Breen, J.E., Green, M.J. and Bradley, A.J. (2009a) An investigation of quarter and cow risk factors associated with the occurrence of clinical mastitis in UK dairy cows. *Journal of Dairy Science* 92, 2551–2561.

Breen, J.E., Bradley, A.J. and Green, M.J. (2009b) An investigation of quarter and cow risk factors associated with a somatic cell count greater than 199,000 cells per millilitre in UK dairy cows. *Journal of Dairy Science* 92, 3106–3115.

Ceballos-Marquez, A., Barkema, H.W., Stryhn, H., Wichtel, J.J., Neumann, J., Mella, A. *et al.* (2010) The effect of selenium supplementation before calving on early-lactation udder health in pastured dairy heifers. *Journal of Dairy Science* 93, 4602–4612.

Chew, B.P., Hollen, L.L., Hillers, J.K. and Hergulson, M.L. (1982) Relationshop between vitamin A and β-carotene in blood plasma and milk and mastitis in Holsteins. *Journal of Dairy Science* 65, 2111–2118.

Cook, N.B., Mentink, R.L., Bennett, T.B. and Burgi, K. (2007) The effect of heat stress and lameness on time budgets of lactating dairy cows. *Journal of Dairy Science* 90, 1674–1682.

de Haas, Y., de Jong, G. and Lam, T.J. (2008) Udder health: breeding. *Dutch Veterinary Journal* 133, 464–468.

De Vliegher, S., Opsomer, G., Vanrolleghem, A., Devriese, L.A., Sampimon, O.C., Sol, J., Barkema, H.W., Haesebrouck, F. and de Kruif, A. (2004) In vitro growth inhibition of major mastitis pathogens by Staphylococcus chromogenes originating from teat apices of dairy heifers. *Veterinary Microbiology* 101, 215-221.

Dingwell, R., Leslie, K.E., Schukken, Y.H., Sargeant, J.M., Timms, L.L., Duffield, T.F. *et al.* (2004) Association of cow and quarter-level factors at drying-off with new intra-mammary infections during the dry period. *Preventive Veterinary Medicine* 63, 75–89.

Dinsmore, R.P., English, P.B., Gonzalez, R.N., Sears, P.M. and Schulte, H.F. (1991) Evaluation of methods for the diagnosis of *Streptococcus agalactiae* intra-mammary infections in dairy cattle. *Journal of Dairy Science* 74, 1521–1526.

do Amaral, B.C., Connor, E.E., Tao, S., Haven, M.J., Bubolz, J.W. and Dahl, G.E. (2011) Heat stress abatement during the dry period influences metabolic gene expression and improves immune status in the transition period of dairy cows. *Journal of Dairy Science* 94, 86–96.

Dodd, F.H., Westgarth, D.R., Neave, F.K. and Kingwill, R.G. (1969) Mastitis – the strategy of control. *Journal of Dairy Science* 52, 689–695.

Dohoo, I.R. and Leslie, K.E. (1991) Evaluation of changes in somatic cell counts as indicators of new intra-mammary infections. *Preventive Veterinary Medicine* 10, 225–237.

Döpfer, D., Barkema, H.W., Lam, T.J., Schukken, Y.H. and Gaastra, W. (1999) Recurrent clinical mastitis caused by *Escherichia coli* in dairy cows. *Journal of Dairy Science* 82, 80–85.

Green, M.J., Green, L.E. and Cripps, P.J. (1996) Low bulk milk somatic cell counts and endotoxin-associated (toxic) mastitis. *Veterinary Record* 138, 305–306.

Green, M.J., Burton, P.R., Green, L.E., Schukken, Y.H., Bradley, A.J., Peeler, E.J. *et al.* (2004) The use of Markov chain Monte Carlo for analysis of correlated binary data: patterns of somatic cells in milk and the risk of clinical mastitis in dairy cows. *Preventive Veterinary Medicine* 64, 157–174.

Green, M.J., Leach, K.A., Breen, J.E., Green, L.E. and Bradley, A.J. (2007a) A national intervention study of mastitis control on dairy herds in England and Wales. *Veterinary Record* 160, 287–293.

Green, M.J., Bradley, A.J., Medley, G.F. and Browne, W.J. (2007b) Cow, farm and management factors during the dry period that determine the rate of clinical mastitis after calving. *Journal of Dairy Science* 90, 3764–3776.

Heringstad, B. and Larsgard, A.G. (2010) Correlated selection responses for female fertility after selection for high protein yield or low mastitis frequency in Norwegian Red cows. *Journal of Dairy Science* 93, 5970–5976.

Heringstad, B., Klemetsdal, G. and Steine, T. (2003) Selection responses for clinical mastitis and protein yield in two Norwegian dairy cattle selection experiments. *Journal of Dairy Science* 86, 2990–2999.

Hillerton, J. (2000) *Proceedings of National Mastitis Council Annual Meeting*, pp. 48–53.

Hogan, J.S., Smith, K.L., Todhunter, D.D. and Schoenberger, P.S. (1992) Field trial to determine efficacy of an *Escherichia coli* J5 mastitis vaccine. *Journal of Dairy Science* 75, 78–84.

Huijps, K., Hogeveen, H., Lam T.J.G.M. and Oude Lansink, A.G.J.M. (2010) Costs and efficacy of management measures to improve udder health on Dutch dairy farms. *Journal of Dairy Science* 93, 115–124.

Hulsen, J. and Lam, T.J. (2006) *Udder Health. A Practical Guide to First-rate Udder Health*. Roodbont Publishers, Zutphen, The Netherlands.

Huxley, J.N., Green, M.J., Green, L.E. and Bradley, A.J. (2002) Evaluation of the efficacy of an internal teat sealant during the dry period. *Journal of Dairy Science* 85, 551–561.

Huxley, J.N., Green, M.J. and Bradley, A.J. (2003) *Corynebacterium bovis* - friend or foe? In: *British Mastitis Conference*, pp. 23–34.

Jansen, J., Renes, R.J. and Lam, T.J. (2010) Evaluation of two communication strategies to improve udder health management. *Journal of Dairy Science* 93, 604–612.

Jayarao, B.M., Pillai, S.R., Sawant, A.A., Wolfgang, D.R. and Hegde, N.V. (2004) Guidelines for monitoring bulk tank milk somatic cell and bacterial counts. *Journal of Dairy Science* 87, 3561–3573.

Kemp, M.H., Nolan, A.M., Cripps, P.J. and Fitzpatrick, J.L. (2008) Animal-based measurements of the severity of mastitis in dairy cows. *Veterinary Record* 163, 175–179.

Kossaibati, M.A. and Esslemont, R.J. (1997) The costs of production diseases in dairy herds in England. *Veterinary Journal* 154, 41–51.

Krömker, V. and Friedrich J. (2009) Teat canal closure in non-lactating heifers and its association with udder health in consecutive lactation. *Veterinary Microbiology* 134, 37–44.

Lam, T.J., van Wuijckhuise, L.A., Franken, P., Morselt, M.L., Hartman, E.G. and Schukken, Y.H. (1996a) Use of composite milk samples for diagnosis of *Staphylococcus aureus* mastitis in dairy cattle. *Journal of the American Veterinary Medical Association* 208, 1705–1708.

Lam, T.J., Lipman, L.J., Schukken, Y.H., Gaastra, W. and Brand, A. (1996b) Epidemiological characteristics of bovine clinical mastitis caused by *Staphylococcus aureus* and *Escherichia coli* studied by DNA finger-printing. *American Journal of Veterinary Research* 57, 39–42.

Lam, T.J., van Vliet, J.H., Schukken, Y.H., Grommers, F.J., van Velden-Russcher, A., Barkema, H.W. and Brand, A. (1997) The effect of discontinuation of postmilking teat disinfection in low somatic cell count herds. I. Incidence of clinical mastitis. *Veterinary Quarterly* 19, 41–47.

Lam, T.J., Jansen, J., van den Borne, B.H., Renes, R.J. and Hogeveen, H. (2011) What veterinarians need to know to optimize their role as udder health advisors in dairy herds. *New Zealand Veterinary Journal* 59, 8–15.

Lievaart, J., Barkema, H.W., Hogeveen, H. and Kremer, W.D. (2009) Reliability of the bulk milk somatic cell count as an indication of average herd somatic cell count. *Journal of Dairy Research* 76, 490–496.

Lopez-Benavides, M.G., Williamson, J.H., Lacy-Hulbert, S.J. and Cursons, R.T. (2009) Heifer teats sprayed in the dry period with an iodine teat sanitizer have reduced *Streptococcus uberis* teat-end contamination and less *Streptococcus uberis* intra-mammary infections at calving. *Veterinary Microbiology* 16, 186–191.

Neijenhuis, F., Barkema, H.W., Hogeveen, H. and Noordhuizen, J.P. (2001) Relationship between teat-end callosity and occurrence of clinical mastitis. *Journal of Dairy Science* 84, 2664–2672.

Newton, H.T., Green, M.J. and Bradley, A.J. (2006) A novel approach to the treatment of subclinical intra-mammary infection in UK dairy cows: Preliminary findings from a recent research project. *Cattle Practice* 14, 77–84.

Newton, H.T., Green, M.J., Benchaoui, H., Cracknell, V., Rowan, T. and Bradley, A.J. (2008) Comparison of the efficacy of cloxacillin alone and cloxacillin combined with an internal teat sealant for dry cow therapy. *Veterinary Record* 162, 678–683.

NMC (2011) *Recommended Mastitis Control Program*. National Mastitis Council, Verona, Wisconsin.

O'Brien, C.N., Guidry, A.J., Fattom, A., Shepherd, S., Douglass, L.W. and Westhoff, D.C. (2000) Production of antibodies to *Staphylococcus aureus* serotypes 5, 8 and 336 using poly (DL-lactide-co-glycolide) micro-spheres. *Journal of Dairy Science* 83, 1758–1766.

Olde Riekerink, R.G., Barkema, H.W., Veenstra, W., Berg, F.E., Stryhn, H. and Zadoks R.N. (2007a) Somatic cell count during and between milkings. *Journal of Dairy Science* 90, 3733–3741.

Olde Riekerink, R.G., Barkema, H.W. and Stryhn, H. (2007b) The effect of season on somatic cell count and the incidence of clinical mastitis. *Journal of Dairy Science* 90, 1704–1715.

Olde Riekerink, R.G., Barkema, H.W., Kelton, D.F. and Scholl, D.T. (2008) Incidence rate of clinical mastitis on Canadian dairy farms. *Journal of Dairy Science* 91, 1366–1377.

Østerås, O. and Sølverød, L. (2009) Norwegian mastitis control programme. *Irish Veterinary Journal* 62, 26–33.

Parker, K.I., Compton, C.W., Anniss, F.M., Heuer, C. and McDougall, S. (2008) Quarter-level analysis of sub-clinical and clinical mastitis in primiparous heifers following the use of a teat sealant or an injectable antibiotic, or both, pre-calving. *Journal of Dairy Science* 91, 169–181.

Passey, S., Bradley, A.J. and Mellor, H. (2008) *Escherichia coli* isolated form bovine mastitis invade mammary cells by a modified endocytic pathway. *Veterinary Microbiology* 130, 151–164.

Peeler, E.J., Green, M.J., Fitzpatrick, J.L. and Green, L.E. (2003) The association between quarter somatic-cell counts and clinical mastitis in three British dairy herds. *Preventive Veterinary Medicine* 59, 169–180.

Petrovski, K.R., Heuer, C., Parkinson, T.J. and Williamson, N.B. (2009) The incidence and aetiology of clinical bovine mastitis on 14 farms in Northland, New Zealand. *New Zealand Veterinary Journal* 57, 109–115.

Piepers, S., Peeters, K., Opsomer, G., Barkema, H.W., Frankena, K. and De Vliegher, S. (2011) Pathogen group-specific risk factors at herd, heifer and quarter levels for intra-mammary infections in early lactat-ing dairy heifers. *Preventive Veterinary Medicine* 99, 91–101.

Sampimon, O.C., De Vliegher, S., Barkema, H.W., Sol, J. and Lam, T.J. (2009) Effect of prepartum dry cow antibiotic treatment in dairy heifers on udder health and milk production. *Journal of Dairy Science* 92, 4395–4403.

Sanford, C.J., Keefe, G.P., Dohoo, I.R., Leslie, K.E., Dingwell, R.T., DesCoteaux, L. *et al.* (2006) Efficacy of using an internal teat sealer to prevent new intra-mammary infections in non-lactating dairy cattle. *Journal of the American Veterinary Medical Association* 228, 1565–1573.

Santman-Berends, I.M., Hage, J.J., Lam, T.J., Sampimon, O.C. and van Schaik, G. (2011) The effect of blue-tongue virus serotype 8 on milk production and somatic cell count in Dutch dairy cattle in 2008. *Journal of Dairy Science* 94, 1347–1354.

Sargeant, J.M., Scott, H.M., Leslie, K.E., Ireland, M.J. and Bashiri, A. (1998) Clinical mastitis in dairy cattle in Ontario: frequency of occurrence and bacteriological isolates. *Canadian Veterinary Journal* 39, 33–38.

Sargeant J.M., Leslie K.E., Shirley J.E., Pulkrabek B.J. and Lim G.H. (2001) Sensitivity and specificity of somatic cell count and California mastitis test for identifying intra-mammary infection in early lactation. *Journal of Dairy Science* 84, 2018–2024.

Scarletti, R.W., Trammell, D.S., Smith, B.A. and Harmon, R.J. (2003) Role of dietary copper in enhancing resistance to *Escherichia coli* mastitis. *Journal of Dairy Science* 86, 1240–1249.

Schalm, O.W., Lasmanis, J. and Carroll, E.J. (1964) Effects of pre-exisiting leukocytosis on experimental coliform (*Aerobacter aerogenes*) mastitis in cattle. *American Journal of Veterinary Research* 25, 83.

Schreiner, A. and Ruegg, P.L. (2003) Relationship between udder and leg hygiene scores and subclinical mastitis. *Journal of Dairy Science* 86, 3460–3465.

Sears, P.M., Wilson, D.J., Gonzalez, R.N. and Hancock, D.D. (1991) Microbiological results from milk samples obtained pre-milking and post-milking for the diagnosis of bovine intra-mammary infections. *Journal of Dairy Science* 74, 4183–4188.

Shuster, D.E., Lee, E.K. and Kehrli, M.E., Jr (1996) Bacterial growth, inflammatory cytokine production, and neutrophil recruitment during coliform mastitis in cows within ten days after calving, compared with cows at midlactation. *American Journal of Veterinary Research* 57, 1569–1575.

Smith, K.L., Todhunter, D.A. and Schoenberger, P.S. (1985). Environmental pathogens and intra-mammary infection during the dry period. *Journal of Dairy Science* 68, 402–417.

Sol, J. 2002. Cure of Staphylococcus aureus mastitis in Dutch dairy cows. PhD thesis; Utrecht University, The Netherlands.

Sommerhäusera, J., Klopperta, B., Woltera, W., Zschöcka, M., Sobirajb, A. and Failing, K. (2003) The epidemiology of *Staphylococcus aureus* infections from subclinical mastitis in dairy cows during a control programme. *Veterinary Microbiology* 96, 91–102.

Sordillo, L.M., ShaferWeaver, K. and DeRosa, D. (1997) Immunobiology of the mammary gland. *Journal of Dairy Science* 80, 1851–1865.

Suriyasathaporn, W., Schukken, Y.H., Nielen, M. and Brand, A. (2000) Low somatic cell count: A risk factor for subsequent clinical mastitis in a dairy herd. *Journal of Dairy Science* 83, 1248–1255.

Tadich, N.A., Carey, A., Porter, R., Ridley, J., Green, M.J. and Green, L.E. (1998) Case control study of risk factors for toxic mastitis in 26 dairy herds. *Veterinary Record* 143, 362–365.

Valeeva, N.I., Lam, T.J. and Hogeveen, H. (2007) Motivation of dairy farmers to improve mastitis management. *Journal of Dairy Science* 90, 4466–4477.

Van Werven, T. (1999) The role of leukocytes in bovine *Escherichia coli* mastitis. PhD Thesis, Utrecht, The Netherlands.

Weiss, W.P., Hogan, J.S., Smith, K.L. and Hoblet, K.H. (1990) Relationship among selenium, vitamin E, and mammary gland health in commercial dairy herds. *Journal of Dairy Science* 73, 381–390.

Weiss, W.P., Hogan, J.S. and Smith, K.L. (2004) Changes in vitamin C concentrations in plasma and milk from dairy cows after an intra-mammary infusion of *Escherichia coli*. *Journal of Dairy Science* 87, 32–37.

Wheelock, J.B., Rhoads, R.P., VanBaale, M.J., Sanders, S.R. and Baumgard, L.H. (2010) Effects of heat stress on energetic metabolism in lactating Holstein cows. *Journal of Dairy Science* 93, 644–655.

Wilesmith, J.W., Francis, P.G. and Wilson, C.D. (1986) Incidence of clinical mastitis in a cohort of British dairy herds. *Veterinary Record* 118, 199–204.

Wilson, D.J., Gröhn, Y.T., Bennett, G.J., González, R.N., Schukken, Y.H. and Spatz, J. (2007) Comparison of J5 vaccinates and controls for incidence, etiologic agent, clinical severity, and survival in the herd following naturally occurring cases of clinical mastitis. *Journal of Dairy Science* 90, 4282–4288.

Windig, J.J., Ouweltjes, W., ten Napel, J., de Jong, G., Veerkamp, R.F. and de Haas, Y. (2010) Combining somatic cell count traits for optimal selection against mastitis. *Journal of Dairy Science* 93, 1690–1701.

Zadoks, R.N., Gillespie, B.E., Barkema, H.W., Sampimon, O.C., Oliver, S.P. and Schukken, Y.H. (2003) Clinical, epidemiological and molecular characteristics of *Streptococcus uberis* infections in dairy herds. *Epidemiology and Infection* 130, 335–349.

# 6 Control of Lameness

Jon Huxley,[1] Simon Archer,[1] Nick Bell,[2] Mark Burnell,[3] Laura Green,[4]
Sarah Potterton[5] and Jon Reader[3]

[1]*School of Veterinary Medicine and Science, University of Nottingham, Sutton
Bonington, Leicestershire LE12 5RD, UK;* [2]*Royal Veterinary College, Hawkshead
Lane, North Mymms, Hatfield, Hertfordshire AL9 7TA, UK;* [3]*Synergy Farm
Health, West Hill Barns, Evershot, Dorset DT2 0LD, UK;* [4]*School of Life Sciences,
The University of Warwick, Coventry CV4 7AL, UK;* [5]*School of Biosciences, University
of Nottingham, Sutton Bonington, Leicestershire LE12 5RD, UK*

---

## Introduction

Lameness is a serious problem in many dairy herds worldwide. The condition has an impact on welfare, milk production and herd profitability. Many farm assurance schemes and milk-buying contracts require that farmers monitor lameness and have control programmes in place. Thus the control of lameness is an important area for the herd health advisor. Before we describe the key features of lameness and its control, it is worth considering what is 'normal': what is a healthy foot and normal locomotion in the dairy cow.

### Healthy feet and normal locomotion

In a well-managed herd with low levels of lameness, most cattle have healthy feet and limbs and walk with normal locomotion. Healthy feet are dry and clean and the hoof horn is hard with tightly packed horn tubules and good-quality inter-tubular horn. Ideally, hoof horn wears at the same rate that it grows and replaces weight-bearing horn as it is worn away.

When a cow takes a step the heel strikes the ground first; the soft, spongy horn in this area cushions the initial impact and the internal elastic, digital cushion acts as a shock absorber. As the claw rolls forward the rigid wall bears the weight of the animal while the sole horn reduces the jarring of the impact to higher joints by flexing (rather like a trampoline). From this description it is clear that the anatomy of a normally shaped claw is such that the wall is proud of the sole and the wall horn is of a quite different consistency (harder and less flexible) from the sole horn.

During movement, the cow's head carriage is low and relaxed and she scrutinizes the walking surface ahead, placing her front feet carefully to avoid obstacles. Strides are long and fluid and the hind feet are placed where the front feet were located (cattle cannot see their hind claw placement so this ensures that the risk of damage to hind claws is minimized). Weight bearing between left and right feet is even and the back is flat. When moving at their own pace, herds of cows walk in columns and follow one another closely. Over time, cattle form tracks when they walk the same route repeatedly, reducing the risk of stumbling and injury by clearing vegetation and debris and compacting the walking surface.

## Definition of lameness

Lameness is the clinical presentation of impaired locomotion (O'Callaghan, 2002). It is usually detected by observation of cows when walking, although mechanical sensors to detect lameness are under development and are used on a small number of farms. Locomotion is scored using a linear scale that is open to intra- and inter-observer variation (Channon *et al.*, 2009; see later section on monitoring).

The vast majority of lameness occurs in the hind feet (Murray *et al.*, 1996; Whay *et al.*, 1997, 1998) and is caused by claw lesions (~90%), with the remainder caused by limb lesions. There are many causes of foot lameness: sole ulcer, white line disease, digital dermatitis and interdigital necrobacillosis (foul-in-the-foot, interdigital phlegmon) are the most common causes globally, although the relative importance of each condition varies by management system and country.

## Incidence and prevalence of lameness

Lameness is an important disease in all developed dairy nations where animals are bred for high milk yields whether they are managed indoors, at pasture or a combination of both systems. For example, the incidence of lameness in UK dairy cows was reported at 70 cases per 100 cows per year during a study with the incentive of free veterinary treatment (Hedges *et al.*, 2001). During winter, the mean herd prevalence of lameness in UK dairy cows was estimated at 36.8% (range, 0–79.2)

based on data from 227 herds (Barker *et al.*, 2010). In contrast, the prevalence of lameness was estimated at 5.1% (0–33) for Swedish dairy herds (Manske *et al.*, 2002). In US studies, prevalence of lameness up to 21.1% in summer and 23.9% in winter were recorded (Cook, 2003), although a period prevalence of 65.3% over 13 months was reported in one study (Sprecher *et al.*, 1997).

## The impact of lameness

### *Farm economics*

The largest financial losses associated with lameness arise from infertility, culling and reduction in milk yield, although costs vary between country and in different economic climates. In addition to reduced milk yield, direct costs of lameness include treatment costs (medicines, depreciation on foot-trimming equipment and discarded milk from cows under treatment), herdsman's time and professional fees. Indirect costs, including the effect of lameness on infertility and culling, are harder to estimate. Depreciation costs associated with culling an average and a high-yielding cow were reported as £575 and £681, respectively, in UK dairy herds (Esslemont, 2003). Time also has an indirect opportunity cost because alternative uses are foregone – for example, time spent dealing with a lame cow may make less time available for preventive foot trimming of non-lame cows.

The costs of lameness in the UK have recently been reviewed (Willshire and Bell, 2009) and are illustrated in Fig. 6.1. Claw

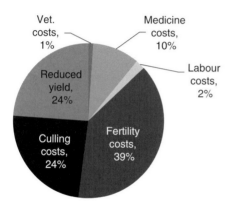
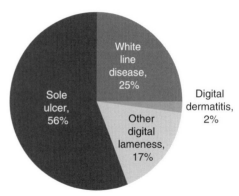

**Fig. 6.1.** Breakdown of lameness costs by category and lesion type in a typical UK herd (Willshire and Bell, 2009).

horn lesions lead to greater losses than other lesions, with sole ulcer resulting in the largest losses. In this example, the average cost of a case of lameness was £323, leading to a total cost for an average UK herd of approximately £7500 per year, £70 per cow or 1.0 pence per litre of milk. In contrast, partial budgeting models applied to Dutch data gave losses due to digital disease equivalent to £88 per year per lame cow or £19 per cow in the herd (Enting et al., 1997). Such numbers can be useful to highlight herd level losses to farmers, although are less useful for making decisions about individual cows. Costs associated with different foot lesions in cows of different parities and months of lactation have been estimated (Cha et al., 2010), and may be useful to inform decisions on treatment, breeding or replacement of lame cows.

### Milk yield

Lame cows produce less milk than if they had not become lame (Green et al., 2002; Amory et al., 2008; Archer et al., 2010a), and higher-yielding cows in a herd are more likely to become lame than their lower-yielding herd-mates. A consequence of this is that farmers might not realize that a lame cow is less productive because she might be yielding a similar volume of milk to non-lame cows in the herd. Milk yield falls before a cow is visibly lame (Reader et al., 2011) and remains low for some time after treatment. Total milk lost varies by lesion but, for example, approximately 600 kg per lactation is lost from a case of sole ulcer.

### Fertility

The link between lameness and infertility is unequivocal. Lame cows have reduced cyclicity (Garbarino et al., 2004) because of anoestrus (Hultgren et al., 2004) or cystic ovarian disease (Melendez et al., 2003) and, once cyclicity occurs, lame cows stand less frequently to be mounted compared with their sound herd-mates (Sood and Nanda, 2006). Lame cows that are served are less likely to conceive (Harman et al.,

1996; Hernandez et al., 2001; Hultgren et al., 2004), have a lower conception rate (Suriyasathaporn et al., 1998; Melendez et al., 2003), an increased risk of conception failure (Hernandez et al., 2005a) and require more services per pregnancy (Sprecher et al., 1997). Unsurprisingly, as a result, lame cows have long calving to first service intervals (Barkema et al., 1994; Sprecher et al., 1997), calving to conception intervals (Hernandez et al., 2001, 2005), numbers of days open (Argaez Rodriguez et al., 1997; Sprecher et al., 1997) and long calving intervals (Enting et al., 1997; Hultgren et al., 2004).

### Welfare

The very fact that cattle alter their gait indicates that lameness is painful. Cows with chronic claw horn disruption have raised levels of cortisol (Belge et al., 2004) and lame cows given local anaesthetic increase weight bearing on the affected leg (Rushen et al., 2007; Flower et al., 2008). Lesions of the claw horn and interdigital skin can lead to hyperalgesia (Whay et al., 1997, 1998), i.e. an increased sensitivity to pain. Lameness leads to a range of behavioural changes; lame cows are less active (O'Callaghan et al., 2003), have reduced total eating time, reduced numbers of meals per day and reduced dry matter intake (Bach et al., 2007), they lie down for longer and get up and down less frequently (Cook et al., 2004). Therefore, lameness is a major welfare issue for dairy cows.

## Heritability of lameness

Milk yield and lameness have a heritable component; however, it is possible to select for cows that both produce more milk and are less likely to become lame. The rate of increase in milk production per generation would reduce slightly if lameness was included in genetic selection. There are often insufficient records of lameness in data used for genetic evaluations and thus selection against lameness is often incomplete. Until this changes,

herds are likely to become even more susceptible to lameness. Unless herd level control is
developed to compensate for this increased
susceptibility, the deteriorating trend in lameness prevalence is likely to continue.

### Causes of foot lameness

The four most common lesions associated
with lameness are outlined in Fig. 6.2. The
reader is referred to other texts and papers
for further information in this area (e.g.
Blowey, 2008; Archer *et al.*, 2010b).
     Claw diseases can be categorized into
claw horn lesions comprising principally
sole ulcers (ranging from sole haemorrhage
through to complete ulcer formation) and
white line disease (encompassing white line
haemorrhage and white line separation),
and infectious diseases, namely digital dermatitis and interdigital necrobacillosis
(interdigital phlegmon or foul-in-the-foot).

#### Claw horn diseases

The aetiologies of sole and wall horn diseases (sole haemorrhage and ulcers, and
white line haemorrhage and separation) are
still not completely understood. The long-
standing proposed aetiology of subacute
ruminal acidosis leading to 'laminitis' has
proved difficult to substantiate in experimental research. Possible predisposing factors are dietary imbalance of vitamins such
as biotin (Hedges *et al.*, 2001), weakening of
collagen in the foot allowing increased
movement of the pedal bone (Tarlton *et al.*,
2002) and thinning of the digital cushion, a
fat pad that runs beneath the distal phalanx
(Räber *et al.*, 2004, 2006; Bicalho *et al.*,
2009). Once at risk, if the farm environment
causes increased trauma on the hoof capsule and the internal structures of the foot,
claw horn disease can result.
     Sole haemorrhage and ulcers are consid-
ered the result of contusions and damage to the
tissues lying under the distal phalanx. White
line haemorrhage and separation may have a
similar cause, although movement of the wall
during weight bearing may predispose to white
line separation. Herd-level control of these

lesions, therefore, revolves around controlling
the factors that increase the risk of contusions
under the distal phalanx; these are described
in detail in the later section on control. While
the aetiology of the various claw lesions is not
clear, some studies have identified management practices associated with an increased
prevalence of different types of claw horn
lesions (see section on control). However,
many of these have not been tested in rigorous
clinical trials to provide good evidence of
cause and effect.

#### Infectious claw diseases

Digital dermatitis is caused by bacteria,
a combination of *Treponema* spp. is implicated. The bacteria are in lesions on diseased feet (Carter *et al.*, 2009), and cow-
to-cow transmission via the environment is
likely to be the most important route of
infection. Disease is likely to enter a herd
following the purchase of infected cattle,
although transmission on fomites (e.g. claw-
trimming equipment) may also occur. Once
infection enters a herd it spreads rapidly.
The authors are not aware of any diseased
herds where digital dermatitis has been
completely eliminated once it has become
established.
     Interdigital necrobacillosis is caused
by *Fusobacterium necrophorum*, which is
present in cattle faeces and shed into the
environment. Other species of bacteria may
facilitate disease, although this is uncertain, and there is little doubt that disease
occurs more frequently when cattle stand
in faeces.
     Digital dermatitis is the more common
and important of these two infectious claw
diseases. Despite the differences between
them, broadly speaking a control programme
designed to control the risks associated with
digital dermatitis will be adequate to control interdigital necrobacillosis.

### Farmer attitudes to lameness

Farmers that manage lameness well generally
have empathy with the welfare of their cattle
and maintain high standards of physical

| Foot lesion | Description of lesion | Typical appearance |
|---|---|---|
| **White line disease,** also known as white line separation or white line haemorrhage | Diseased horn affecting the junction between the sole and wall, including bruising (haemorrhage), separation (fissuring) and the formation of abscesses | 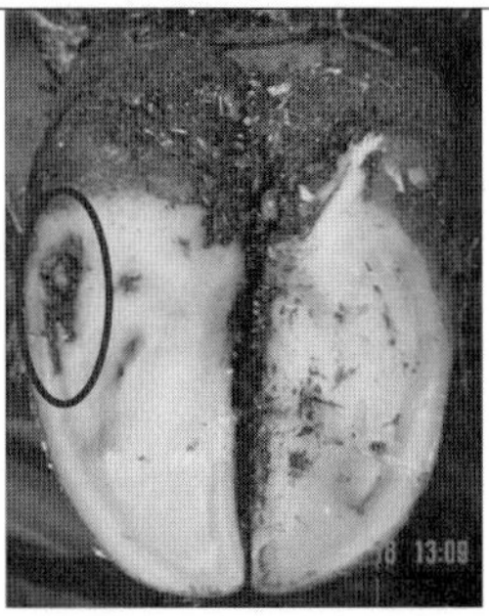 |
| **Sole ulcer,** also known as pododermatitis circumscripta or Rusterholz disease | Exposed corium at the site below the flexor process of the pedal bone | 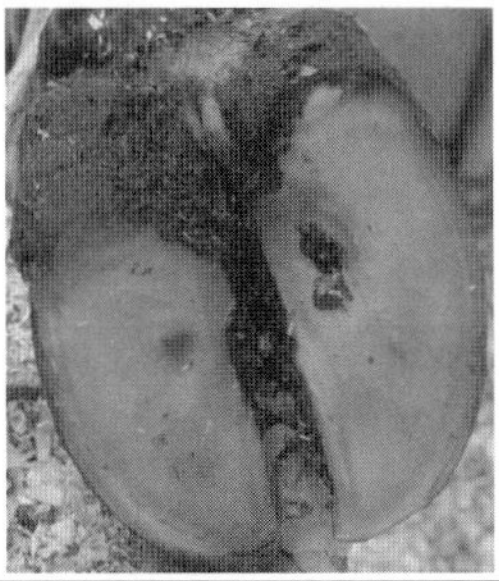 |
| **Digital dermatitis,** also known as hairy heel warts or Mortellaro disease | A well-circumscribed infection of the skin, often between the heel bulbs or palmar/plantar pastern area. Lesions usually start as exudative epithelial erosions/ulceration, progressing to granulation, followed by hyperkeratosis and scab formation | 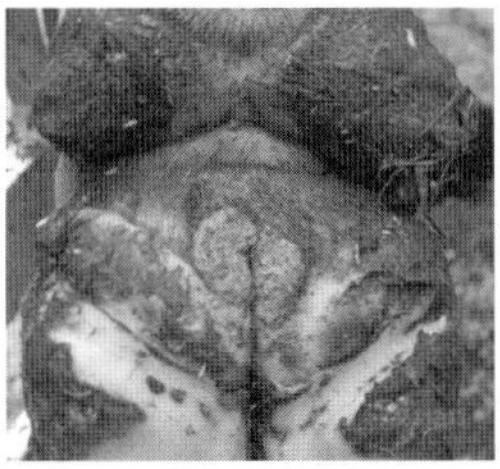 |
| **Interdigital necrobacillosis,** also known as foul-in-the-foot, foot rot, foul or interdigital phlegmon | An acute bacterial infection of the subcutaneous tissues of the interdigital space characterized by symmetrical swelling, separation of the claws and interdigital skin necrosis, with a pungent odour | 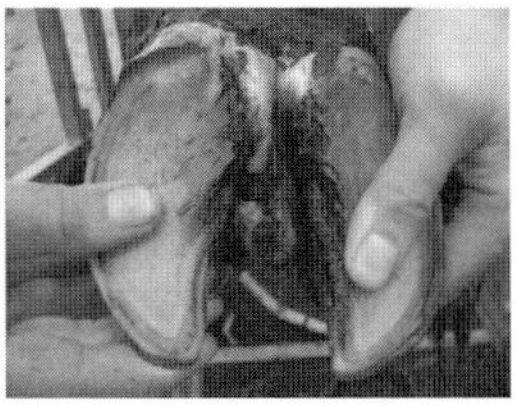 |

**Fig. 6.2.** Common causes of lameness in cattle.

comfort for their cows with low stocking densities, clean, soft bedding (straw or sand), generous nutrition that keeps cows in good body condition, good routine foot care and rapid treatment of lame cows. Cows in such herds are often contented and have short flight distances.

There are, however, many farms where the prevalence and incidence of lameness is high and it is worth considering why this occurs. We know that many farmers are not able to recognize lameness, or become tolerant to the levels of lameness in their herd. In addition, farmers might assume that the level of lameness in their herd is normal because it is consistent (untreated cows often remain lame for a considerable time) and similar to that of other herds they know (this is termed a 'social norm' – see Chapter 2). On most farms several people including foot trimmers, herdsmen, farmers and veterinarians are involved in the management of foot health and lame cows, and this might result in no single person feeling responsible or sufficiently powerful to implement a control programme. Finally, unlike mastitis and infertility, from the farmer's viewpoint, lameness does not overtly impact on farm economics – lame cows continue to produce milk. In these herds farmers are often very busy and attending to lame cows is low down in a long list of things to do. Motivation to improve lameness may not always be financial, however, and cannot necessarily be valued in financial terms (e.g. farmers' pride in a healthy herd (Leach *et al.*, 2010b)). Overall, many dairy farmers find it difficult to accurately estimate the prevalence of lameness in their herds; when compared with an independent observer using a scoring system, farmers do not appear to assess accurately which of their own cows are lame (Mill and Ward, 1994; Whay *et al.*, 2003; Leach *et al.*, 2010a).

## Evaluating and Monitoring Lameness

### The importance of good farm records

Historically, lameness has been monitored and recorded poorly on many farms in com-

parison with mastitis and fertility. This may in part explain why lameness control has lagged behind that of other endemic diseases. Access to good-quality data is a vital first step in monitoring and controlling lameness. At a minimum, the herd health advisor will require access to treatment records and routine herd locomotion (mobility) score data. Treatment records can be used to estimate the incidence and causes of lameness (and therefore assist with risk factor control, see section 'Control of lameness') and the success of treatment. Locomotion score data can be used to estimate the prevalence of lameness, to identify animals for treatment and to measure the success of control programmes over time.

Currently, much recording is performed as a consequence of the requirements of industry assurance schemes. Many farmers in the UK only record a case of lameness when antibiotic is used (although this may not include cases of digital dermatitis treated topically). Lame cows treated solely by trimming may go unrecorded, although this has improved in recent years as a consequence of the increased use of professional foot trimmers, who record such data.

Consequently, on many farms existing lameness records should be interpreted with caution and one of the first roles of the advisor is to initiate a reliable, structured, standardized system of data recording. A suitable recording system on farm includes:

- Regular herd locomotion scoring using a recognized and repeatable system carried out by a trained operator.
- Data from treatment of lame cows, to include at least cow identity, date of examination, affected claw, diagnosis (correct identification of primary lesion(s) ideally with all secondary lesions included) and treatment given. More precise data on lesion location and/or an assessment of lesion severity are secondary requirements.
- Data on lesions observed during routine trimming of non-lame cows. These should be kept separately to the data from treatment of lame cows.

## Setting up a locomotion scoring system on the farm

The first step in setting up a recording system is to ensure that all those involved in the detection of lame cows use the same definition. Farmers and farm staff should be trained in a system to score the locomotion of each cow in the herd. Many locomotion scoring systems have been described; the two most commonly used are those of (i) Sprecher *et al.* (1997; Table 6.1), who proposed a five-point scale from not lame through to barely able to stand; and (ii) Whay *et al.* (1997, 2003), who proposed a four-point scale that has been accepted as the industry standard in the UK (and is often referred to as the DairyCo Mobility Score, see Fig. 6.3). For routine on-farm monitoring we recommend the four-point scale for its simplicity and versatility; consequently, the DairyCo Mobility Scoring system will be used throughout this chapter. In this system, cows with a score of 2 or 3 are defined as lame and cows with a score of 0 or 1 are not lame. It is essential that scorers are trained initially and then undergo refresher sessions with other operators to ensure consistency. While initially locomotion scoring can be perceived negatively by farmers, particularly for those who have not spent time observing cows walk, the majority of clients find the process useful once they have learned the technique.

A single trained observer should perform all assessments on a unit because inter-observer differences in scoring can occur. Any member of farm staff can be trained; in many cases it is good to use someone who does not have daily contact with the cows because they are more detached and will not be biased by knowing particular cows, although they might have more difficulty identifying individuals. The observer should position themselves to avoid affecting cow flow. Cows should be observed from the side and the rear.

When carrying out mobility scoring, cattle should be observed on a flat, hard, non-slip surface with no impediments to cow flow for a minimum of four uninterrupted strides. On most farms cows can be scored after they exit the milking parlour. If this is not practical (e.g. in automated milking systems) the whole herd can be walked past the observer in a steady and controlled manner. It is recommended that cows are scored in a wide passage where flow is uninhibited, to limit bunching and shadowing which can make identification and scoring difficult. Animals should be scored on a day when no other management procedures are taking place that might interfere with either cow flow or the score (e.g. foot bathing).

Data collected from each cow should include its unique identification, a mobility score, the identity of the lame leg(s) and any other pertinent information (e.g. any indication that the lameness is not caused by a foot lesion; a suspicion of bilateral lameness). It is also possible to collect other useful information (e.g. body condition score) at the same time, providing this does not interfere with the primary objective. Scores can be entered on to a paper recording sheet, a PDA, a ruggedized laptop or spoken into a

**Table 6.1.** The mobility scoring system described by Sprecher *et al.* (1997).

| Score | Description |
|---|---|
| 1 | Stands and walks with a level back posture; gait is normal |
| 2 | Stands with level back but arched back when walking; gait is normal |
| 3 | Arches back when walking and standing; gait is affected |
| 4 | Arched back posture always evident; gait shows deliberate steps |
| 5 | Inability or extreme reluctance to bear weight on one or more limbs |

Many other scoring systems have been described; see also Manson and Leaver (1988a, a nine-point scale); Tranter and Morris (1991, a five-point scale); Wells *et al.* (1993, a five-point scale); Winckler and Willen (2001, a five-point scale); and Cook (2003, a four-point scale).

# DairyCo Mobility Score

| Category of score | Score | Description of cow behaviour | Suggested action |
|---|---|---|---|
| **Good mobility** | 0 | Walks with even weight bearing and rhythm on all four feet, with a flat back<br><br>Long, fluid strides possible | • no action needed;<br>• routine (preventive) foot trimming when/if required; and<br>• record mobility at next scoring session |
| **Imperfect mobility** | 1 | Steps uneven (rhythm or weight bearing) or strides shortened; affected limb or limbs not immediately identifiable | • could benefit from routine (preventive) foot trimming when/if required; and<br>• further observation recommended |
| **Impaired mobility** | 2 | Uneven weight bearing on a limb that is immediately identifiable and/or obviously shortened strides (usually with an arch to the centre of the back) | • lame and likely to benefit from treatment;<br>• foot should be lifted to establish the cause of lameness before treatment; and<br>• should be attended to as soon as practically possible |
| **Severely impaired mobility** | 3 | Unable to walk as fast as a brisk human pace (cannot keep up with the healthy herd) and signs of score 2 | • very lame;<br>• cow will benefit from treatment;<br>• cow requires urgent attention, nursing and further professional advice;<br>• cow should not be made to walk far and kept on a straw yard or at grass; and<br>• in the most severe cases, culling may be the only possible solution |

**Fig. 6.3.** The DairyCo Mobility Score (www.dairyco.net/library/farming-info-centre/health-welfare/mobility-score-instructions.aspx).

dictaphone. The herd should be scored at least monthly and ideally every two weeks, especially if scoring is the primary method used to identify lame animals in need of treatment. Importantly, once lame cows have been identified, they should be examined, diagnosed and treated as soon as possible.

### Recognizing foot lesions

One of the key roles of the herd health advisor is to provide training on the correct identification of lesions and ongoing motivation for data recording (Table 6.2 and Fig. 6.4). Digital cameras or mobile phones can be used to photograph lesions that farmers are unsure of and sent to the veterinarian for discussion. Sole ulcer, sole haemorrhage, white line haemorrhage, white line separation, digital dermatitis, interdigital necrobacillosis, interdigital hyperplasia and heel horn erosion are the lesions that are a minimum for farmers to recognise and record.

Extension of training to less common lesions can be used to maintain the interest of experienced operators. Identifying the cause of lameness is sometimes complicated. Not all lesions cause lameness and lame cows often have more than one type of lesion. Researchers have reported that sole ulcer and interdigital phlegmon, when present (Manske *et al.*, 2002; Tadich *et al.*, 2010) are likely to be the cause of lameness while white line separation and digital dermatitis can be highly prevalent in non-lame cows. It is best to encourage farmers to record all lesions with a probable cause of lameness (i.e. what they consider to be the primary lesion), and the mobility score of the cow. As stated previously, the reason for

the examination should be recorded so that lesion data from lame and non-lame cows can be analysed separately.

While accurate lesion identification alone is adequate for most purposes, the addition of an indication of the severity of lesions can help to assess response to treatment and give an indication of the relative importance of different lesions to both the individual animal and the herd lameness profile. To date, most lesion scoring systems have been used for research purposes but they are increasingly being used on the farm, particularly by professional hoof trimmers. Digital dermatitis is perhaps the easiest and most important lesion to grade; the use of the system described by Dopfer *et al.* (1997, Table 6.2) should be encouraged as recent work has suggested that, within endemically infected herds, M4.1 lesions (chronic with a subacute component; Fig. 6.4) may be important in driving infection.

### Methods of recording locomotion and lesions

Historically, lameness recording has generally been in paper format (Fig. 6.5) and this remains the preferred method for many farmers and foot trimmers. The lesion(s) are recorded alongside the appropriate foot (Fig. 6.5). More recently, there has been a trend towards computerized recording with hardware and software available that allow cow-side recording on to a PDA or ruggedized laptop. To optimize speed and decision making, paper records should be entered into standard herd data software for further analysis. Data from electronic recording systems can be analysed *in situ*

**Table 6.2.** A lesion recording system for digital dermatitis (Dopfer *et al.*, 1997).

| | |
|---|---|
| M1 | Small (2 cm), circumscribed red or grey erosion (focal bacterial keratolysis) |
| M2 | Acute ulcerative or granulomatous lesion |
| M3 | Healing scab |
| M4 | Chronic dyskeratotic or proliferative lesion |
| M4.1 | Chronic with subacute component |

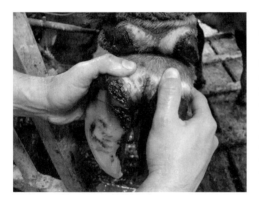

**Fig. 6.4.** Digital dermatitis score M4.1 (chronic with subacute component; Dopfer *et al.*, 1997).

giving virtually instantaneous results, or exported and incorporated directly into other software programs. Whatever system is used to record lesions, the most important issue is that the data are analysed and used. Too often foot trimming and mobility recording sheets are left 'floating' in the farm office and are never used again. This is a waste of a valuable resource.

### Practical use of lameness data

#### *Overview of herd lameness*

When the herd health advisor starts working with a dairy farmer to facilitate the control of lameness on farm there are three key pieces of information required to begin the process:

**1.** The current prevalence and incidence of lameness in the herd.
**2.** The lesions that are the major causes of lameness in the herd.
**3.** The animals that need immediate treatment.

Regular, consistent locomotion scoring of all the cows in the herd allows the farmer to create an action list of lame cows for treatment and to conduct important analyses. Basic herd analysis should include monitoring the prevalence of clinical lameness over time, with further analysis of mobility scores to examine patterns in management groups, by days in milk and parity (see below). Between-herd analyses allows benchmarking

against other farms (e.g. farms within a veterinary practice or buying group; Fig. 6.6). Benchmarking in this way can help motivate change and demonstrate what is achieved on other units. When benchmarking mobility data between farms, it is important to consider the groups of cows that have been assessed to ensure that comparisons are fair. Most farms score the entire milking herd, but this should also include dry cows and the 'sick pen' cows, which often includes convalescent lame cows.

After collection of a herd locomotion score, one of the following indices should be calculated:

- Mobility index = number cows not lame/number in herd.
- Lameness score = number of cows lame/number in herd (Bell and Huxley, 2009a).

Clearly these two indices are related, but some farmers prefer mobility index as it has more positive connotations (i.e. the proportion not lame rather than the proportion lame). Either can be used providing the terminology is correct, especially if comparisons are made between farms.

#### *Calculation of further lameness indices*

More information about the underlying reasons for lameness on a dairy unit can be obtained from a more detailed analysis of lameness data, particularly the estimation of incidence rates of lameness at different times and in different groups of cows. Incidence rate is the number of new cases of lameness in a group of individuals at risk over a specified time period, and is usually expressed as cases per 100 cows per year. Lameness incidence rates can be calculated either using data from cows individually identified and treated, or from sequential herd mobility scoring. These two methods are described below.

ANALYSIS OF DATA FROM COWS TREATED FOR LAMENESS. The incidence rate of lameness cases can be calculated on a monthly, rolling three-monthly or rolling annual basis. The incidence rate of lameness should be evaluated for different

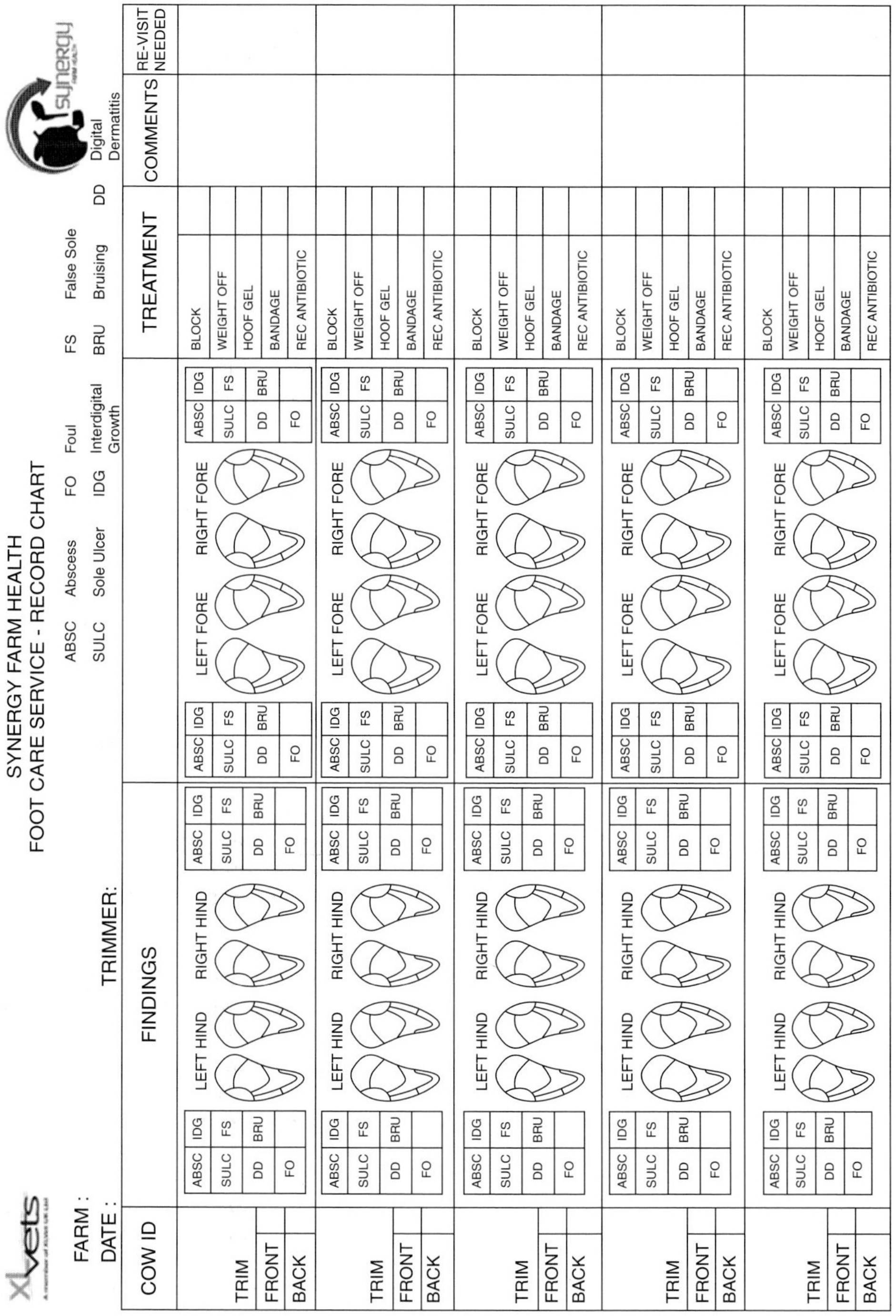
XLvets
SYNERGY FARM HEALTH
FOOT CARE SERVICE - RECORD CHART
synergy
FARM :
DATE :
TRIMMER:
ABSC Abscess
SULC Sole Ulcer
FO Foul
IDG Interdigital Growth
FS False Sole
BRU Bruising
DD Digital Dermatitis
COW ID
FINDINGS
TREATMENT
COMMENTS
RE-VISIT NEEDED
TRIM
FRONT
BACK
LEFT HIND
RIGHT HIND
LEFT FORE
RIGHT FORE
ABSC IDG
SULC FS
DD BRU
FO
BLOCK
WEIGHT OFF
HOOF GEL
BANDAGE
REC ANTIBIOTIC

**Fig. 6.5.** An example of a paper-based lameness recording sheet.

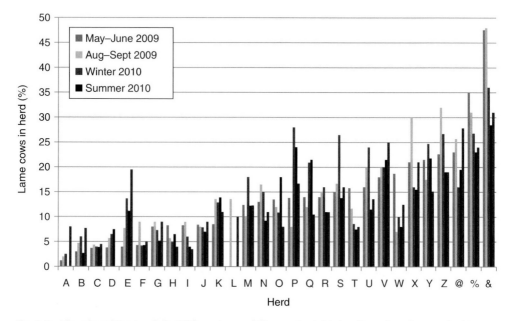

**Fig. 6.6.** A benchmarking graph for 29 farms in a mobility-scoring initiative. Farms have been ranked to allow anonymous comparisons to be made among them (bars indicate the herd lameness score (proportion of lame animals)).

stages of lactation, for cows of different parity, in different groups of cows within the herd, at different times of the year (or at times associated with specific management changes such as turnout) and for different lesion types and severities. The incidence rates of first cases of lameness during a lactation should be analysed separately from all cases (i.e. those including recurrent cases). Rates of recurrence following treatment of different types of lesion should also be evaluated.

ANALYSIS OF DATA FROM MOBILITY SCORES. The regular collection of mobility score data allows a range of month-to-month analyses (in a similar way that SCC data are used – see Chapter 5) to provide trends in lameness over time. Locomotion scores are used to classify cows as 'Not lame' and 'Lame' ('Not lame' = scores 0 and 1 and 'Lame' = scores 2 and 3 using the DairyCo system), and then cows are categorized into one of four groups, based on scores in consecutive assessments:

- 'Not lame' (not lame at both scores);
- 'New case' (moving from non-lame to lame);

- 'Recovered case' (moving from lame to non-lame); and
- 'Chronic case' (lame at both scores).

Using these categories, mobility score changes can be used to estimate an incidence rate of lameness (i.e. cows that move into the lame category as a proportion of those in the non-lame category at the previous mobility score recording). This estimated incidence rate of lameness can be assessed over a two-weekly, monthly, or three-monthly period (depending on the frequency of scoring) and evaluated for different groups of cows and for different times of the year, as described for data from treated cases of lameness (see above).

A net lameness index (NLI) can also be calculated for mobility scores (Archer *et al.*, 2009), similar to the net transmission index in mastitis analysis, by dividing the number of new cases by the number of recovered cases. NLI values < 1 indicate an improvement in lameness while an NLI > 1 indicates deterioration. Interpretation of mobility score data requires a degree of caution, however, because of its relatively dynamic nature (compared with SCC data, for example). On some farms, cows on the borderline frequently move between non-lame and lame categories and thus indices such as NLI can fluctuate.

### Practical limitations of evaluating lameness data

If the goal is to monitor and reduce the number of new cases of lameness, then the incidence rate is generally a more useful measure than prevalence. Importantly however, poor lameness detection can affect estimates of the incidence rate in the following ways:

- reduction in the number of new cases identified (numerator) due to the poor sensitivity of diagnosis; and
- increase in the denominator because some lame cows are incorrectly included in the population at risk.

Therefore, poor-quality clinical records will result in a significant underestimation of the true lameness situation in the herd. The denominator is often approximated to the number of cows in the herd, but this simplification is only appropriate if lameness prevalence is low and cases do not become chronic. Practically speaking, this means that one of the ways for a farm to have a low recorded incidence of lameness is to be poor at identifying lame cows and to treat what cases they do identify ineffectively! Therefore, incidence rates should be calculated and used with great care and should never be used to benchmark or draw conclusions about lameness in a herd unless strict supervision of recording is undertaken.

The relative difficulty of generating good-quality incidence data and the relative ease of measuring the prevalence of lameness in herds using mobility scoring have led to the latter being the method commonly used to monitor lameness. While this is a pragmatic solution to a less than ideal situation, it is vital that the herd health advisor appreciates the difficulties of using lameness prevalence data alone so that incorrect conclusions are not drawn. For example, a herd with a relatively high prevalence of lameness may be in any one of a range of situations; to

illustrate this, three points on this spectrum are outlined below.

- High incidence with rapid resolution of lameness: new cases occur all the time but animals recover quickly. The high prevalence is driven by new cases (e.g. a herd in which digital dermatitis is the predominant cause of lameness).
- Low incidence with prolonged recovery: new cases are infrequent but when they do occur animals remain lame for long periods. The high prevalence is driven by chronic cases (e.g. a herd in which sole ulcers are the predominant cause of lameness).
- Medium incidence with variable resolution of lameness: the high prevalence is driven by a combination of some new cases and other cases becoming chronic (e.g. a herd where lameness is caused by a range of diseases).

Similarly and importantly, a herd with a low prevalence of lameness can have a relatively high incidence rate of new lameness cases, but of short duration. In this case monitoring prevalence will not identify the herd problem and thus can be misleading in terms of the overall lameness picture.

In conclusion, to quantify and monitor lameness in a herd, complete records of clinical cases (including treatments), regular mobility scores and lesions identified at routine foot trimming are all important. Data need careful interpretation based on a thorough understanding of how they have been collected, but analysis of the data provides a useful insight into the main causes of lameness on a unit and areas to target control measures (see later section on control of lameness).

### Lameness targets

National and transnational organizations have been quick to put targets on levels of lameness that are 'acceptable'; however, these can often be ambiguous. For example, the European Food Safety Authority (EFSA, 2009) highlighted among its recommendations that 'there should be systems for monitoring the prevalence of lameness by scoring locomotion and foot lesions every 3 to 6 months in all dairy herds'. It goes on to say that the intervention level should be 10%. However, there is no explanation of what this means and to which scoring system it relates.

Key indices and targets recommended for lameness control are outlined in Table 6.3; all targets set by the advisor should be 'SMART' (farm-specific, measurable, attainable, realistic and time-based) and therefore these will need adjusting for individual herds over time. To put these target levels in context, recent results from a large sample of UK farms reported a median herd prevalence of DairyCo mobility score 2 and 3 cows as 32.7% (range 0–48%) and 3.3% (range 0–31.2%) respectively. Thus, on the average farm, 36% of cows were lame (score 2 or 3) on the day they were assessed. The top 25% of farms had a prevalence of lameness (scores 2 and 3) of ≤22%.

### The future of monitoring lameness in dairy herds

Locomotion scoring is time consuming, can only be performed by trained operators and even then has large inter-observer variability (which makes comparisons between farms difficult). A number of automated methods for detection of lameness are under development. Lame animals alter their weight distribution and force plates and sensor platforms that measure the rate of limb placement are available (Rajkondawar *et al.*, 2006). Kinematic gait analysis (the study of motion) also shows potential as a tool to monitor lameness. Whilst differences in stride length, foot height and the speed of various stride phases can be identified between lame and sound cows, automated systems for on-farm use are still under development. Finally, both walking speed and behaviour (e.g. increased lying times) have been suggested as indirect indicators of lameness. While it is unlikely that these methods will ever be sufficiently sensitive or specific in their own right, it may become possible to remotely monitor levels of activity and/or types of behaviour and to use these as an indicator of cows likely to be or to become lame and therefore in need of examination.

**Table 6.3.** Outline of targets to evaluate herd lameness.

| Index | Description | Target |
| --- | --- | --- |
| Incidence rate of lameness for treated cases (i.e. calculated from cows treated for lameness) | Cases/100 cows at risk/year (equivalent rate is applicable when used on a monthly or three-monthly basis) | <10–20[a] |
| Recurrence rate of lameness for treated cases (i.e. calculated from cows treated for lameness) | Percentage of cows treated for lameness in which the lameness recurs in a six-month period | <25 |
| Lameness index (calculated from mobility score data at a herd recording) | Percentage lame (scores 2 and 3) Percentage severely lame (score 3) | <10–15 <1–2 |
| Monthly incidence rate of lameness defined by mobility score (calculated from mobility score data at consecutive two-weekly or monthly herd recordings) | Cows moving into a lame category as a percentage of those in the non-lame category at the previous recording | <1–5 |
| Monthly recovery rate of lameness defined by mobility score (calculated from mobility score data at consecutive two-weekly or monthly herd recordings) | Cows moving into a non-lame category as a percentage of those in the lame category at the previous recording | >75 |
| Frequency of mobility scoring | | 2–4-weekly |
| Time between identification and treatment of lame cows (h) | Lame (score 2) Severely lame (score 3) | Maximum 48 Maximum 24 |

[a] Relevant only if complete recording takes place; see text for further details.

## Summary

One of the key roles for the herd health advisor is to institute a reliable, structured and standardized system of recording lameness data on the farm. This may include working with clients to develop suitable processes, training and ongoing motivation for farm staff and demonstrating value by using data to illustrate trends and generate key performance indicators that can be used to monitor lameness in the herd.

Ideally, once all data have been collected and recorded accurately, a period of time (e.g. 6–12 months) would elapse before a herd-level lameness control programme was instituted using the accurate and complete data as a starting point. In reality, control programmes almost invariably begin alongside, not after, improved data recording because of the necessity to begin reducing the levels of lameness in the herd. In this situation the authors recommend the following approach to investigation of the current situation on the farm.

- Locomotion score the entire herd and institute routine locomotion scoring by a trained member of staff.
- Analyse foot trimming data to identify commonly reported lesions.
- Analyse farm clinical lameness (treatment) records to identify commonly reported lesions.
- Ask farmers and farm staff to point out lesions they commonly see on a photographic foot lesions atlas (this can help avoid incorrect diagnosis or inappropriate nomenclature).
- Institute a reliable, structured and standardized system of recording lameness data (as described above).

## Control of Lameness

Lameness is not a single disease, rather it is a presenting sign for a wide range of conditions. While the majority of lameness is caused by four different conditions of the foot (sole haemorrhage/ulcers, white line disease, digital dermatitis and, to a lesser extent, interdigital necrobacillosis), other causes exist. Importantly, our understanding of these four common conditions is far from complete; for example, the aetiology of claw horn lesions, sole ulcers and white line disease is still not established. Furthermore, the impact of herd-level lameness control has proved difficult to demonstrate.

There are several reasons why lameness control measures are not yet clearly established. First, many of the suggested herd-level interventions are complicated or expensive to implement and this makes a 'trial and error' approach difficult in practice. Secondly, since claw horn lesions take many months to develop (it is increasingly recognized that the feet can become irretrievably damaged in the first lactation) evaluation of the cause and effect of interventions is difficult. Therefore, even if appropriate management changes are made, it may take many months or years before levels of lameness are reduced by identifiable amounts. There is, however, increasing evidence from both research and clinical observation that herd-level lameness control programmes can deliver real and sustained reductions in lameness on commercial farms. A herd example is shown in Fig. 6.7, in which lameness prevalence was reduced from nearly 60% to under 20% in the first 18 months of an ongoing control programme, based on the principles outlined later in this section.

Despite the fact that there are few controlled trials showing cause and effect of interventions to reduce lameness, there is broad agreement on likely factors to decrease the incidence of lameness. Generally speaking, control measures for sole haemorrhage/ulcers and white line disease are related and, similarly, measures designed to control digital dermatitis will also control interdigital necrobacillosis. Therefore, we divide farm control strategies into two broad categories, those designed to control claw horn disease (comprising sole haemorrhage/ulcers and white line haemorrhage and separation; Table 6.4) and those designed to control infectious disease (digital dermatitis and interdigital necrobacillosis; Table 6.5). If claw horn disease predominates, control measures should be concentrated in this area and vice versa.

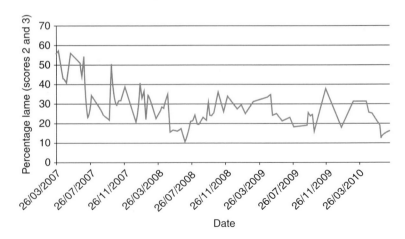

**Fig. 6.7.** Mobility score data from one farm engaged in a lameness control programme.

**Table 6.4.** Categories and examples of specific risks associated with claw horn disease.

| General category of risk | Examples of specific risks that can be addressed in control programmes |
|---|---|
| Prolonged standing on hard surfaces (e.g. concrete/slats) | Poor cubicle comfort or inadequate numbers of cubicles (leading to decreased lying time) <br> Prolonged standing in the collecting yard before milking <br> Inadequate feed space <br> Heifers not trained to use cubicles before they calve |
| Poor-quality standing and walking surfaces | Areas of broken or rough/abrasive concrete in yards and walkways <br> Presence of loose stones and debris in the environment <br> Poor-quality/inappropriate tracks to pasture |
| Concussive and shearing forces (e.g. turning sharply on concrete) | Poor building design leading to poor cow flow (e.g. bottlenecks and dead-ends causing pushing and bullying) <br> Forcing animals (e.g. with a quad bike, goad or dog) <br> Sharp turns on concrete (e.g. at the parlour exit) <br> Unnecessary mixing or changing of groups causing aggressive interactions and bullying |
| Foot conformation and claw function | Claw horn overgrowth <br> Excessive wear from abrasive walking surfaces causing thin soles <br> Inappropriate or excessive trimming causing poor conformation or thin soles |
| Poor-quality, less resilient claw horn | Dirty, wet environment softening horn as water is absorbed <br> Walking on abrasive surfaces causing excessive wear <br> Inadequate nutrition, particularly vitamin and mineral supply |
| Inadequate digital cushion function | Excessive body condition score loss in early lactation[a] |
| Peri-parturient loss of strength in claw support structures | Recently calved cows in a high-risk environment[a] |

[a] Recent research has suggested this may be a key area of risk; however, more information is required before these risks can be considered definitive.

**Table 6.5.** Categories and examples of specific risks associated with infectious foot disease.

| General category of risk | Examples of specific risks that can be addressed in control programmes |
|---|---|
| Environmental hygiene | Inadequate slurry management – cows standing in slurry for prolonged periods |
| | Wet, unhygienic conditions due to inadequate cleaning, ventilation and poor building design |
| | Rough underfoot conditions increasing the risk of damage to the interdigital space and increasing the risk of interdigital necrobacillosis |
| | Overstocked housing |
| | Poorly maintained yards, tracks and walkways leading to pooling of water and slurry |
| Poor foot conformation and claw function | Inadequate trimming leading to claw overgrowth |
| Reservoir of infection | Clinical cases of dermatitis left untreated (presence of M4.1 lesions; see Table 6.2 and Fig. 6.4). |
| | Inadequate, inappropriate or ineffective foot bathing protocols leaving subclinical cases of dermatitis untreated |
| | Inadequate preventive measures in dry cows and heifers |
| Biosecurity | Inadequate biosecurity protocols increasing the chance of digital dermatitis entering a disease-free herd |
| | Inadequate biosecurity increasing the chance of more pathogenic biotypes entering already infected herds |
| | Unnecessary mixing or changing of groups promoting transmission of disease between animals |

A lameness control programme is made up of four broad steps:

**1.** Evaluate and monitor the disease situation on the farm (described in the previous section) to identify the predominant cause(s) of lameness.
**2.** Categorize the cause(s) as either claw horn disease, infectious causes or both.
**3.** Identify key risks present on the farm for the identified cause(s).
**4.** Facilitate the implementation of appropriate management changes to reduce or eliminate the hazards identified.

Where good-quality lesion data are already available, risk assessment and control measures can focus on those areas most likely to lead to a reduction for that disease(s). On the majority of farms engaging in control programmes for the first time, these data can take time to generate. In this situation we recommend initially concentrating on generic measures such as early and effective treatment of clinical cases or assuming that all predominant lesions types are present (a reasonably safe assumption on most units, and which can be validated

further by examining a random selection of 10–15 lame cows). If this assumption is made it is vital that lesion-specific control measures requiring substantial effort or investment are delayed until accurate lesion data become available, at which point the control programme can be reassessed.

The following section concentrates on some of the key risk areas and suggests practical methods of addressing them. Lameness control requires an understanding of many different aspects of dairy farm construction, engineering and management including building and cubicle design. Some of these areas are large subjects in their own right and consequently we highlight and discuss the key principles. Where necessary, we refer the reader to comprehensive sources for further information.

### Treatment of clinical cases

Early and effective treatment of lame cows is an important component of any proactive lameness control programme; in two UK studies, delayed treatment was a management factor associated with higher levels of lameness (Bell *et al.*, 2009; Barker *et al.*, 2010) and another study demonstrated that animals that are lame in the first lactation are more likely to become lame in subsequent lactations (Hirst *et al.*, 2002). Early and accurate identification and effective treatment reduce the prevalence of lameness directly by shortening the length of time an animal is lame. This is also likely to lead to a reduction in the incidence of future lameness by reducing the number of repeat cases (if permanent damage to hoof structures is avoided).

In developed dairy nations, the veterinarian is now less involved in the day-to-day treatment of lame cows. This role is increasingly undertaken by paraprofessional cattle foot trimmers or designated farm staff. The role of the veterinarian is becoming, and should be seen as, one of working with farm management to oversee the appropriate treatment as well as prevention of lame cows. This role has a number of facets, including (i) training and guidance on treatment; (ii) treatment of unresponsive and difficult individual cases; (iii) collation and analysis of lesion-specific incidence to direct and support other herd-level interventions; and (iv) motivating/mentoring staff with responsibility in this area.

Training staff to treat lame cows appropriately is a key role. Often farm staff have received no formal training or have been taught 'on the job' by other staff members. Consequently, in some situations, treatment can be inappropriate or, in the worst cases, damaging. Running training courses for farm staff builds the working relationship between farm staff and the veterinarian and is an excellent first step in developing on-farm lameness control programmes. Following appropriate training on the diagnosis and treatment of lameness, the veterinary practitioner can work with farm staff to develop standard recording and treatment protocols and develop a route for referral back to the veterinarian for more complicated cases and those that fail to respond to treatment. Mentoring and overseeing of treatment should also include ensuring that farm staff have the appropriate facilities and equipment

to treat lame cows efficiently and effectively, and providing positive feedback and encouragement to maintain enthusiasm.

Where treatment of lame cows is conducted by a paraprofessional hoof trimmer, the veterinarian should ensure the use of fully trained and accredited personnel (for example, in the UK, fully licensed 1 trimmers as accredited by the National Association of Cattle Foot Trimmers) and work with the paraprofessional to integrate their data into the farm's lameness control programme and again establish a referral route back to the veterinarian for difficult and unresponsive cases.

While description of the treatment of individual lesions and individual lame cows is outwith the remit of this book, it is worth noting that various reference texts describe a variety of different treatment options, particularly for sole ulcers and white line disease. Despite their duration of use and the number of animals these protocols have been used to treat, the research literature underpinning effective treatment options for these diseases is sparse. That is not to say that current treatment protocols are ineffective, rather that they have not been rigorously evaluated and compared to identify the most efficacious regimes.

In summary, lameness is a complex and challenging issue and one where the evidence for treatment and prevention is far from complete. Despite this, much can be done to reduce the prevalence of lameness and this includes attending to lame cows as soon as possible. We recommend that severely lame cows (DairyCo mobility score 3) are treated as soon as they are identified and lame cows (DairyCo mobility score 2) within 2 days. The most successful farms maintain regular mobility scoring (every 14 days) and treat all lame cows as they are identified (Fig. 6.8). A combination of early detection and effective treatment may have a number of benefits to the cow, herd and farm. The early stages of foot disease are usually easier to treat, respond more quickly and fully to treatment (better cure rates) and are less likely to recur. Consequently, treatment interventions are likely to reduce lameness severity, duration and prevalence. However,

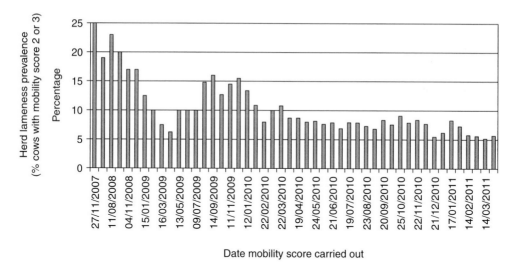

**Fig. 6.8.** Reduction in prevalence of lameness in a herd where regular scoring and immediate action were instituted. Cows are scored on a 2-weekly basis, with all lame cows being presented to the foot trimmer on the following day.

if foot trimming and treatment are carried out inadequately, then early intervention can potentially have the opposite effect.

### Routine foot trimming

In situations where claw overgrowth, foot imbalance (mediolateral claw imbalance) or lameness are not a problem, foot trimming is unnecessary. Foot trimming may be described as preventive, corrective or a combination of the two (although routine foot trimming should not be an alternative to the prompt treatment of lame cows). The most widely accepted method of cattle foot trimming is the Dutch five-step method (Toussaint Raven, 1985), with some minor refinements. This five-step procedure requires that functional shape is restored before corrective measures are started. Lesions to be treated are carefully prioritized and individualized to the cow, which requires some degree of experience and mentoring to allow effective interpretation of the simple rules. Certain parts of the claws are not trimmed to ensure that cows without problems are not compromised by over-trimming. Hence, foot trimming is a skilled job and should be performed by a trained member of farm staff, trained veterinary surgeon or a trained paraprofessional. Regular training sessions are recommended to ensure that foot trimming methods remain optimal.

Given that most animals have naturally larger lateral hind claws, it has been proposed that 2–3 mm extra thickness of sole should be left on the lateral claw to prevent over-trimming, especially in older cows (Nuss and Paulus, 2006). These authors proposed that dishing of the typical sole ulcer site (removing sole thickness in this area to decrease weight bearing) should be extended more widely across the sole to increase weight bearing on the wall. Burgi and Cook (2008) also suggested that dishing in the lateral hind claw should be twice that of the medial hind claw, that the target foot angle should be 52° and that the flat, weight-bearing surface of the sole of the medial claw should be 80 mm to provide stability and prevent pivoting on to the back of the heel when walking. When implemented and interpreted correctly, the Dutch method of foot trimming can improve the locomotion and mobility of cows and can reduce the incidence and duration of lameness (Manson and Leaver, 1986, 1987, 1988b).

Foot-trimming intervals should vary according to need. All cows that are lame or have overgrown claws (>9 cm of the dorsal wall for Holsteins) should be examined and trimmed as soon as practically possible. Preventive trimming regimes should occur before overgrowth contributes to lameness. Given that most claw lesions develop in the weeks following calving, preventive trimming immediately before or soon after drying off is an appropriate time for many herds. When maiden heifers have overgrown claws, trimming 60 days before calving may be beneficial. In housed animals, a further examination may be warranted in mid-lactation (Hernandez *et al.*, 2007). Many producers intervene earlier than this (60–100 days), to correct the sole and toe overgrowth associated with sole bruising that, in some cases, progresses to a sole ulcer. Since primiparous heifers develop lesions earlier in lactation than multiparous cows, it is sensible to examine heifers closer to 60 days into lactation.

Horn wear is known to exceed horn growth in early lactation. Therefore, apart from the treatment of lameness, foot trimming is not recommended in the first 60 days of lactation. Additionally, in dairy systems based on a combination of housing and pasture, the periods around turnout and housing are high-risk periods for stone penetration and sole bruising. Therefore, foot trimming should not coincide with these events, but there may be benefits to examining feet a few weeks before or after these risk periods. A summary of the recommended times for routine foot trimming is provided in Table 6.6.

## Foot bathing and disinfection

Assisting clients with key aspects of foot bath design, treatment regimes and practical implementation is an important component of lameness control. Foot bathing is one of the principle measures for controlling lameness associated with digital dermatitis, both as a primary disease and when it is secondary to other lesions (Evans *et al.*, 2011). Effective control of digital dermatitis also appears to reduce lameness associated with interdigital hyperplasia, and regular foot bathing can help control this. It should be noted that if performed badly (i.e. with poor standards of hygiene or infrequent changes of solution), foot bathing can increase outbreaks of both digital dermatitis and interdigital necrobacillosis. Ensuring that foot bathing is routinely and effectively implemented is a key role for the herd

**Table 6.6.** Recommended times for routine foot trimming.

| Time of trim | Group of animals | Comments |
|---|---|---|
| Drying off | All cows | Core recommendation for most units; care with handling, do not trim heavily pregnant animals if foot-trimming facilities are unsuitable or of poor quality; do not trim and administer dry cow therapy at the same time |
| 60–100 days in milk | All cows | Helps to prevent progression of claw horn lesions: consider on units with a high incidence of these diseases; trim heifers closer to 60 days in milk; do not trim at <60 days in milk |
| Heifers ~60 days before calving | All heifers | Consider on units where the feet are visibly overgrown before calving; care with handling |
| When overgrowth recognized | As identified | Only animals with visible overgrowth are trimmed; however, some animals that are not overgrown but would benefit from trimming are missed |
| Regular scheduled trimming (e.g. every 6 months) | Whole herd | Preferred by some contract trimmers, and may reduce overall costs; depending on their stage of lactation, some animals may not be trimmed at the most appropriate time; avoid scheduling trimming close to housing or turnout |

health advisor, and often involves assisting clients to overcome practical problems with its implementation.

Numerous chemicals with disinfectant qualities have been experimentally evaluated as foot bath solutions for dairy cattle (Laven and Logue, 2006), including formalin (~5%, range 2–10%), copper sulfate (5%, range 2–6%), peracetic acid (1–2%) and hypochlorite (2%). Research has demonstrated that all are effective in controlling digital dermatitis (Laven and Hunt, 2002), although the results of one recent study suggest that formalin is superior to hypochlorite (Speijers *et al.*, 2010). Formalin and copper sulfate are probably the most widely used agents, but the use of formalin requires appropriate health and safety precautions (e.g. gloves, eye/face shield and handling in well-ventilated areas only) and is not recommended for animals with painful, ulcerated lesions. Its long-term availability has been questioned, and its use may become illegal in some countries. Long-term use of copper sulfate can lead to high levels accumulating on the land (once slurry is spread), and some countries prohibit its use because of possible environmental toxicity. If permitted, copper solutions can be acidified (various commercial products are available) to reduce the concentration of copper required to 2% or less. Soil and forage copper levels should be monitored on farms using copper products regularly. A wide range of other chemicals and proprietary products are used, with variable amounts of trial work to support their efficacy. Parlour washings (the cleaning solutions remaining following circulation-cleaning of the plant at the end of milking) are increasingly commonly used but have limited efficacy beyond cleaning feet, and so, if used, should form only part of a rotation involving agents with known efficacy. It is worth noting that the herd health advisor can usefully provide assistance by calculating correct dosage rates (i.e. measuring footbath volume and recording the exact quantity of product to be added).

A range of antibiotic solutions are also used to treat digital dermatitis (Watson, 1997; Laven and Logue, 2006), although the prescribing veterinarian must ensure their use complies with national prescribing regulations (e.g. in the UK, as their use constitutes 'off licence use of a prescription product', minimum milk and meat withhold periods are required) and they are considerably more expensive than disinfectants. We recommend their use in the initial phase of a control programme, to reduce the prevalence of digital dermatitis (particularly if levels of the ulcerative form are high), before instituting routine bathing with a disinfectant.

There is little research work on the most effective frequency of foot bathing. In endemically infected herds, experience suggests that foot bathing must be considered routine throughout the year. Initially, we recommend foot bathing after 4–6 milkings each week (either consecutive milkings or consecutive days), which can then be adjusted up or down depending on the prevalence of dermatitis lesions. Few data exist on when to change spent solutions; we suggest changing the solution after one cow passage per litre (i.e. a 250 l bath should be changed after 250 cow passages). Routine bathing should include dry cows (to prevent them calving with active lesions following a period without treatment) and heifers prior to first calving, if they are infected. In situations where this is difficult to implement they can be treated individually (see later).

In order to make routine foot bathing practical, foot baths should be easy to fill and simple to clean out. Practical recommendations on foot bath construction are available (see Box 6.1, and more detail is available at www.dairyco.org.uk, under the 'Healthy Feet Programme'), but are not based on robust science. Foot bath construction is often a compromise to accommodate many factors such as cost of filling, convenient location and ensuring good cow flow so that milking is not slowed down as cows exit the parlour. A rinse bath followed by a treatment bath reduces contamination in the treatment bath (alternatively, feet can be washed in the parlour). Adding a biocide to both the rinse bath and treatment bath is prudent but increases costs. Hypochlorite should be avoided in the rinse bath if formalin is

---

**Box 6.1.** Key aspects of foot bath design.

- at least 3 m long – cows take several steps;
- solution 10 cm deep – completely covers feet above the coronary band;
- single-cow (~1.1 m) or double-cow width (~1.8 m) – trade-off between volume (and therefore expense) and cow flow;
- easy to fill – volume washer close to hand or mount a header tank with wide bore (~10 cm) outflow above the bath;
- easy to drain – fit with a ~10 cm bung plug;
- single- (treatment only) or double- (prewash and treatment) bath system – trade-off between being cleaner before entering treatment bath and cost and space problems with a double bath;
- position is paramount – ensure the location allows good cow flow (can be problematic on some units). Use plastic bath and movable gates to 'test' location before building permanent set-up;
- ensure design does not allow animals to walk along one or both edges of the bath; and
- calculate volume and amount of agent required – attach to or paint instructions on the wall above the bath.

---

being used as a treatment, to avoid chemical interactions. The bath should be deep enough to fully immerse the foot to the coronary band and should be long enough to deter cows from jumping through. Cow comfort is paramount, so cows should walk slowly with minimal splashing.

The practice of mass-spraying of feet with licensed or unlicensed antibiotics or disinfectants as cows stand (either at the feed face or in the parlour) has emerged as an alternative to foot bathing. It has not been the subject of research and may not adequately treat lesions extending between the heel bulbs. However, practical experience suggests it can work well in some situations, particularly as an alternative to foot bathing for dry cows and heifers that are kept in buildings or yards away from the foot-bathing facilities. Animals can be sprayed using a 'knapsack'-style sprayer, once or twice per week whilst feeding; the wand can safely be directed between the claws from a standing position.

## Management of cow groups and movements

Cattle are highly social herd animals and engage in complex social interactions to establish dominance and herd bonding. Herds have a predominantly linear hierarchy in which social rank is largely predicted by age and stature. When individuals first meet they compete to establish rank. Once the hierarchy is established within a group, negative interactions become less common except when animals compete for a limited resource, e.g. access to feed (see Chapter 8) or lying areas, or when closely ranked animals seek to re-establish the dominance order. Aggression between animals of very different rank is uncommon, because subordinate animals acknowledge the more dominant individual by surrendering control of the resource. In order to maximize productivity and control disease in a group, the environment should be designed and herds managed to limit the impacts on subordinate animals. If animals have to compete for limited resources, subordinate animals are forced to wait to use the resource. This is particularly pertinent for control of lameness, where standing time on concrete is now thought to be a key risk factor in the development of claw horn lesions.

### Standing time at milking

Many dairy farms have increased cow numbers (in an attempt to improve profitability) without making proportionate changes to parlour capacity. Cows enter the milking parlour in a very similar order each milking. Consequently, subordinate animals are forced to wait by standing on concrete in the collecting yard, sometimes for many hours each milking. Where practical, the best solution is to increase the number of groups within the herd (see section 'Fresh cow and heifer groups'), thereby reducing the number of animals in each group and limiting the maximum waiting time to a target of one hour or less at each milking. Unfortunately, producers are often resistant to this change because it increases the complexity of their management system: first by increasing the time required to perform routine tasks and secondly because of the limitation of buildings (e.g. it is often difficult to split groups without interfering with cow flow). In these situations laying rubber matting in the collecting yard (see section 'Standing time and concrete surfaces') to soften the standing surface is a feasible alternative.

## Management at the feed face

Trough access is a valued resource and cows tend to feed as a herd (Grant and Albright, 2001). This is particularly true in total mixed ration fed herds where the provision of fresh feed encourages all animals to eat together. Consequently, animals will compete for access; if feed space is inadequate, bullying forces subordinate animals to wait, increasing their standing time. For example, increasing feeding space per cow from 0.5 to 1.0 m resulted in a 57% reduction in aggressive interactions; this was particularly true for subordinate animals (DeVries et al., 2004). One row of feed face for every two rows of standard-width cubicles (~120 cm) provides approximately 60 cm of space per cow (i.e. the absolute minimum), and 75 cm is much preferred. Many modern sheds are designed with three rows of cubicles per row of feed face, reducing space to approximately 40 cm/cow. This is likely to limit both dry matter intake and increase standing time in subordinate animals. There is also evidence that feed face design can influence aggressive behaviour; cows were displaced more frequently from a post and rail barrier, compared with a barrier composed of headlocks (Huzzey et al., 2006), although these systems are more expensive

to install. Lastly, the feed face is considered one of the priority areas for rubber matting (see section 'Standing time and concrete surfaces') to mitigate the effects of extended feeding times, particularly for high-yielding animals (~4–6 h/day).

## Fresh cow and heifer groups

Recent changes in our understanding of the aetiology of claw horn disease suggest that the peri-parturient period is a time of particular risk. Fresh cow groups (grouping all recently calved cows separately for a period of approximately 1–2 months) have grown in popularity and appear particularly pertinent for lameness control. These allow the targeted reallocation of farm resources and investment to early-lactation animals most at risk of disease (late-lactation animals are more resilient and can be proportionately disadvantaged if necessary). The advantages, for lameness control, of a fresh cow group are:

- Access to the most comfortable cubicles (see section 'Lying time and cubicle comfort') at a low stocking rate (at least 10% more cubicles than cows and ideally 20% more) to maximize lying times and reduce standing time. The group can be operated on a 'one in, one out' basis or through the instigation of a weekly group exit routine.
- Provision of at least 80 cm of feed face per cow (although we recommend 100 cm/cow with rubber matting) to maximize dry matter intake and reduce competition to minimize unnecessary standing.
- The group should be milked first to reduce standing time (its relatively small size helps in this respect) and reduce exposure to slurry (digital dermatitis risk) as it builds up during the milking process.

Heifer groups work on similar principles. Housing all first-lactation animals together reduces bullying and competition by mature cows, particularly during critical periods such as early lactation. Although the practical difficulties of maintaining multiple groups on the farm can be challenging, the health and production benefits reported by farms that have changed systems can be substantial.

## Lying time and cubicle comfort

Both research and field findings have demonstrated over many decades that animals housed in cubicle-based systems suffer more lameness compared with animals kept in straw yards (e.g. Barker *et al.*, 2010), and this is particularly true for the claw horn lesions. Increased standing time has been linked directly to an increase in the number of sole lesions (Galindo and Broom, 2000). Optimizing cubicle comfort and maximizing lying times is now considered one of the key interventions to reduce the risk of lameness, particularly claw horn lesions. Lying times at pasture are replicated by most straw yards. In these herds the space requirements in straw yards for controlling diseases such as mastitis will be adequate for lameness control (see Chapter 5). In well-designed cubicle housing, lying times can be very similar to those achieved at pasture and in straw yards, but all too often they are not.

The key aspects of cubicle comfort are design, dimensions, stocking rate and lying surface. All of these factors can act cumulatively to restrict the willingness of animals to use the cubicle, and therefore will reduce lying time.

A stocking rate of at least one cubicle per cow should be provided, but we recommend providing 10% more cubicles than cows; this is especially important in fresh cow groups where a 20% surplus is recommended (see section 'Fresh cow and heifer groups'). As the stocking rate increases above 100%, lying times decrease and animals are more likely to be displaced from their cubicle (Fregonesi *et al.*, 2007).

Design and appropriate dimensions (e.g. see Fig. 6.9) must allow animals to enter and stand in the stall, lie down, rise and exit the stall with minimum hindrance. Above all, adult cows need approximately 1 m of unrestricted lunge space in front of them (the chin almost reaches the floor as they bob forward) in order to stand unhindered. Without adequate lunge space, cows collide with the stanchions as they attempt to rise or are forced to shuffle around on the cubicle surface causing abrasions (e.g. hock lesions) and

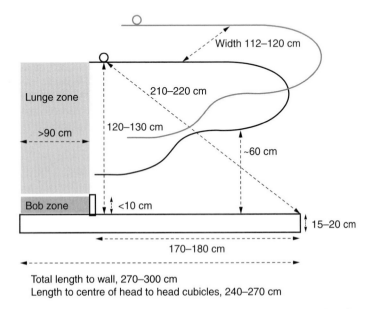

**Fig. 6.9.** Cubicle dimensions appropriate for a 700 kg Holstein-Friesian cow. Fine-tuning from these approximate values is often necessary depending on how animals interact with the environment once the cubicles are installed.

injuries as they strive to create enough room to stand. While animals can alter their behaviour to some extent to compensate for cubicle inadequacies (e.g. if space at the front is limited, cows can lunge sideways into the adjacent stall), inappropriate design can increase lameness. For example, lameness scores were reported to be higher and the number of lame cows increased in cubicles with a restrictive neck rail (Bernardi *et al.*, 2009).

Many lying surfaces can be used, ranging from deep straw on a concrete base through to mats, mattresses and water beds. Unfortunately none are perfect and all have both advantages and disadvantages (see Table 6.7). From an animal health perspective, including lameness control, deep sand beds are best but can be difficult to manage (e.g. slurry management can be difficult on units not originally designed to house cows on sand). For further detail on cow bedding, the reader is referred to the practical material held by DairyCo (www.dairyco.org.uk, under the 'Healthy Feet Programme').

In older buildings, optimizing cow comfort need not mean that dated sheds require demolition (an unrealistic suggestion on many units) – many cubicles and buildings can be modified and substantially improved, at relatively low cost, if the basic requirements of the cow are taken into account (see Fig. 6.10). When new buildings or renovations are planned, it is vital that the herd health advisor provides input to prevent all building design being driven by agricultural engineers who may have limited experience and expertise in animal health and welfare. Even in new cubicles, finding the correct set-up for the cows is an iterative process (e.g. partitions are set initially at standard values and then altered depending on how the animals respond to the set-up). Therefore, it is important that the expectations of the client are managed so that they anticipate having to make changes but, more importantly, cubicle infrastructure *must* be joined with adjustable fittings to allow alterations to be made both in the initial set-up phase and in the future if cow stature in the herd changes.

One of the difficulties with optimizing cubicle design and set-up is the 'one size fits all' approach. Cubicle dimensions should be specified for the larger animals in the herd, rather than the average. This approach maximizes comfort for all animals but is disliked by some farmers because it increases the amount of cleaning required (and possibly the risk of mastitis), because small animals may defaecate on the back of the stall. However, this is preferable to large cows having reduced lying times because of uncomfortable cubicles. Ultimately, it is impossible to optimally design housing for a herd of animals of disparate sizes. Breeding policy should be altered to reduce variation in the medium term or, in some cases, the only solution is to divide cows into groups of different stature (e.g. heifer groups; see 'Fresh cow and heifer groups') and provide cubicles of appropriate dimensions (this works particularly well on farms that have old cubicles that are too small for the modern mature Holstein cow and new accommodation with larger cubicles).

To aid the clinician or advisor, a number of indices have been described that provide an estimate of cubicle comfort (e.g. cow comfort and stall use indices) by counting the proportion of animals engaged in a variety of behaviours (e.g. lying in cubicles). However, recent research has demonstrated that neither index is associated with the actual daily lying time of the animals (Ito *et al.*, 2009). Instead, subjective assessments of how cows interact with the cubicle may be preferable – for example, the ease with which cows get up and lie down in the stalls or whether the neck rail impairs entry to the stall (in which case it should be raised).

Finally, whilst direct research is lacking, experience suggests that 'training' heifers to use cubicles before first calving (so they do not experience cubicles for the first time during the high-risk period immediately after calving) is a sensible procedure. On many units this is best achieved by housing in-calf heifers in the cubicle accommodation for a few weeks during the summer when the adult cows are at pasture.

## Standing times and concrete surfaces

Standing times on concrete and the quality of the concrete surface can influence the incidence

**Table 6.7.** Advantages and disadvantages of different cubicle bedding systems.

| Cubicle bedding system | Advantages | Disadvantages | Notes |
|---|---|---|---|
| Deep sand | Gold standard for comfort, lying times and animal health (good for both mastitis and lameness) Improves grip in alleyways | Management can be problematic, does not suit many slurry handling systems and very wearing on any pumps used to move slurry Teats may require more cleaning at milking Requires a sand spreader to dispense sand | Washed sand best, some unwashed sands can set hard in the bed Various sources available including beach sand, water treatment works and commercial suppliers ~2.0–2.5 t/cow/year ~£10–15/t including delivery |
| Mattress (rubber crumb- or foam-filled) usually with light bedding (e.g. sawdust, chopped straw, paper waste, power station ash) | Second only to deep-bed sand for cubicle comfort in most trials | Combination of abrasive surface (to prevent slips) and abrasive substrate can cause painful hock lesions | ~£40–60 per mattress Additional cost of bedding, which varies depending on choice and location |
| Mat (varying from thin to thick and cushioned), usually with light bedding (e.g. sawdust, chopped straw, paper waste, power station ash) | May be more durable than mattress Slightly cheaper than mattress | Less comfortable than mattress Combination of abrasive surface (to prevent slips) and abrasive substrate can cause painful hock lesions | ~£30–50 per mat Additional cost of bedding, which varies depending on choice and location |
| Solid base (e.g. concrete, tarmac, hardcore, clay, limestone), usually deep-bedded with straw or paper | Good cow comfort if deep straw bed provided | Poor cow comfort unless a deep bed provided Major mastitis risk if deep straw bed provided Straw and paper do not suit all slurry handling systems | Initially cheap to install but ongoing cost of bedding The cost of straw can fluctuate widely by year and farm location |

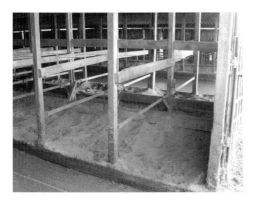

**Fig. 6.10.** An example of cubicle renovation. All woodwork has been removed from the front of the cubicle and the lower dividing rail has been replaced by a tensioned strap allowing cows to share space and lunge both sideways and forwards. Cows are positioned by a brisket board and a new neck rail (of tensioned rope) set far forward in the stall. The old bed has been replaced by deep sand. While the cubicles remain short, cow comfort has been dramatically improved and the functional life of the building extended at relatively low cost.

of sole ulcers, sole bruising and white line lesions and can indirectly increase exposure to wet and unhygienic conditions leading to digital dermatitis and foul-in-the-foot.

Forcing cows to stand for more than 2 h/day while waiting for milking, artificial insemination, pregnancy diagnosis or other routine management activities can predispose to foot lesions. Similarly, poor lying comfort or overstocked buildings can also lead to prolonged standing (see 'Lying time and cubicle comfort'). On units where standing time is considered a significant risk, there is great value in calculating approximate time budgets for cows. Calculations should concentrate on the 'worst' 25% of cows (i.e. those likely to have the longest standing times), particularly around milking, on various days in the week and at different times of the year. Time budget calculations should include walking as well as standing times and should factor in time for feeding, drinking, lying down and moving between these activities (Cook et al., 2007; Cook and Nordlund, 2009). Calculating time budgets can highlight instances when cows are needlessly penned away from lying areas. For example, the common practice of penning

the herd after milking to allow teat end closure may be unnecessary if fresh food is provided after milking, bed hygiene is optimal and mastitis control is good.

Prolonged standing times are more hazardous if the standing surface is rough, uneven, wet or contaminated with slurry. Areas of broken concrete contain stale slurry (as they are never scraped clean) and can damage claws. These should be filled and repaired as soon as practically possible, particularly if they occur in areas of high cow flow (e.g. the collecting yard). Wet, slurry-contaminated surfaces are major risk factors for digital dermatitis and foul, but also predispose cows to heel erosion, soft claw horn, sole bruising, sole ulcers and possibly white line lesions. Wet concrete is also less abrasive, and if concrete surfaces are too smooth, then claw overgrowth may become a problem. Therefore, concrete should be dry and provide good grip without being sharp or allowing pooling of slurry. Stocking rates, foot-bathing regimes and foot-trimming frequency can be adjusted to decrease the risk from poor flooring to some extent.

While it represents a low risk for foot lameness, smooth concrete will need correcting to reduce the risk of cows slipping and to increase natural activities such as feeding and oestrous behaviour. Several options exist, including grooving, scabbling (mechanically roughening the surface by pounding it with a series of steel tips) or fitting rubber yard matting. There is little published evidence to indicate which approach is superior, although there is a body of evidence showing the benefits of rubber matting (Bell and Huxley, 2009b). Unpublished recommendations from work conducted by a UK advisory body specified that grooving should be diamond-cut (not flailed) and should be 6–10 mm deep, 10 mm wide with 40 mm between lines. Grooves are usually cut to form squares or diamonds to provide grip in all directions. Scabbling is an alternative approach that produces a roughened surface without grooves or ridges, and we recommend it as potentially superior for grip without gross unevenness, while still providing some claw horn wear.

Excessively abrasive surfaces are a major hazard for claw horn lesions, particularly thin soles and sole bruising, and can be a problem with eroded or excessively scabbled concrete. There are a number of practical solutions, few of which have been investigated scientifically. Options include concrete planing (mechanically removing the abrasive top surface which, whilst possible, is practically difficult), rubbing cement mixes into the surface and resurfacing with resins, bitumen or rubber matting. Old, broken concrete may require replacement. For small areas where cows turn, small sections of targeted rubber matting are the easiest and most cost-effective solution.

Rubber matting in the parlour exit lanes (Fig. 6.11) and collecting yard has benefits for foot health and speed of cow flow (cows walk more confidently on rubber matting (Telezhenko and Bergsten, 2005)). Rubber matting in housing, particularly where cows stand, such as the feed face, can be used when the lying comfort is good (otherwise cows choose to lie on the rubber floors rather than uncomfortable cubicles). While the benefits of rubber matting in terms of lameness reduction are still equivocal, cows prefer to stand on rubber (Telzhenko *et al.*, 2007), and hence at a very minimum it improves welfare and cow movement. Rubber matting can be particularly beneficial when slats are present in the housing, the latter helping by preventing pooling of water, urine and slurry, although the same benefit can be achieved with wide alleys (ideally, 4–5 m), slopes of 2% and good ventilation. Cost remains the biggest problem

with rubber matting; for example, proprietary products cost in the region of £30/m² (including fitting), in the UK.

For new buildings, tamping concrete produces a surface with better traction than floated concrete with grooves (Albutt *et al.*, 1990). The direction of tamping is largely a practical consideration, as tamping provides grip in all directions. Tamping becomes impractical in large buildings, and alternatives include a brush finish or imprints with lines or patterns. Very little information is available on the benefits of achieving these effects. While again scientific evidence is lacking, the use of 40 mm-diameter hexagonal imprints with grooving 6–10 mm deep and 10 mm wide engraved into floated concrete appears to provide a safe finish.

### Cleanliness and slurry management

Exposure to slurry has been associated with a high prevalence of digital dermatitis (Rodriguez-Lainz *et al.*, 1996; Wells *et al.*, 1999). Trigger factors for interdigital necrobacillosis are less clear and may relate more to stage of lactation, breed and risk of skin trauma than previously thought (Alban *et al.*, 1996). Research on slurry management has been somewhat limited by the methods used to evaluate it – for example, the extent to which cleanliness can be measured over time. The prevalence and severity of heel horn erosion are strongly correlated with wet, unhygienic conditions, but the importance of hygiene in the development of other claw horn lesions remains uncertain (although probably poor hygiene softens horn). Increased claw horn moisture has been associated with thin soles in housed dairy cattle (van Amstel *et al.*, 2004) and consequential lesions such as bruising, white line disease and sole ulcer. Similarly, there is seasonality in the occurrence of white line lesions related to rainfall. Heel horn erosion is often used as a marker for poor environmental hygiene, and has been correlated to sole ulcers, digital dermatitis and abnormal claw shape (Manske *et al.*, 2002). Further work is required to establish the causal relationships and details of pathogenesis of lesions in wet, unhygienic environments.

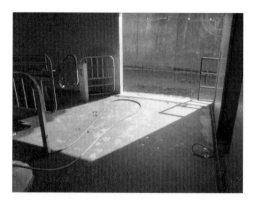

**Fig. 6.11.** Rubber matting fitted in the parlour and on right-angled turns at the parlour exit.

Generally the greatest exposure to wet, unhygienic conditions occurs during housing, although well-managed housing systems can perform well compared with extended grazing systems in wet climatic conditions. Numerous housing management factors can increase the amount of slurry in the environment, reduce the cleanliness of the foot and increase the amount of foot lameness. These include (i) the use of automatic scrapers (animals must step through a 'bow wave' of slurry as the scraper passes); (ii) scraping too infrequently; (iii) incomplete scraping (particularly hand-scraping in areas where cows congregate and that cannot be reached using a tractor, such as around water troughs and out-of-parlour feeders); (iv) overstocked housing; (v) inadequate drainage or inadequate falls on surfaces; (vi) areas of broken or pot-holed concrete that accumulate stale slurry, dirty foot baths or raceways; (vii) insufficient bedding; (viii) inadequate scraping of, or prolonged time for cows in the collecting yard prior to milking; and (ix) the use of bedding materials that adheres to wet feet.

In this context the role of the veterinary advisor is to identify and highlight risks so that they can be addressed and to provide advice if new buildings or substantial management changes are required. Ideally, to gain a true picture of slurry contamination, the environment should be assessed at its worst (i.e. just before it is next cleaned). Most veterinary visits are conducted in the morning just after the morning clean, which can give a false impression of the true situation.

## Tracks and walkways

Good-quality cow tracks, walkways and cow flow are important for the prevention of white line disease, thin soles and sole penetrations. It may be possible that stony tracks help identify cows with pre-existing lesions because of the increased risk of stones penetrating diseased sole horn. Wet muddy tracks are a risk factor for digital infections such as digital dermatitis (Rodriguez-Lainz et al., 1996).

Good cow track construction is particularly important for large herds on extended grazing systems, and technical guidance on this subject has been published (Chesterton, 1989). A range of materials can be used (Table 6.8); the reader is referred to the practical material held

**Table 6.8.** Relative merits of materials that can be used for cow tracks.

| Material | Cow comfort | Dryness | Grit-free | Cost of laying | Suitable for vehicular use | Maintenance |
|---|---|---|---|---|---|---|
| Cow carpet | +++ | ++ | ++ | H | ++ | L – replace after 5 years |
| Pine peelings | +++ | – – | +++ | L–M | – – | H – top up twice per year |
| Crushed hard stone | ++ | ++ | – – – | M | ++ | L – patch every 2 years |
| Chalk | ++ | – | ++ | M | – | L – patch every 2 years |
| Fine stone (e.g. basalt, quarry dust) | ++ | – | – – – | M | – | M – top up every year |
| Oolitic limestone | ++ | ++ | ++ | M | ++ | L – patch every 2 years |
| Sand | ++ | – | ++ | M–H | – | M – top up regularly |
| Shellet (or similar) | ++ | – | ++ | L | – | M – top up every year |
| Concrete | + | + | – – – | H | + | M – sweep monthly |
| Tarmac | + | ++ | – – – | L | ++ | M – sweep monthly |
| Concrete railway sleepers | – to + | + | – | M | + | M – sweep monthly |

– – –, very poor; – –, poor; –, mediocre; +, good; ++, very good; +++, excellent; L, low; M, medium; H, high.

by DairyCo (www.dairyco.org.uk, under the 'Healthy Feet Programme') for more extensive information. The most appropriate material to use depends on what is available locally and the cost of these materials, including transportation. All tracks require maintenance: maintenance can be minimized by ensuring (i) good drainage (track raised above surrounding ground, 5% camber, drainage ditches and cross-channels across steeply sloped areas); (ii) optimal natural drying (avoid shading from wind or sun – e.g. keep hedges well trimmed if they are next to tracks); and (iii) that tracks run in straight lines and that heavy vehicles do not use them. Frequency of resurfacing varies enormously with the nature of surface material, rainfall and degree of use. Generally speaking, organic surfaces (woodchip, pine peelings or straw) require topping up twice yearly, soft stone tracks in high-rainfall areas generally require some resurfacing every 2–4 years and hard stone stabilized with cement often lasts longer. Concrete and concrete sleepers will last many years but require regular sweeping with tractor-mounted brushes.

Speed of cow flow will in part be determined by the comfort of walking for the cow, but other factors can cause bottlenecks such as sharp turns, narrowing of tracks or steep slopes. In general there should be sufficient width to allow subordinate cows to pass around dominant animals. A width of 3–4 m will generally be sufficient, albeit with some possible slowing. Rushing cows at the back of the herd with a dog or vehicle has been shown to increase the risk of lameness (Chesterton *et al.*, 1989), does little to alleviate the causes of slow cow flow and can even reduce flow in the long term if cows become lame.

## Nutrition

The perceived role of nutritional management in the control of lameness has changed substantially over the last few years. Historically, much attention was paid to controlling subacute ruminal acidosis (SARA) because of its proposed link with 'laminitis' and hence claw horn lesions. However, this aetiology has not been substantiated by research. While limiting the effects of SARA remains important from a health and production point of view (see Chapter 8), we now consider this a low priority as part of a lameness control programme. Rather, if recent research evidence proves correct, more attention should be paid to limiting condition score loss in early lactation. Cows with a low body condition score at calving and in early lactation are more likely to suffer from lameness (Hoedemaker *et al.*, 2009); condition score is positively correlated with the thickness of the digital cushion, and the prevalence of sole ulcers and white line disease were significantly associated with the thickness of the digital cushion (Bicalho *et al.*, 2009). It is likely that managing nutrition to reduce the number of thin cows at calving and limit condition score loss in early lactation should be part of controlling claw horn lesions. More details on management of body condition score are provided in Chapter 8.

The results from a number of studies have suggested that heifers reared on diets containing fermented forage (e.g. grass silage) with low dry matter are more likely to suffer claw horn lesions after calving than animals fed diets based on drier, non-fermented forage, e.g. hay or straw (Offer *et al.*, 2001; Leach *et al.*, 2005). The outcome of these and other studies suggests that heifer-rearing diets should be formulated using forages with a dry matter content greater than 25% (e.g. dry grass silage, hay or straw). However, it remains possible that wet faeces (produced by animals on wet diets) are an important factor mediating the effects observed and so environmental hygiene is also likely to be important in the heifer environment. Either way, where possible feeding a high dry matter diet to in-calf heifers is likely to reduce clinical lameness after calving.

There is good evidence that the supplementation of diets with biotin (20 mg/cow/day) leads to a significant reduction in the incidence of white line disease (approximately halving the risk; Hedges *et al.*, 2001; Pötzsch *et al.*, 2003). Data on sole haemorrhage and sole ulcer are equivocal. Higher levels of biotin can be added directly to mixed rations or concentrates can be specifically fortified with the vitamin on request. On farms where white line disease is a significant problem, we recommend supplementation with biotin to these levels. It is worth noting that periods of supplementation of six months or more may be required before a significant benefit is seen; ongoing supplementation is required to maintain the effect (biotin is water soluble), and results from the research suggest that animals on some farms may not benefit from supplementation (Hedges *et al.*, 2001).

A number of studies have investigated the impacts of supplementing diets with methionine, zinc, manganese, copper and cobalt at different levels of inclusion and in different forms (inorganic versus complexed, sulfate or non-sulfate based; Nocek *et al.*, 2006; Siciliano-Jones *et al.*, 2008). There is some evidence that diets supplemented with these trace elements may improve claw health and reduce the incidence of claw horn lesions. The effects seem more likely if minerals are supplied in the forms more available, but it should be stressed that mineral supplementation forms a small part of a holistic lameness control strategy (see Chapter 8 for more information on mineral supplementation).

## Biosecurity

The presence and prevalence of digital dermatitis in a herd has been associated with breaches in biosecurity (Rodriguez-Lainz *et al.*, 1996; ArgaezRodriguez *et al.*, 1997; Wells *et al.*, 1999). The bacteria associated with digital dermatitis are fastidious anaerobic organisms, and therefore the most likely route of entry to a herd is through infected cattle. Contact of uninfected cows with contaminated equipment or contaminated mud or slurry are potential routes for transmission, although this is uncertain. Virulence of the various phylotypes of the causal treponeme may vary, so that herds endemically infected with digital dermatitis may still benefit from strict biosecurity standards. Furthermore, as an infectious disease, any means of reducing spread within the herd through bio-containment within facilities will also improve overall herd control in endemically infected herds.

Consequently, preventing the entry of digital dermatitis through effective biosecurity is essential for farms that are disease free, and is also likely to be of value in herds with infected cows. When formulating biosecurity protocols, it is important to consider (i) policies for personnel, including vets, foot trimmers, relief staff and visitors; (ii) policies for the movement of live animals in and out of groups at all ages; (iii) the use of shared equipment or facilities; and (iv) possible contact with other species. Where practical, providing external workers (e.g. foot trimmers and vets) with appropriate farm-based equipment (e.g. protective clothing, crushes, foot-trimming equipment) rather than allowing kit to be brought on to the unit is prudent. At the very least, any external equipment brought on to the farm should be thoroughly disinfected before use. For digital dermatitis, there is little evidence on which to base isolation protocols for newly purchased animals, but knowing the health status of the herd of origin, examining the feet of purchased animals and the treatment of incoming animals with topical and systemic antibiotics followed by isolation for at least 3 weeks is prudent. Identifying possible risks from contiguous holdings and ensuring good boundary security may also reduce the risk of local spread. In herds free from infection or with low-virulence digital dermatitis, regular foot bathing with a disinfectant may help prevent minor breaches in biosecurity translating into disease outbreak.

## Conclusions

Achieving control of lameness on dairy farms is undoubtedly difficult. The herd health advisor must overcome a number of barriers, including (i) the relative difficulties of establishing and maintaining good-quality monitoring and recording systems; (ii) the practical and financial complications of implementing key aspects of control (particularly for claw horn lesions); and (iii) the lag between implementation of control measures and appreciable improvements in the levels of lameness. These difficulties mean that sustained control will be achieved on units where the herd health advisor works with key farm staff to generate shared ownership of the problem and can maintain enthusiasm and motivation so that staff actively engage with control programmes over the medium term (see Chapter 2). That said, practical experience from around the world has demonstrated that achieving low levels of lameness is possible and that this leads to significant health, welfare and financial returns for the unit as a whole. Lameness control now attracts a high profile in many countries. Consequently, the amount of money being invested in research and control programmes to assist the herd health advisor has increased over the last decade. Results from this investment are already being seen and are likely further to improve both the knowledge base and availability of resources for on-farm use in the next decade.

## References and Further Reading

Alban, L., Agger, J.F. and Lawson, L.G. (1996) Lameness in tied Danish dairy cattle: The possible influence of housing systems, management, milk yield, and prior incidents of lameness. *Preventive Veterinary Medicine* 29, 135–149.

Albutt, R.W., Dumelow, J., Cermak, J.P. and Owen, J.E. (1990) Slip-resistance of solid concrete floors in cattle buildings. *Journal of Agricultural Engineering Research* 45, 137–147.

Amory, J.R., Barker, Z.E., Wright, J.L., Mason, S.A., Blowey, R.W. and Green, L.E. (2008) Associations between sole ulcer, white line disease and digital dermatitis and the milk of 1824 dairy cows on 30 dairy cow farms in England and Wales. *Preventive Veterinary Medicine* 83, 381–391.

Archer, S.C., Green, M.J. and Huxley, J.N. (2009) The dynamics of dairy herd mobility. In: *Proceedings of the Cattle Lameness Conference*, 25 March 2009, University of Nottingham, pp. 49–50.

Archer, S.C., Green, M.J. and Huxley, J.N. (2010a) The association between milk yield and serial locomotion score assessments in UK dairy cows. *Journal of Dairy Science* 93, 4045–4053.

Archer, S.C., Bell, N.J. and Huxley, J.N. (2010b) Lameness in UK dairy cows: a review of the current status. *In Practice* 32, 492–504.

Argaez-Rodriguez, F.D.J., Hird, D.W., deAnda, J.H., Read, D.H. and Rodriguez-Lainz, A. (1997) Papillomatous digital dermatitis on a commercial dairy farm in Mexicali, Mexico: Incidence and effect on reproduction and milk production. *Preventive Veterinary Medicine* 32, 275–286.

Bach, A., Binares, M., Devant, M. and Carre, X. (2007) Associations between lameness and production, feeding and milking attendance of Holstein cows milked with an automatic milking system. *Journal of Dairy Research* 74, 40–46.

Barkema, H.W., Westrik, J.D., van Keulen, K.A.S. and Schukken, Y.H. (1994) The effects of lameness on reproductive performance and culling in Dutch dairy farms. *Preventive Veterinary Medicine* 20, 249–259.

Barker, Z.E., Leach, K.A., Whay, H.R., Bell, N.J. and Main, D.C.J. (2010) Assessment of lameness prevalence and associated risk factors in dairy herds in England and Wales. *Journal of Dairy Science* 93, 932–941.

Belge, F., Bildik, A., Belge, A., Kikcalp, D. and Atasoy, N. (2004) Possible association between chronic laminitis and some biochemical parameters in dairy cattle. *Australian Veterinary Journal* 82, 556–557.

Bell, N.J. and Huxley, J.N. (2009a) Locomotion, lameness and mobility in dairy cows. *Veterinary Record* 164, 726.

Bell, N.J. and Huxley, J.N. (2009b) The use of rubber floor matting on dairy units: a critical review. *Cattle Practice* 17, 142–147.

Bell, N.J., Bell, M.J., Knowles, T.G., Whay, H.R., Main, D.J. and Webster, A.J.F. (2009) The development, implementation and testing of a lameness control programme based on HACCP principles and designed for heifers on dairy farms. *The Veterinary Journal* 180, 178–188.

Bernardi, F., Fregonesi, J., Winckler, C., Veira, D.M., von Keyserlingk, M.A.G. and Weary, D.M. (2009) The stall-design paradox: Neck rails increase lameness but improve udder and stall hygiene. *Journal of Dairy Science* 92, 3074–3080.

Bicalho, R.C., Machado, V.S. and Caixeta, L.S. (2009) Lameness in dairy cattle: A debilitating disease or a disease of debilitated cattle? A cross-sectional study of lameness prevalence and thickness of the digital cushion. *Journal of Dairy Science* 92, 3175–3184.

Blowey, R.W. (2008) *Cattle Lameness and Hoofcare, 2nd edn.* Old Pond Publishing, Ltd, Ipswich, UK.

Burgi, K. and Cook, N.B. (2008) Three adaptions to the functional trimming method. In: *The 15th International Symposium and the 7th Conference on Lameness in Ruminants*, 9–13 June 2008, Kuopio, Finland, pp. 196.

Carter, S., Evans, N., Timofte, D., Brown, J., Blowey, R., Murray, R. *et al.* (2009) Dermatitis – microbial aetiopathogenesis approaches providing opportunities for treatment. In: *Proceedings of the Cattle Lameness Conference*, 25 February 2009, Sutton Bonington, UK, pp. 9–18.

Cha, E., Hertl, J.A., Bar, D. and Grohn, Y.T. (2010) The cost of different types of lameness in dairy cows calculated by dynamic programming. *Preventive Veterinary Medicine* 97, 1–8.

Channon, A.J., Walker, A.M., Pfau, T., Sheldon, I.M. and Wilson, A.M. (2009) Variability of Manson and Leaver locomotion scores assigned to dairy cows by different observers. *The Veterinary Record* 164, 388–392.

Chesterton, R.N. (1989) Examination and control of lameness in dairy herds. *New Zealand Veterinary Journal* 37, 133.

Chesterton, R.N., Pfeiffer, D.U., Morris, R.S. and Tanner, C.M. (1989) Environmental and behavioural factors affecting the prevalence of foot lameness in New Zealand dairy herds – a case-control study. *New Zealand Veterinary Journal* 37, 135–142.

Cook, N.B. (2003) Prevalence of lameness among dairy cattle in Wisconsin as a function of housing type and stall surface. *Journal of the American Veterinary Medical Association* 223, 1324–1328.

Cook, N.B. and Nordlund, K.V. (2009) The influence of the environment on dairy cow behaviour, claw health and herd lameness dynamics. *The Veterinary Journal* 179, 360–369.

Cook, N.B., Bennett, T.B. and Nordlund, K.V. (2004) Effect of free stall surface on daily activity patterns in dairy cows with relevance to lameness prevalence. *Journal of Dairy Science* 87, 2912–2922.

Cook, N.B., Mentink, R.L., Bennett, T.B. and Burgi, K. (2007) The effect of heat stress and lameness on time budgets of lactating dairy cows. *Journal of Dairy Science* 90, 1674–1682.

DeVries, T.J., von Keyserlingk, M.A.G. and Weary, D.M. (2004) Effect of feeding space on the inter-cow distance, aggression and feeding behaviour of free-stall housed lactating dairy cows. *Journal of Dairy Science* 87, 1432–1438.

Dopfer, D., Koopmans, A., Meijer, F.A., Szakall, I., Schukken, Y.H., Klee, W. *et al.* (1997) Histological and bacteriological evaluation of digital dermatitis in cattle, with special reference to spirochetes and *Campylobacter faecalis*. *Veterinary Record* 140, 620–623.

Enting, H., Kooij, D., Kijkhuizen, A.A., Huirne, R.B.M. and NoordhuizenStrassen, E.N. (1997) Economic losses due to clinical lameness in dairy cattle. *Livestock Production Science* 49, 259–267.

Esslemont, R.J. (2003) The costs of poor fertility and what to do about reducing them. *Cattle Practice* 11, 237–250.

European Food Safety Authority (2009) Scientific report on the effects of farming system on dairy cows welfare and disease. Annex to the *EFSA Journal* 1143, 1–38.

Evans, N.J., Blowey, R.W., Timofte, D., Isherwood, D.R., Brown, J.M., Murray, R. *et al.* (2011) Association between bovine digital dermatitis treponemes and a range of 'non-healing' bovine hoof disorders. *Veterinary Record* 168, 214.

Flower, F.C., Sedbauer, M., Carter, E., von Keyserlingk, M.A.G., Sanderson, D.J. and Weary, D.M. (2008) Analgesics improve the gait of lame dairy cows. *Journal of Dairy Science* 91, 3010–3014.

Fregonesi, J.A., Tucker, C.B. and Weary, D.M. (2007) Overstocking reduces lying time in dairy cows. *Journal of Dairy Science* 90, 3349–3354.

Galindo, F. and Broom, D.M. (2000) The relationship between social behaviour of dairy cows and the occurrence of lameness in three herds. *Research in Veterinary Science* 69, 75–79.

Garbarino, E.J., Hernandez, J.A., Shearer, J.K., Risco, C.A. and Thatcher, W.W. (2004) Effect of lameness on ovarian activity in postpartum Holstein cows. *Journal of Dairy Science* 87, 4123–4131.

Grant, R.J., and Albright, J.L. (2001) Effect of animal grouping on feeding behaviour and intake of dairy cattle. *Journal of Dairy Science* 84(e-Suppl.), E156–E163.

Green, L.E., Hedges, V.J. Schukken, Y.H., Blowey, R.W. and Packington, A.J. (2002) The impact of clinical lameness on the milk yield of dairy cows. *Journal of Dairy Science* 85, 2250–2256.

Harman, J.L., Grohn, Y.T., Erb, H.N. and Casella, G. (1996) Event-time analysis of the effect of season of parturition, parity, and concurrent disease on parturition-to-conception interval in dairy cows. *American Journal of Veterinary Research* 57, 640–645.

Hedges, J., Blowey, R.W., Packington, A.J., O'Callaghan, C.J. and Green, L.E. (2001) A longitudinal field trial of the effect of biotin on lameness in dairy cows. *Journal of Dairy Science* 84, 1969–1975.

Hernandez, J., Shearer J.K. and Webb, D.W. (2001) Effect of lameness on the calving-to-conception interval in dairy cows. *Journal of the American Veterinary Medical Association* 218, 1611–1614.

Hernandez, J.A., Garbarino, E.J., Shearer, J.K., Risco C.A. and Thatcher W.W. (2005) Comparison of the calving-to-conception interval in dairy cows with different degrees of lameness during the prebreeding postpartum period. *Journal of the American Veterinary Medical Association* 227, 1284–1291.

Hernandez, J.A., Garbarino, E.J., Shearer, J.K., Risco, C.A. and Thatcher, W.W. (2007) Evaluation of the efficacy of prophylactic hoof health examination and trimming during midlactation in reducing the incidence of lameness during late lactation in dairy cows. *Journal of the American Veterinary Medical Association* 230, 89–93.

Hirst, W.M., Murray, R.D., Ward, W.R. and French, N.P. (2002) A mixed-effects time-to-event analysis of the relationship between first-lactation lameness and subsequent lameness in dairy cows in the UK. *Preventive Veterinary Medicine* 54, 191–201.

Hoedemaker, M., Prange, D. and Gundelach, Y. (2009) Body condition change ante- and postpartum, health and reproductive performance in German Holstein cows. *Reproduction in Domestic Animals* 44, 167–173.

Hultgren, J., Manske, T. and Bergsten, C. (2004) Associations of sole ulcer at claw trimming with reproductive performance, udder health, milk yield and culling Swedish dairy cattle. *Preventive Veterinary Medicine* 62, 233–251.

Huzzey, J.M., DeVries, T.J., Valois, P. and von Keyserlingk, M.A.G. (2006) Stocking density and feed barrier design affect the feeding and social behaviour of dairy cattle. *Journal of Dairy Science* 89, 126–133.

Ito, K., Weary, D.M. and von Keyserlingk, M.A.G. (2009) Lying behaviour. Assessing within- and between-herd variation in free-stall-housed dairy cows. *Journal of Dairy Science* 93, 4412–4420.

Laven, R.A. and Hunt, H. (2002) Evaluation of copper sulphate, formalin and peracetic acid in footbaths for the treatment of digital dermatitis in cattle. *Veterinary Record* 151, 144–146.

Laven, R.A. and Logue, D.N. (2006) Treatment strategies for digital dermatitis for the UK. *Veterinary Journal* 171, 79–88.

Leach, K.A., Offer, J.E., Svoboda, I. and Logue, D.N. (2005) Effects of type of forage fed to dairy heifers: Associations between claw characteristics, clinical lameness, environment and behaviour. *The Veterinary Journal* 169, 427–436.

Leach, K.A., Whay, H.R., Maggs, C.M., Barker, Z.E., Paul, E.S., Bell, A.K. *et al.* (2010a) Working towards a reduction in cattle lameness: 1. Understanding barriers to lameness control on dairy farms. *Research in Veterinary Science* 89, 311–317.

Leach, K.A., Whay, H.R., Maggs, C.M., Barker, Z.E., Paul, E.S., Bell, A.K. *et al.* (2010b) Working towards a reduction in cattle lameness: 2. Understanding dairy farmers' motivations. *Research in Veterinary Science* 89, 318–323.

Manske, T., Hultgren, J. and Bergsten, C. (2002) Prevalence and interrelationship of hoof lesions and lameness in Swedish dairy cows. *Preventive Veterinary Medicine* 54, 247–263.

Manson, F.J. and Leaver, J.D. (1986) Effect of hoof trimming and protein level on lameness in dairy cows. *Animal Production* 42, 451.

Manson, F.J. and Leaver, J.D. (1987) Effect of concentrate to silage ratio and hoof trimming on lameness in dairy-cows. *Animal Production* 44, 469.

Manson F.J. and Leaver J.D. (1988a) The influence of concentrate amount on locomotion and clinical lameness in dairy-cattle. *Animal Production* 47, 185–190.

Manson, F.J. and Leaver, J.D. (1988b) The influence of dietary-protein intake and of hoof trimming on lameness in dairy-cattle. *Animal Production* 47, 191–199.

Melendez, P., Bartolome, J., Archbald, L.F. and Donovan, A. (2003) The association between lameness, ovarian cysts and fertility in lactating dairy cattle. *Theriogenology* 59, 927–937.

Mill, J.M. and Ward, W.R. (1994) Lameness in dairy cows and farmers' knowledge, training and awareness. *Veterinary Record* 134, 162–164.

Murray, R.D., Downham, D.Y., Clarkson, M.J., Faull, W.B., Hughes, J.W., Manson, F.J. *et al.* (1996) Epidemiology of lameness in dairy cattle: Description and analysis of foot lesions. *Veterinary Record* 138, 586–591.

Nocek, J.E., Socha, M.T. and Tomlinson, D.J. (2006) The effect of trace mineral fortification level and source on performance of dairy cattle. *Journal of Dairy Science* 89, 2679–2693.

Nuss, K. and Paulus, N. (2006) Measurements of claw dimensions in cows before and after functional trimming: a post mortem study. *The Veterinary Journal* 172, 284–292.

O'Callaghan, K.A. (2002) Lameness and associated pain in cattle – Challenging traditional perceptions. *In Practice* 24, 212–219.

O'Callaghan, K.A., Cripps, P.J., Downham, D.Y. and Murray, R.D. (2003) Subjective and objective assessment of pain and discomfort due to lameness in dairy cattle. *Animal Welfare* 12, 605–610.

Offer, J.E., Fisher, G.E.J., Kempson, S.A. and Logue, D.N. (2001) The effect of feeding grass silage in early pregnancy on claw health during first lactation. *The Veterinary Journal* 161, 186–193.

Pötzsch, C.J., Collis, V.J., Blowey, R.W., Packington, A.J. and Green, L.E. (2003) The impact of parity and duration of biotin supplementation on white line disease lameness in dairy cattle. *Journal of Dairy Science* 86, 2577–2582.

Räber, M., Lischer, Ch.J., Geyer, H. and Ossent, P. (2004) The bovine digital cushion – a descriptive anatomical study. *The Veterinary Journal* 167, 258–264.

Räber, M., Scheeder, M.R.L., Ossent, P., Lischer, Ch.J. and Geyer, H. (2006) The content and composition of lipids in the digital cushion of the bovine claw with respect to age and location – A preliminary report. *The Veterinary Journal* 172, 173–177.

Rajkondawar, P.G., Liu, M., Dyer, R.M., Neerchal, N.K., Tasch, U., Lefcourt, A.M. *et al.* (2006) Comparison of models to identify lame cows based on gait and lesion scores, and limb movement variables. *Journal of Dairy Science* 89, 4267–4275.

Reader, J.D., Green, M.J., Kaler, J., Mason, S.A. and Green, L.E. (2011) Effect of mobility score on milk yield and activity in dairy cattle. *Journal of Dairy Science* 94, 5045–5052.

Rodriguez-Lainz, A., David, W.H., Carpenter, T.E. and Read, D.H. (1996) Case-control study of papillomatous digital dermatitis in southern California dairy farms. *Preventive Veterinary Medicine* 28, 117–131.

Rodriguez-Lainz, A., Melednez-Retamal, P., Hird, D.W., Read, D.H. and Walker, R.L. (1999) Farm and host-level risk factors for papillomatous digital dermatitis in Chilean dairy cattle. *Preventive Veterinary Medicine* 42, 87–97.

Rushen, J., Pombourcq, E. and de Passile, A.M. (2007) Validation of two measures of lameness in dairy cows. *Applied Animal Behaviour Science* 106, 173–177.

Siciliano-Jones, J.L., Socha, M.T., Tomlinson, D.J. and DeFrain J.M. (2008) Effect of trace mineral source on lactation performance, claw integrity and fertility of dairy cattle. *Journal of Dairy Science* 91, 1985–1995.

Sood, P. and Nanda, A.S. (2006) Effect of lameness on oestrus behaviour in crossbred cows. *Theriogenology* 66, 1375–1380.

Speijers, M.H.M., Baird, L.G., Finney, G.A., McBride, J., Kilpatrick, D.J., Logue, D.J. *et al.* (2010) Effectiveness of different footbath solutions in the treatment of digital dermatitis in dairy cows. *Journal of Dairy Science* 93, 5782–5791.

Sprecher, D.J., Hostetler, D.E. and Kaneene, J.B. (1997) A lameness scoring system that uses posture and gait to predict dairy cattle reproductive performance. *Theriogenology* 47, 1179–1187.

Suriyasathaporn, W., Nielen, M., Dieleman, S.J., Brand, A., Noordhuizen-Stassen, E.N. and Schukken, Y.H. (1998) A Cox proportional-hazards model with time-dependent covariates to evaluate the relationship between body-condition score and the risks of first insemination and pregnancy in a high-producing dairy herd. *Preventive Veterinary Medicine* 37, 159–172.

Tadich, N., Flor, E. and Green, L.E. (2010) Associations between hoof lesions and locomotion score in 1098 unsound dairy cows. *The Veterinary Journal* 184, 60–65.

Tarlton, J.F., Holah, D.E., Evans, K.M., Jones, S., Pearson, G.R. and Webster, A.J.F. (2002) Biomechanical and histopathological changes in the support structures of bovine hooves around the time of first calving. *Veterinary Journal* 163, 196–204.

Telzhenko, E. and Bergsten, C. (2005) Influence of floor type on the locomotion of dairy cows. *Applied Animal Behaviour Science* 93, 183–197.

Telzhenko, E., Lidfors, L. and Bergsten, C. (2007) Dairy cow preferences for soft or hard flooring when standing or walking. *Journal of Dairy Science* 90, 3716–3724.

Toussaint Raven, E. (1985) *Cattle Footcare and Claw Trimming*. Farming Press, Ltd, Ipswich, UK.

Tranter, W.P. and Morris, R.S. (1991) A case-study of lameness in 3 dairy herds. *New Zealand Veterinary Journal* 39, 88–96.

Van Amstel, S.R., Shearer, J.K. and Palin, F.L. (2004) Moisture content, thickness, and lesions of sole horn associated with thin soles in dairy cattle. *Journal of Dairy Science* 87, 757–763.

Watson, C.L. (1997) The role of antibiotics in arthritis and foot diseases. *Cattle Practice* 5, 109.

Wells, S.J., Trent, A.M., Marsh, W.E. and Robinson, R.A. (1993) Prevalence and severity of lameness in lactating dairy cows in a sample of Minnesota and Wisconsin herds. *Journal of the Veterinary Medical Association* 202, 78–82.

Wells, S.J., Garber, L.P. and Wagner, B.A. (1999) Papillomatous digital dermatitis and associated risk factors in US dairy herds. *Preventive Veterinary Medicine* 38, 11–24.

Whay, H.R., Waterman, A.E. and Webster, A.J.F. (1997) Associations between locomotion, claw lesion and nociceptive threshold in dairy heifers during the peri-partum period. *The Veterinary Journal* 154, 155–161.

Whay, H.R., Waterman, A.E., Webster, A.J.F. and O'Brien, J.K. (1998) The influence of lesion type on the duration of hyperalgesia associated with hindlimb lameness in dairy cattle. *The Veterinary Journal* 156, 23–29.

Whay, H.R., Main, D.C.J., Green, L.E. and Webster, A.J.F. (2003) Assessment of the welfare of dairy cattle using animal-based measurements: direct observations and investigation of farm records. *Veterinary Record* 153, 197–202.

Willshire, J.A. and Bell, N.J. (2009) An economic review of cattle lameness. *Cattle Practice* 17, 136–141.

Winckler, C. and Willen, S. (2001) The reliability and repeatability of a lameness scoring system for use as an indicator of welfare in dairy cattle. *Acta Agriculturae Scandinavica, Section A - Animal Science* 51, 103–107.

# 7 Control of Infectious Disease

**Laura Green,[1] Simon Archer,[2] Andrew Biggs,[5] Andrew Bradley,[2,3]**
**James Breen,[2,3] Peter Down,[2] Martin Green,[2] Mike Kerby,[4]**
**Gerdien van Schaik[6] and Wendela Wapenaar[2]**

[1]*School of Life Sciences, Gibbet Hill Campus, The University of Warwick, Coventry
CV4 7AL, UK;* [2]*School of Veterinary Medicine and Science, University of Nottingham,
Sutton Bonington Campus, Leicestershire LE12 5RD, UK;* [3]*QMMS Limited, Cedar Barn,
Easton Hill, Caston, Wells BA5 IDU, UK;* [4]*Delaware Veterinary Group, Fulford House,
Torbay Road, Castle Cary, Somerset BA7 7DT, UK;* [5]*The Vale Veterinary Centre, The
Laurels, Tiverton, Devon EX16 4LF, UK;* [6]*GD Animal Health Service, PO Box 9, 7400
AA, Deventer, The Netherlands*

## Introduction

This chapter focuses on the control of infectious diseases in dairy herds. It is beyond the scope of the book to describe in detail the entire collection of infectious agents and their aetiology, pathogenesis, treatment and control. Instead, our aim is to highlight the key principles of infectious disease control that apply to all endemic infectious diseases when conducting herd health. As examples of the application of these principles, throughout this chapter we consider the control of the following important infectious diseases: mycobacterium paratuberculosis (MAP or Johne's disease), bovine viral diarrhoea (BVD), infectious bovine rhinotracheitis (IBR), bovine leptospirosis, bovine tuberculosis (bTB) and neosporosis.

## Principles of infectious disease control

No herd can ever be free from all disease and it is crucial that whole-herd management is not an alternative to the care of individual sick animals in the herd requiring treatment to optimize health and welfare. In addition, rapid treatment of an individual sick animal with an infectious disease can reduce the period of infectiousness and so reduce transmission from the diseased individual to herd-mates. Isolation of infectious animals while they are treated can further reduce transmission of the pathogen if the individual is infectious. Therefore, individual cow treatment and isolation contribute to herd control of infectious diseases.

An appreciation of how infectious diseases are transmitted between cows is essential in deciding the best methods for control of each disease. Important aspects of disease dynamics are described below.

## Introduction of a new pathogen

A new pathogen can be introduced into a naïve herd via infectious cows, other host species or host products, such as hide or milk. It can also enter through vectors such as insects, or via fomites such as vehicles or boots. However, conspecifics (cows) are often the most likely source of infection for other cows and therefore a closed herd is the best way to prevent introduction of an infection. When cattle are purchased, they should preferably originate from a herd free from specific pathogens or the animal itself should be diagnosed as being free from the infection. Additionally, cattle should be kept in quarantine until proved free from the infection. Note that quarantine facilities need to be sufficiently far from the herd, with separate care for quarantined cows, to prevent infection transmitting to the main herd. To ensure that quarantine is successful it needs to be of a sufficiently long duration to prevent introduction of the pathogen. In quarantine, the pathogen will either die out or the disease will manifest when affected cows should be managed accordingly (treatment, culling, delayed entry to the herd). There are certain pathogens for which a single-animal test result or quarantine is unlikely to prevent introduction of disease, because of either long incubation period or poor test sensitivity (e.g. MAP).

All of the above also holds true for the *reintroduction* of an existing pathogen. Although we might not notice reintroduction if a pathogen is already present on a farm, it is worth noting that intermittent reintroduction is an important route for persistence of pathogens within a population (e.g. bTB). In this case, pathogens are moving in a metapopulation, that is, herds of cows linked by some degree of contact.

### Spread of a new pathogen within a herd

Once in a herd, the pathogen spreads through susceptible cows by one or more routes (e.g. respiratory, oral-faecal, vector). The average number of secondary cases from one infectious individual in a naïve population is termed the reproduction number, Ro, (Anderson and May, 1991). While Ro is specific to pathogen, time and place (i.e. the value of Ro might vary between herds infected with the same pathogen), it can also be used as a guide to tell us whether on average one infectious host infects many or few cows. However, it does not tell us the time over which this occurs, and for this we

need the average infectious period (e.g. for BVD this is relatively short in adult cattle while for MAP it is relatively long).

Hosts move through a variety of states in relation to a pathogen. They may be susceptible, then infectious and then, depending on the nature of the pathogen and host, the host might die, become resistant, partially resistant (i.e. can be infected again), a carrier or become susceptible again. The susceptible, infective, recovered (SIR) model is a framework used to describe this process for infectious diseases with lifelong immunity. There are very few endemic diseases with such simple transmission process and host immunity, and modifications of the SIR model have therefore been developed. Mathematical models are specific for a particular pathogen and can be used to further our understanding of the transmission process (Green and Medley, 2002). In many countries mathematical and statistical models of disease are increasingly being used to inform policy decisions when managing an incursion of an exotic disease and to understand endemic diseases (Carslake *et al.*, 2011).

### Persistence of a pathogen within a herd

As a new pathogen spreads through a herd, cows become infected and the number of susceptible cows declines. Persistence of a pathogen arises when the pathogen remains sufficiently long in a population to encounter new susceptible hosts (arising through purchase, birth or waning immunity). Pathogens have several strategies that facilitate persistence: they can persist in the host (e.g. herpes viruses such as IBR), in another host species (e.g. bTB in wildlife) or in the environment (e.g. *Salmonella* spp.). Over time a disease may become endemic in a herd or metapopulation (see below), with each infectious individual infecting on average one susceptible individual and the prevalence of the disease becoming stable. In addition, the disease often becomes less severe, and this also aids persistence: it is in the pathogen's interest for the host to survive for sufficiently long to transmit the pathogen to other susceptible hosts.

Routes for persistence of a pathogen are an important consideration when deciding whether to eliminate or control a disease, because pathogens that persist in several host species (e.g. bTB, MAP) or in the environment (e.g. MAP) are much more difficult to eliminate from a herd than pathogens that are host specific (e.g. BVD, IBR).

## The spread of infectious diseases between herds

Cows are typically kept in fairly small herds or populations (50–1000). Generally, infectious diseases cluster within herds, i.e. they occur at a higher or lower incidence than by chance when compared with the population average. The risk of introduction of a new pathogen or reintroduction of an existing pathogen into a herd is dependent on how the pathogen spreads (as described above) and on how the populations are connected. This connection of herds is a metapopulation and the contact between herds determines the pattern of transmission of a pathogen between herds. Determining herd contacts is a critical element of disease control, and for dairy herds common contacts are purchased cows, cows or cow products from neighbouring farms, buying and sharing bulls, movements of cows to and from markets and shows and movement of people between herds (friends, relatives, neighbours and professionals such as vets or hoof trimmers).

The total proportion of herds in a metapopulation infected with a specific pathogen is an important consideration when deciding whether to eliminate or control a disease, because herds where a disease has been eliminated are at high risk of reintroduction of the pathogen if that herd is in a metapopulation where most herds are infected.

## Principles of Infectious Disease Control

Management of infectious diseases can include maintaining freedom from disease by preventing introduction, elimination (removal from the herd, region, country/ state or larger area, e.g. EU), eradication (removal worldwide, e.g. rinderpest) or control (minimizing impact on host health). Freedom from disease is an ideal that is achieved for some diseases and is an aspiration for others; the European Union (EU) has a list of diseases that have been eliminated or are targeted for elimination in the EU (e.g. foot-and-mouth disease (FMD), bTB). However, such a policy comes at a cost – incursions of exotic diseases are expensive because populations are entirely susceptible and therefore the impact of disease on the health of the animals is severe, and also because of the costs incurred in stamping out the incursion (e.g. FMD in the UK in 2000–2001). Management of endemic diseases to achieve elimination is also expensive – the UK currently spends over half its animal health budget on control of bTB, with the aim of elimination. Elimination of BVD and IBR has been achieved by some countries through nationwide programmes of testing, segregation of diseased and healthy herds and ultimately compulsory removal of persistently infected herds. Scotland has recently started a BVD elimination programme. Such programmes receive investment from the state and/or farmers and have a body to oversee the process. It is unlikely that a voluntary programme, where individual farmers opt into a scheme to eliminate a disease, would be successful because free-riders (farmers benefitting from other farmers investing in elimination) arise. An external organization, monitoring and standard setting are required.

## Elimination of a disease from a herd

It is possible for farmers to eliminate certain pathogens from their herd although the metapopulation prevalence needs to be considered, as explained above. We need to understand how a pathogen spreads and persists in order to be able to deliver control strategies. The nature of the pathogen, host range, transmission routes, environment, accuracy of diagnostic tests, vaccines available and herd attributes need to be considered before deciding to eliminate a disease.

We can eliminate disease by culling the whole herd if the pathogen persists only in the cows, rather than in the environment or other hosts, and if the replacement herd can be sourced from known disease-free stock. We can also eliminate disease, more cost effectively, by removing infected individuals through a test-and-cull strategy. These are effective when the inter-test interval is shorter than the latent period (time from infection to infectiousness) such that all infected individuals are removed before they become infectious. At a minimum, a test-and-cull interval has to result on average in one infectious individual infecting fewer than one other individual. One issue with the test-and-cull strategy for bTB in the UK is that the latent period is highly variable and therefore some individuals are likely to become infectious in the inter-test interval, especially as this increases to 4 years in perceived low-risk areas. It is important to note that, when successful, restocking or test-and-cull strategies lead to a totally susceptible population and so the herd is very vulnerable to reintroduction of disease.

Elimination of a disease can also be achieved by ensuring that there are no susceptible hosts until the pathogen has died out. This is usually done by vaccination. A vaccine that prevents transmission of the pathogen removes susceptible individuals and raises herd immunity, which might be sufficient to eliminate the pathogen and ultimately lead to cessation of vaccine use. Some vaccines control disease, but cattle still shed the pathogen and so elimination is not possible using these vaccines. Even quite poor vaccines can be effective if used strategically; the aim is to ensure that a sufficient proportion of a herd is protected against

disease at all times, in order to protect the herd at a level that provides herd immunity.

### Control of a disease in a herd

Control of disease starts with excellent husbandry to ensure that hosts are healthy and well fed and kept in hygienic conditions (fields or buildings), and that their exposure to the pathogen is minimized or timed to lead to good immunity without disease. In addition, vaccination, strategic culling and other management methods can be used for further control of disease. This is discussed further using examples of common endemic diseases (see final section on disease control).

There are certain measurements that contribute information when deciding how to control an infectious disease, and these are discussed below.

MEASURING DISEASE.    The two most important measures of disease in the context of herd health are prevalence and incidence rate (see equations at bottom of page).

These two measures are linked by the duration of disease such that

Prevalence = incidence × duration.

For example, in practice, a herd might have fewer than two cases of mastitis per 100 cows on one day (prevalence) but the incidence rate might be 50 cases/100 cows/ year. This means that the average duration of mastitis would be estimated as 0.04 years (~14 days) per case. Similarly, the prevalence of MAP might be two cases per 100 cows on one day but the incidence rate might be one case/100 cows/year, and this means that the average duration of disease would be 2 years.

---

$$\text{Prevalence} = \frac{\text{number of diseased individuals at a point or period of time}}{\text{number of animals in the population}}$$

$$\text{Incidence rate} = \frac{\text{number of new cases of disease}}{\text{number of animals at risk (i.e. susceptible)}} \text{ per unit time}$$

Incidence rate can be a challenging measurement in dairy herds because denominators are often small (50–200) and the number of cattle in a particular risk group even smaller (e.g. in a herd with BVD there might be 80% of cattle immune, and so the denominator is the remaining 20% of susceptible cattle). This means that incidence rates can become very large (e.g. 5 new cases out of 20 susceptible cattle = an incidence rate of 25/100 cattle/time unit).

It is important to consider both incidence and prevalence when thinking about disease control, because these measure different properties of the disease process: prevalence relates to the pool of diseased animals (the potential reservoir of infection) whereas incidence rate provides information on the rate of new cases.

The relative risk can be calculated from the incidence rate (see equation at bottom of page) (e.g. Exposure might be to an infectious individual, a field, a diet or at a stage of production, etc.).

For example, if 5 cows/100 develop mastitis in the first week after calving and 2/95 develop mastitis in the second week after calving then the relative risk = (5/100) ÷ (2/95) ~ 2.5. We can conclude that cattle have a 2.5-fold risk of developing mastitis in the first week after calving compared with the second. We cannot conclude that this is causal (indeed it is highly unlikely to be directly causal) but that there is an association, and we can then evaluate why this risk is occurring.

We can also calculate an attributable risk – this is a useful measure when estimating the possible impact of a change in management:

Attributable risk = incidence rate of disease in cattle exposed
− incidence rate in cattle unexposed

Using the example above, if the risk of developing mastitis in the first week after calving could be reduced to a risk similar to that two weeks after calving, then ~3 cases of mastitis would be prevented (NB: not all 5 cases).

## Diagnostic Tests

To measure a disease, we need an accurate case definition for that disease and this is often supported by diagnostic tests. It is common to make decisions on the results of diagnostic tests (whether clinical signs, laboratory tests or a combination of both) without reflecting on their accuracy. A perfect test that correctly identifies all diseased cattle as diseased and all non-diseased cattle as non-diseased is termed the gold standard. For many diseases there is no gold standard and we use tests that do not always produce the correct results. This arises for a variety of reasons: (i) some diseases do not lead to development of antibodies in all hosts or until late in the disease process, which lowers their sensitivity (e.g. bTB, MAP); and (ii) some tests cross-react with other antibodies, which lowers their specificity (e.g. MAP vaccine and bTB). There are several measures that we need to be aware of, in order to assess the usefulness and appropriateness of a diagnostic test, two of which are its sensitivity and specificity.

### Test sensitivity and specificity

The sensitivity is the proportion of truly positive (either infected or diseased) cows that are defined as positive by the test.

The specificity is the proportion of truly negative (not infected) cows that are defined as negative by the test.

For most practical purposes, the sensitivity and specificity of a test are independent

$$\text{Relative risk} = \frac{\text{incidence rate of disease in cattle exposed}}{\text{incidence rate in cattle unexposed}}$$

from the prevalence of disease and are consistent across populations. Manufacturers of a diagnostic test should provide its sensitivity (tested on known infected individuals) and specificity (tested on known uninfected individuals) and a reference as to how these were estimated.

When the test results arrive we do not know which animals are correctly classified and which are incorrectly classified. For example, if we have a (fictitious) test for MAP with a sensitivity of 40% and a specificity of 90%, and if some cows in a herd *truly* have MAP, then we can expect the test to identify 40% of the *truly* infected cows and 90% of the *truly* uninfected cows: 60% of infected cows would be defined as uninfected (i.e. false-negatives) and 10% of uninfected cows would be defined as infected (i.e. false-positives). If we forget to consider test sensitivity and specificity, we might make an incorrect decision about the management of an individual or a herd. For example, if we suspect that there is MAP in a herd and we test one cow that truly has MAP with our fictitious test above, then there is a 60% chance that the test result would be negative. By testing two cows, this error reduces to 36% (0.60 × 0.60); by testing ten cows, there is >0.1% risk of incorrectly identifying all ten cows as negative ($0.6^{10}$). For an individual cow, by retesting with the same test (assuming that the test error is due to chance rather than a host-specific characteristic), we can increase our chance of identifying a true positive from 40 to 64% (i.e. 100–36%).

Similarly, a cow that is *truly* negative will, at the first test, have a 10% chance of testing positive. The chance that a cow tests negative twice when she is positive is 1% (0.1 × 0.1); thus we have a 1% chance that we can claim that a truly negative cow is positive for MAP.

What do we do when a cow tests positive to one test and negative to another? We have to decide whether we want to raise the sensitivity (define a cow as infected if any test is positive) or specificity (define a cow as uninfected if any test is negative). We can also use a different second test with a different sensitivity and specificity. For example,

we might choose a sensitive test initially to ensure that all truly positive cows are identified, accepting that some cows that are false-positives will be included, then use a more specific test to identify the truly negative cows.

*Test sensitivity and specificity are linked*

For most tests with a cut-off value that determines a positive or negative result, as sensitivity increases specificity decreases. If we have this information, we can use it to our advantage. We can alter a diagnostic test's sensitivity and specificity by altering the cut-off value used to define positive and negative test results. For example, if we want to select only disease-free individuals, we can choose a cut-off that makes a test highly sensitive, so that all truly affected individuals are indeed test-positive (i.e. 100% sensitivity). Inevitably, test specificity will be low and there will be individuals that are false-positives. However, we can select our disease-negative cows from the group that are test-negative with a high degree of confidence that they are truly negative. Conversely, there are occasions when we would want a highly specific test. If we decide to cull pedigree cows with a disease, we might not wish to cull cows that are true negatives for this disease because of the economic losses, so we might choose a specific test. This does of course raise the concern that we might fail to eliminate the disease because a high specificity (associated with a relatively low sensitivity) will mean that some truly positive animals are not identified. A useful example here is the use of somatic cell count (SCC) as a measure of intra-mammary infection (see Chapter 5). When purchasing a cow where we need to be sure that no intra-mammary infection is present, it is usually wise to increase test sensitivity by using a relatively low threshold for SCC (e.g. <50,000 or 100,000 cells/ml). This reduces the chance that the cow will have an intra-mammary infection (i.e. is a false-negative) but at the cost of discarding cows with a higher SCC (e.g. 100,000–200,000 cells/ml) that may be uninfected. Conversely, when considering culling a cow with an intra-mammary infection, a higher SCC threshold would be used to increase test specificity (e.g. several tests might be used with a threshold of 200,000–400,000 cells/ ml), and this minimizes the removal of truly uninfected (false-positive) cows.

## Predictive value of a test

Repeating a test or using a second test on a subset of cows to improve decision making is effective, because by taking a group of cows already positive to a test we are increasing the proportion of the sample that are test-positive, i.e. we 'increase' the prevalence of the disease. The result of this is that we increase the positive predictive value of the test.

• The positive predictive value of a test is the probability that a cow has a disease given that it has a positive test result. The positive predictive value of a diagnostic test increases as prevalence increases for a given test sensitivity.
• The negative predictive value of a test is the probability that a cow without a disease has a negative test result, and this increases as the prevalence of the disease decreases.

If disease prevalence is very low, then the positive predictive value of a test is low and vice versa. After some consideration, this becomes intuitive. Considering a test that is 97% specific (i.e. 3% false-positives), we will get 3% positive test results even in a population free from disease. This is important in decisions on disease control. Let us consider our test for MAP above with a sensitivity of 40% and specificity of 90%. If the prevalence of disease is 2%, then <10% of test-positive individuals will be true positives. If the prevalence is 30%, the positive predictive value of the test will be >60%; fewer test-positive cows will be false-positives. This has implications for control: if our decision is to remove test-positive individuals from the herd, most test-positive cattle will be truly negative if the prevalence of disease is very low. We can reduce the

proportion of false-positive cows culled if we use several tests, but it is unwise to use an imprecise test in such a situation because it is not possible to know which of the test positives are truly negative.

In the UK, by the 1960s bTB had become controlled to a level where <1% herds were considered infected. As well as great celebrations at the success of the control programme, a decision was made to test herds less often and to remove restrictions that prevented the selling of cattle from infected herds to uninfected herds. This change was made because the control measures were expensive, and most cows positive to the skin test were false-positives; however, bTB had not been eliminated and one explanation for the increase in herd break down seen from the 1960s onwards is likely to be the increase in inter-test interval and the ability to move cattle from infected to uninfected herds.

It is worth noting here that care should be taken in relation to the interpretation of a test-positive result because this will vary by disease. For example, an adult cow that has antibodies to BVD is immune to the disease, while one with antibodies to MAP or neosporosis is infected and possibly infectious.

## Estimating the presence and prevalence of disease

One question of interest for herd health programmes is whether a disease is present or absent from a herd and, if present, at what prevalence. If we wish to be confident that a disease is absent from a herd, we could test every individual in the herd. This is usually prohibitively expensive and unnecessary if we are prepared to compromise slightly. We can use statistical theory to estimate how many cows we need to sample to decide, with a given certainty, whether a disease is present, or present at a specified prevalence. This is an important concept in herd health and defines the number of animals to test to establish the presence or prevalence of disease. We refer the reader to Appendix 1, where we provide further details and a method for estimating the number of cows to be tested in different herd scenarios.

## Monitoring Infectious Disease

The veterinary herd health advisor needs to work with clients to develop a farm-specific protocol to monitor infectious diseases, alongside routine monitoring of fertility performance, udder health, foot health and metabolic disease.

The first indication of a new disease is likely to be individual cows presenting with unusual or unexpected clinical signs, and farmers need to be aware that they should alert their advisor immediately rather than waiting for several animals to become ill. Prompt recognition of an unusual presentation might indicate an epidemic of an endemic or exotic disease. Thorough evaluation of individual sick cows represents a form of monitoring for infectious disease that should not be overlooked. This can be extended to dead cows at post-mortem and cull cows at meat inspection (where a farmer receives feedback from the abattoir); for example, subclinical or clinical disease such as a thickened intestine in MAP might be identified and this might lead to further herd testing.

Veterinary practitioners often recognize clinical presentations indicative of endemic infectious diseases in individual cows, such as chronic diarrhoea and weight loss in MAP or abortion suggestive of BVD. In a herd health context, however, it is important to establish the prevalence of infectious diseases within a herd where there are no obvious signs of disease and to decide whether a disease is present and how the disease should be managed (prevention, control or elimination). Farmer compliance with such management will vary, and a monitoring and control programme will be farm specific unless there are compulsory control programmes set by region or country.

### Principles of detecting infectious diseases

There are many ways to detect infection in dairy herds. These include measuring antigen or antibody in individual or pooled blood or faeces samples or individual or bulk milk samples and, most recently, antigen in tissue samples. The development of new diagnostics is rapid and advisors need to keep abreast of new developments. This is often best achieved through consultation with a specialist laboratory that will be able to supply details of the best current testing methods (as well as test characteristics such as sensitivity and specificity).

### Which common infectious diseases should be considered?

Deciding which infectious diseases to monitor in a herd health programme is not straightforward and should be regularly re-evaluated. It will depend on factors including (i) the infectious diseases present in a country or region; (ii) the risk of a new infectious disease entering a location; (iii) the importance of specific diseases to the market place (e.g. a requirement to be free from certain diseases); (iv) farm-specific management/policies (e.g. an open or closed herd); and (v) the farm history of specific infectious diseases. We consider six example diseases in detail at the end of this chapter: MAP, BVD, IBR, bovine leptospirosis, neosporosis and bTB, and in Table 7.1 we list the common infectious diseases of cattle that may require monitoring in a herd health programme.

### Detecting infectious diseases

Infectious diseases can be monitored by detecting antigen (micro parasites such as viruses, bacteria, protozoa or macroparasites such as fluke, worm eggs or adults, and external parasites such as ticks or lice) or an immune response to the antigen, typically antibody, but for some diseases specific interferon gamma. Detection of antigen clearly indicates current infection and usually infectiousness. Detection of antibody can indicate vaccination (unless a marker vaccine and test is available), exposure (past or present) and might also indicate immunity or infection, depending on the pathogen. For example, an adult cow with

**Table 7.1.** Infectious diseases of cattle that may require monitoring in a herd health programme.[a]

| Agent | Disease |
|---|---|
| Viral | Bovine viral diarrhoea (see later section on control) |
| | Infectious bovine rhinotracheitis (see later section on control) |
| | Infectious teat lesions (e.g. bovine papilloma virus, pseudocowpox virus, bovine herpesvirus 2; visual assessment or virus isolation) |
| Bacterial | Leptospirosis (see later section on control) |
| | Salmonellosis |
| | Johne's disease (see later section on control) |
| | Bovine tuberculosis (see later section on control) |
| | Digital dermatitis (see Chapter 6) |
| | Contagious intra-mammary pathogens (see Chapter 5) |
| | *Campylobacter venerealis* (see Chapter 5) |
| | Clostridial diseases |
| Protozoal | Neosporosis (see later section on control) |
| Parasitic | *Fasciola hepatica* (see Chapter 3) |
| | Parasitic gastroenteritis (see Chapter 3) |
| | *Dictyocaulus* (see Chapter 3) |
| | Lice/mange |
| Fungal | Dermatophytosis (ringworm) |
| Mixed | Calf pneumonia complex (see Chapter 3) |
| | Calf diarrhoea (see Chapter 3) |

[a] Depending on local disease status, monitoring might also include anaplasmosis, Aujeszky's disease, babesiosis, besnoitiosis, bovine leucosis, blue tongue virus, brucellosis, contagious bovine pleuropneumonia, enzootic disease, foot-and-mouth disease, infectious bovine keratoconjunctivitis, Lyme disease, parafilaria, rabies, Schmallenberg virus, tick-borne fever and warble fly.

antibodies to BVD has been exposed to BVD virus (BVDV) and has developed immunity, while one with detectable antigen is currently infected with BVDV (either transiently or as a persistently infected animal). Cattle with antibodies to *Mycobacterium avium* subsp. *paratuberculosis* or *Neospora caninum* are infected with these pathogens and are not immune.

Several methods are available for the detection of infectious diseases in individuals or the herd, and each has advantages and disadvantages. Testing individual cows is necessary to detect seroconversion or recent infection, with paired samples demonstrating a rise in antibody titre. This can be done using blood samples, but is relatively expensive compared with using milk samples and, where the test allows, milk is an efficient alternative to blood.

Individual and bulk milk samples provide an easily accessible route for monitoring lactating cows. There is generally good correlation between serum and milk antibodies,

and testing is simple and cheap to perform. Individual cow samples can be tested when milk is collected for other routine procedures, e.g. SCC. By pooling milk the antibody status of a particular group can be tested cheaply (e.g. a group of purchased cattle or cattle in a particular age group). Milk antibody can be used to test whether a cow/herd has been exposed to a particular disease (i.e. positive or negative) and to assess disease prevalence/transmission over time.

Bulk milk testing (BMT) is often used in regional control programmes for specific diseases, e.g. BVD. It can be used to detect antibody or antigen and to categorize herds as having a negative, low, medium or high prevalence of infection. For regional programmes and individual herds, samples over time ensure that the current herd status is known and that changes in status are detected (e.g. BVD antibodies might increase after newly calved heifers start lactating). Bulk milk testing is not reliable as a one-off test, and patterns over time are needed to identify trends and avoid over-interpretation of sudden changes – the population of lactating cows changes over time and a spike or drop in bulk milk antibody might arise from newly calved individual cows contributing large or small amounts of antibody. Bulk milk testing cannot be used in isolation to monitor diseases: in large herds, antibodies from small numbers of infected cows might not be detected because of dilution in the bulk milk. Finally, only lactating animals contribute to the pool; non-lactating cows or lactating cows under treatment milked separately are just as important when monitoring infectious disease.

Individual or pooled faeces samples for PCR or bacterial culture are easy and cheap to obtain, but test sensitivities are often well below 100%. As with serum or milk, pooled samples do not identify individually infected animals and culture can be slow compared with antibody tests.

Most recently, tests have been developed to detect antigen in tissue, and currently this is used to detect calves persistently infected with BVDV. When calves are identified with an ear tag a small sample of tissue is collected into a pot from the tag site. This can then be used to test for the presence of BVDV RNA.

## Control of Infectious Disease: General Concepts

The general approach to control of infectious disease in dairy herd health is similar to that of non-infectious disease (see Fig. 1.1, Chapter 1): evaluate herd goals, assess current disease status, set up control measures, monitor and re-evaluate. However, with infectious diseases, cows not only succumb to a condition (as, for example, with sole ulcer or subacute ruminal acidosis), they also contribute to disease dynamics. Therefore, for infectious diseases, management of cows according to infection status forms a key component of disease control. This means that herd screening, culling, treatment, isolation, vaccination, external and internal

biosecurity and continuous monitoring and re-evaluation all play pivotal roles. A summary of a general approach to the management of infectious disease in dairy herds is provided in Fig. 7.1. Biosecurity is of particular importance for control of infectious disease, and this is described in detail in the next section.

### Biosecurity in dairy herds

Biosecurity refers to measures that prevent the transmission of pathogens to individuals or groups of animals between and within herds. It is a central component of infectious disease control.

The herd health advisor should investigate herd biosecurity measures and evaluate their efficacy. Appropriate biosecurity might change over time, and regular reappraisal as herd circumstances change is recommended.

Important routes of introduction of pathogens into a herd are:

- purchased cattle;
- cattle returning to the farm (e.g. growing heifers);
- contact with cattle from neighbouring farms;
- contact with cattle products (e.g. slurry from neighbouring farms);
- contamination of feedstuffs and water;
- vectors (e.g. flies); and
- fomites (e.g. vehicles, stockpersons).

Important routes for persistence of pathogens within a herd are:

- contact with infectious cattle (clinically and subclinically diseased and treated and untreated);
- contact with feedstuffs and water contaminated by infectious cattle;
- contact with infectious cattle products (e.g. faeces, milk);
- contact between infectious cattle/products and susceptible animals arising from birth, purchase or cattle returning to the farm (e.g. growing heifers);
- vectors (e.g. flies) spreading disease;

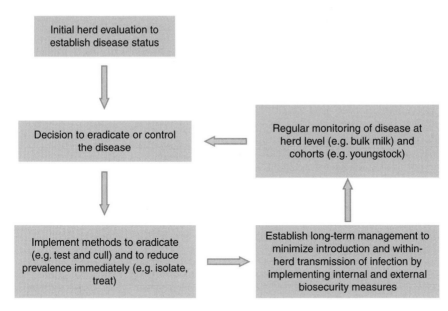

**Fig. 7.1.** Outline of a general approach to the control of infectious disease in dairy herd health.

- fomites (e.g. vehicles, stockpersons) spreading disease; and
- reintroduction of a pathogen from brought-in cattle.

Because each herd has different disease status, goals and ambitions and levels of stockmanship, a herd-specific biosecurity plan is important. Farmers are increasingly familiar with phrases such as biosecurity and closed herd, but might not use these words to mean the same as a trained advisor. It is worth probing and asking precise questions to ensure that you and your client understand each other, to avoid errors that lead to the introduction or reintroduction of disease. For example, many cattle farmers in the UK state that their herd is closed but, when specifically asked whether they buy or borrow bulls, state that they do. In addition, in some areas it is customary to purchase some of a neighbour's cows or equipment when a farm is sold, and farmers do this despite biosecurity risks.

A recommended strategy to develop a herd biosecurity plan is described in Box 7.1.

## Practical Implementation of Infectious Disease Control: Disease Examples

While it is not possible to describe the control of every infectious disease, we use the framework described earlier in the chapter to compare and contrast the control of six common diseases of dairy cows, to illustrate how this framework can be applied to diseases with a range of routes for transmission and persistence and varying diagnostic test accuracy. As before, the example diseases are MAP, BVD, IBR, bovine leptospirosis, bTB and neosporosis. We assume a basic knowledge of the diseases and outline key features of transmission and control in Tables 7.2, 7.3 and 7.4.

### Control or eradication?

It is worth highlighting that national or regional control programmes override a farmer's individual management of certain diseases (e.g. bTB, BVD, IBR and MAP in some countries) and must be followed.

---

**Box 7.1.** A strategy to develop a biosecurity plan for infectious disease control in a dairy herd.

Step 1: Decide which infectious diseases are important for the herd (see Table 7.1)
Step 2: Define current herd status
   Use antibody and antigen testing to determine whether the herd is infected or naïve and whether infection is active or historical.
Step 3: Evaluate major transmission routes between herds for diseases specified in Step 1 and establish biosecurity measures to address risk. Common measures are:

**1.** Maintain a closed herd.
   • Avoid introduction of any cattle. No introduction of young animals, adult cows or bulls from other herds of cattle should be allowed and no contact with cattle from other herds should be possible (e.g. via cattle returning from shows or markets).
**2.** Where a herd is not closed:
   • Source cattle from herds known to be free from the infections of concern.
   • Isolate and test purchased animals: this may involve a complex testing protocol that should be fully discussed with the herd manager or owner *before* the animal(s) are purchased.
   • Vaccinate against common diseases with a dead vaccine (see individual disease sections).
**3.** Ensure the farm boundaries are secure with regard to other cattle (e.g. double fence, no shared access or pathways with other livestock).
**4.** Ensure that visitors moving onto the farm are kept to a minimum. Provide visitors with disposable overalls and disinfectant boot dips.
**5.** Ensure that equipment shared between farms is kept to a minimum and disinfected before being brought on to the farm.
**6.** Monitor feed and water quality, including manure spread onto pasture (e.g. MAP and *Clostridium botulinum*) and clamp silage quality (e.g. aspergillosis, *Listeria* spp.).
**7.** Ensure that vehicles unload in designated areas and are washed/disinfected before leaving the farm.
**8.** Minimize contact between other domestic species (e.g. dogs, to reduce neosporosis) and wildlife and the cattle herd.

Step 4: Internal biosecurity (to reduce within-herd transmission – 'biocontainment')

**1.** Vaccinate cattle against diseases present if possible (e.g. BVD, IBR).
**2.** Keep cattle in small group sizes to reduce spread of disease throughout the herd.
**3.** Avoid overstocking and potential increased risk of spread of pathogens.
**4.** Keep youngstock separate from the main herd and with the same external biosecurity measures applied.
**5.** Isolate diseased and infectious cattle: physically feed, house and manage animals separately; disinfect equipment such as milking clusters/liners.
**6.** Practise good parlour hygiene and management of cattle with mastitis (see Chapter 5).
**7.** Minimize contact between cattle and slurry.
**8.** Reduce environmental reservoirs of infection (slurry management, bedding management, remove stale air by improved ventilation).
**9.** Identify disease-specific measures (e.g. cull cattle with MAP, avoid keeping replacements from cattle with neosporosis (see later for details on individual diseases).

---

Otherwise, endemic diseases can be managed by the farmer and veterinary advisor, with advice from specialized laboratories as required.

Most endemic diseases are difficult to eliminate – if they were easy to eliminate then farmers would have already done so.

Elimination of a disease is possible when all locations of a pathogen can be detected and the pathogen can be removed from every location. It is more feasible when the pathogen is cattle-specific (e.g. BVD, IBR) and there is no alternative host (as there is for neosporosis and TB) or environmental

**Table 7.2.** Outline of disease testing/monitoring methods relevant for control of bovine viral diarrhoea (BVD), infectious bovine rhinotracheitis (IBR), leptospirosis, neosporosis and MAP (paratuberculosis, Johne's disease).

| | Diseases in order of decreasing ease of eradication | | | | |
| --- | --- | --- | --- | --- | --- |
| | BVD | IBR | Leptospirosis | Neosporosis | MAP |
| Samples available | Blood, tissue, milk, abortion products | Blood, milk, ocular/nasal swabs, bronchoalveolar lavage, abortion products | Blood, milk, urine, abortion products | Blood, abortion products | Blood, milk, faeces |
| Antigen/ pathogen identification | Tissue samples, milk, blood (care with maternal immunity in calves <6–8 months old) | Ocular/nasal secretions | Abortion products, urine | Abortion products | Faecal PCR |
| Testing for antibody | Blood, milk | Blood, milk | Blood, milk | Blood, milk | Blood, milk |
| Monitoring | Youngstock cohorts (test each batch for antibody – and antigen if antibody-positive animals are present), pooled or bulk milk (~3-monthly) | Age cohorts (to determine extent of spread within herd), pooled or bulk milk (~3-monthly) | Age cohorts (to determine extent of spread within herd), pooled or bulk milk (~3-monthly) | Blood test adult cows and calves (ideally pre-colostral); bulk milk serology | Regular (1–6-monthly) individual cow milk antibody testing; bulk milk antibody provides a guide to presence of disease but only a poor approximation of prevalence |
| Individual animal test sensitivity | Good | Good | Good | Good | Poor |
| Individual animal test specificity | Good | Good | Good | Good | Good |

reservoir (as there is for MAP, TB and leptospirosis). Test accuracy affects the ability to correctly identify infected/infectious hosts, and so imprecise tests (TB, MAP) greatly hinder elimination.

After a herd has been screened over a period of time, the prevalence of an endemic disease will be known with some degree of certainty. The nature of the disease, together with the prevalence of infection and incidence rate of disease, can be used to decide on the best strategy – this might be elimination or control. The economic impact of the disease versus the economic costs of control or elimination needs to be evaluated. It is worth remembering that the costs of control

**Table 7.3.** Summary of the features of disease transmission relevant in the control of bovine viral diarrhoea (BVD), infectious bovine rhinotracheitis (IBR), leptospirosis, neosporosis and MAP (paratuberculosis, Johne's disease).

| | Diseases in order of decreasing ease of eradication | | | | |
| --- | --- | --- | --- | --- | --- |
| | BVD | IBR | Leptospirosis | Neosporosis | MAP |
| Infectious cattle | Transient acutely infected adults + long-term shedding from persistently infected (PI) cattle | Shedding from carrier cattle – shedding can recur after a latent period | Infected cattle, mainly adults | Infected cows (vertical transmission) | Adults + transient shedding from young calves |
| Duration of infectiousness | PIs – lifelong; acute infections, up to 14 days | Generally short-term, (days) | Several months to >1 year | Lifelong | Adults, months–years; calves, days–weeks |
| Sources of pathogen | Shed in many body fluids (including saliva, semen, faeces, urine and milk), abortion products | Shed in many body fluids | Urine, abortion products | Infected cows (vertical transmission) + via canid faeces + placental tissues at calving | Faeces + milk |
| Sources of infection | Direct from cattle, environment for ~2 weeks | Direct from cattle + via semen | Direct from cattle + infected water | Vertical transmission from infected cows to calf + via canid faeces + possibly horizontal; via placental tissues | Infected milk and colostrum + survives 18 months in slurry |
| Long-term persistence in environment | No | No | Yes | No | Yes |
| Persists in host | Yes, PIs | Yes, carriers | Yes, long-term shedders | Yes | Yes, long-term shedders |
| Other host species significant | No | No | Possibly, sheep | Dogs and wild canids | Possibly other host species |
| Zoonotic | No | No | Yes | No | Uncertain |

**Table 7.4.** Summary of control options for bovine viral diarrhoea (BVD), infectious bovine rhinotracheitis (IBR), leptospirosis, neosporosis and MAP (paratuberculosis, Johne's disease).

| | Diseases in order of decreasing ease of eradication | | | | |
|---|---|---|---|---|---|
| | BVD | IBR | Leptospirosis | Neosporosis | MAP |
| Elimination from herd feasible | Yes | Yes | Controversial | Unlikely | Unlikely/no |
| Treatment of sick individuals | Palliative (not PIs) | Palliative | Dihydrostreptomycin | Not applicable | No, cull |
| Vaccination | Yes | Yes | Yes | No | Not commonly available |
| Breaking transmission cycles | Remove PIs, vaccinate, clean up after abortions | Vaccinate, avoid infected bulls, reduce stressors, clean up after abortions | Avoid urine contamination, avoid infected bulls, clean up after abortions | See Box 7.3 | See Box 7.2 |
| Within-herd control measures after establishing prevalence | Cull PIs, vaccinate, rear youngstock away from adult herd | Avoid mixing different age groups in shared air space; rear youngstock away from adult herd, vaccinate | Vaccinate; isolate and treat affected individuals; use AI rather than natural service; improve drainage (housing and pasture); reduce humidity; ensure excellent ventilation; keep youngstock separate from adults | See Box 7.3 | See Box 7.2 |
| If purchasing cows | Select antigen- and antibody-negative replacements (beware of antibody-positive pregnant cows– possibility of PI calf) | Select antibody-negative replacements | Select antibody-negative replacements | Select antibody-negative replacements | Source replacements from established low-prevalence herds |
| Test and cull | PIs | | | | High-shedders |

are continuous; control is a continuous feature and if control measures are relaxed the disease incidence rate will increase. Similarly, the costs of elimination might be finite over a period of time but the costs to maintain freedom from disease are continuous and there is an extra cost if reintroduction occurs, because all animals are susceptible and an epidemic will occur.

Therefore, when deciding whether to eliminate or control a disease the prevalence of disease in the herd and its impact on health, welfare and economics, and whether this is changing over time, will need to be considered. This might be difficult to evaluate and will depend on the natural history of the pathogen – some pathogens have long incubation and latency periods and covert spread within the herd (e.g. MAP), while others have a short latency period and lead to overt disease. An illustration of how complexity in the host–pathogen–environment interaction

affects the likelihood of eradication, using disease examples, is shown in Fig.7.2.

### Evaluating herd infection status

The control of infectious disease starts with establishing the herd infection status. The frequency of herd testing required for evaluating and monitoring an infectious disease will depend on the current herd disease status, whether the aim is eradication or control, the accuracy of the tests being used for monitoring, and the extent to which monitoring directly informs control (e.g. identification of infectious cows). The frequency of herd testing is determined directly from principles of infectious disease control being applied to a specific pathogen (see Table 7.2), but in practice, herd infection status is often usefully monitored at 1–6-month intervals. A zero (BVD, IBR) or low (MAP, neosporosis) prevalence of infection with no signs of transmission means that

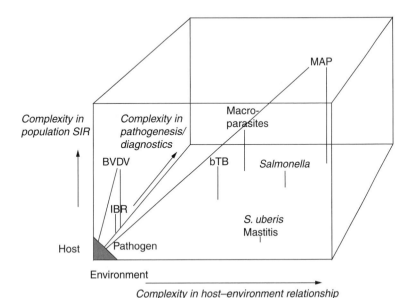

**Fig. 7.2.** A qualitative illustration of the complex host–pathogen–environment relationships that influence the feasibility of elimination of a pathogen. The further a pathogen is from the green corner on account of the roles of environment, diagnostics and persistent host immune response, the greater the difficulty in achieving elimination. For example, BVDV versus MAP is indicated by the pale blue lines. bTB, bovine tuberculosis; BVDV, bovine viral diarrhoea virus; IBR, infectious bovine rhinotracheitis; MAP, paratuberculosis; SIR, population dynamics of susceptible, infectious and resistant cows).

the focus can be on external biosecurity measures (Box 7.1). A high prevalence of infection, or evidence of disease transmission, indicates that internal biosecurity measures and active disease control are required.

In the earlier sections of this chapter we highlighted that it is possible to test a proportion of the herd or even all the herd (with individual milk sampling) and be relatively certain of the presence of disease. This is possible where diagnostic tests are sufficiently sensitive and specific for diseases such as BVD, IBR, leptospirosis and neosporosis, but more problematic where diagnostic tests are less accurate (MAP, bTB). The sensitivity of tests for MAP is low and changes with disease progression; several farmers who have been members of MAP elimination schemes have found that as cattle are tested repeatedly over time in an apparently negative herd, a positive animal arises. This might be an adult becoming positive over time but with a low test sensitivity cattle could test negative several times by chance before

testing positive. Less than 100% specificity also means that some cows will be false positives; the more often cattle are tested the greater the chance of false positives. Research adjusting for the errors in the MAP test has suggested that many herds with a very low prevalence of MAP serum antibody and no clinical cases of MAP are probably free from disease. Cattle that test negative at several bTB tests will subsequently test positive; this could be recent infection but, given that the current estimates for test sensitivity of the intradermal skin test are 50% – 60%, some will be previous false negatives. Consequently, for diseases such as MAP and bTB it is very difficult to define a negative cow or herd from testing alone. The metapopulation then becomes important. If no herds in the metapopulation have bTB then a farmer can be more confident that their herd is free from bTB. This is possible for bTB in some countries and regions, but seems increasingly less possible with MAP.

A summary of testing and monitoring methods, relevant for control of BVD, IBR,

---

**Box 7.2.** Outline of control measures to prevent within-herd transmission of Johne's disease (MAP).

Milk/colostrum management

- Do not allow pooling and/or storage of colostrum from cows of positive or uncertain status.
- Consider 'snatching weaning' of calves immediately after birth (i.e. do not allow colostrum to be fed from cows of positive or *uncertain* status) – use colostrum replacer or that from cows of known negative status.
- Use individual calving pens to prevent cross-suckling.
- Do not feed waste milk to replacement heifers.
- Consider feeding replacement heifer calves with artificial milk.

Calving and youngstock environment

- Clean out and disinfect calving pens between cows.
- Do not allow contamination of calf-rearing areas with slurry from adult cow housing.
- Avoid the spreading of slurry on paddocks used by first-season grazing animals.
- Segregate heifer calves and rear in individual hutches to prevent potential horizontal transmission.

Cow management

- Keep cows of positive, provisionally positive and currently *uncertain* status away from the dry cow and calving cow environment (calve these cows separately and clean out accommodation between calvings).
- Consider breeding known MAP antibody-positive cows to beef (or culling from the herd).
- Consider confirming likely infected cows identified from antibody tests by using faecal PCR to inform a culling policy.

leptospirosis, neosporosis and MAP, is shown in Table 7.2.

## Avoiding introduction or reintroduction of a pathogen

Preventing the introduction of pathogens is essential in the control of infectious disease. Good external biosecurity is important even if a pathogen is already on a farm – reintroduction can cause disease from a new strain or facilitate persistence in the metapopulation. For all six example diseases, pathogens can be introduced into a naïve herd or reintroduced into an infected herd by infected cattle. BVD and IBR are host specific, and since cows are the only animal source of disease and tests are reasonably accurate, testing individual cows to avoid introduction of antigen is possible. bTB and MAP have poor test accuracy and so testing individual cattle is inaccurate and of little worth in preventing introduction.

An important element in the prevention of the introduction of disease from purchased cows is to correctly interpret their infection status from diagnostic (often serological) tests. For example, paired serological tests for BVD give an indication of an animal's status; adult cattle with antibodies to BVD are immune and not carriers, while those with no antibodies are susceptible or possibly persistently infected. The latter should be confirmed with an antigen test. A farmer needs to consider whether to buy cattle susceptible or immune to BVD: if the herd is negative this is not important (assuming that the antibody-positive cow carries no virus on to the farm), but if the herd is positive and there is BVD virus circulating a susceptible cow might become infected with BVD, aid the persistence of the virus and potentially produce a persistently infected (PI) calf. Caution is required when purchasing pregnant cows – an antibody-positive pregnant cow may give birth to a PI calf in the new unit.

In contrast to BVD, adult cattle with antibodies to IBR or neosporosis are infected

and may transmit the pathogens. They should not be introduced to a naïve herd and, in addition, are a risk to positive herds. For IBR, there are different subtypes of the virus and farmers run a risk of introducing a new strain when introducing a positive cow. The stress associated with movement and settling into a new herd might lead to shedding of virus and an epidemic of IBR in the herd.

Adult cattle with antibodies to leptospirosis may or may not be shedding the pathogen. Positive cattle preferably should not be purchased, although treatment with dihydrostreptomycin prior to a 3-week isolation period before entering the herd may be effective.

Testing for MAP or bTB might detect a positive animal, but a negative animal might well be a false-negative. The current tests do not give sufficient confidence that an animal is definitely free from infection. In addition, given the long latent period from initial infection to disease, quarantine is not feasible. A better approach to avoid inadvertent introduction would be to source cattle from a herd known to be free from bTB and with no clinical evidence of MAP (often in a metapopulation that is free from these pathogens). For both MAP and bTB, purchasing cattle from herds where there has been no history of disease for several years and where these herds also source their animals carefully might be the best solution to prevent the inadvertent introduction of disease. This is true for reintroduction as well as introduction into naïve herds.

A summary of the features of disease transmission, relevant for control of BVD, IBR, leptospirosis, neosporosis and MAP, is shown in Table 7.3.

## Preventing spread and persistence of a pathogen within a herd

Once in a herd, direct cattle-to-cattle transmission of pathogens is the most important route of spread for BVD, IBR and leptospirosis, and vaccination is an effective and important control measure for these diseases, to reduce the susceptible population. For BVD, PI cattle shed virus for months or years and so their early detection and removal, alongside vaccination, minimizes the spread of BVDV. For IBR, infected cattle are carriers and shed virus if stressed and so minimizing stress is important. Cattle-to-cattle transmission can occur via vertical transmission *in utero* with BVD, neosporosis and occasionally MAP and, because BVD, IBR, leptospirosis and neosporosis cause abortion, infected calves, placenta and fetal fluids are a risk for spread of infection and so should be removed as soon as possible (Table 7.4).

Indirect transmission of pathogens is common with endemic diseases, and this influences control measures. MAP survives in faeces for many months and so avoiding contact between young cattle and adult faeces is essential. Preventing cattle from drinking from rivers, keeping calving boxes clean and youngstock in clean areas to prevent exposure to infected faeces are key elements in reducing the dose of MAP on farms (Table 7.4). Neosporosis can be spread horizontally if dogs or wild canids eat infectious placentae. MAP and bTB are also not cattle specific and so other reservoir hosts can transmit these diseases to cattle; biosecurity to prevent dogs and wildlife spreading existing diseases on the farm is important.

One key management issue for many diseases is keeping youngstock and adults in separate groups, which prevents transmission between groups. For BVD the risk is a PI calf to a pregnant adult, while for MAP it is the older cattle shedding MAP that are a risk to cattle under 6 months of age.

A summary of control options for BVD, IBR, leptospirosis, neosporosis and MAP is shown in Table 7.4 and, using the examples of MAP and neosporosis, in Boxes 7.2 and 7.3 we highlight specific areas of herd management important in reducing within-herd transmission of these infectious diseases.

## Conclusions

A variety of infectious diseases affect the health and production of dairy cows, and their control is an important component of a herd health programme. While the principles of infectious disease management are known, the behaviour of endemic pathogens, a lack of detailed knowledge of some pathogens and the poor accuracy of some diagnostic tests means that disease eradication is often difficult or impossible – and not necessarily financially viable. Where elimination is not feasible, control is essential and a herd health programme provides an excellent framework to achieve this, through the continual monitoring and re-evaluation of herd and group infection status and farm management policies.

---

**Box 7.3.** Outline of control measures to prevent within-herd transmission of neosporosis.

- Limit access of canids to infected tissues by disposing of aborted foetuses, fetal membranes and other tissues immediately after calving/abortion.
- Limit access of canids to feed areas; 'dog-proof' fencing of appropriate areas.
- Prevent possible factors for disease recrudescence in congenitally infected cattle, such as mouldy feed, exposure to other infectious agents that suppress immunity and other factors such as stress and dietary imbalances (Anthony and Williams, 2001).
- Embryo transfer can be used for valuable *Neosprum caninum*-positive dams; a positive donor will not transmit infection to the early embryo. It is important to ensure that recipients are not infected.
- Limit access of other cows to contaminated material by using individual calving pens (cows may infect themselves by ingesting infected placentae from other cattle).
- The use of beef bull semen for *N. caninum*-positive cattle has been demonstrated to reduce the risk of abortion, possibly due to a favourable effect of crossbreeding on placental function (López-Gatius, 2005)

# References and Further Reading

Ackermann, M. and Engels, M. (2006) Pro and contra IBR-eradication. *Veterinary Microbiology* 113, 293–302.

Anderson, R.M. and May, R.M. (1991) *Infectious Diseases of Humans: Dynamics and Control.* Oxford University Press, Oxford and New York.

Anthony, A. and Williams, N.B. (2001) Recent advances in understanding the epidemiology of *N. caninum* in cattle. *New Zealand Veterinary Journal* 49, 42–47.

Barrett, D.J., Mee, J.F., Mullowney, P., Good, M., McGrath, G., Clegg, T. *et al.* (2011) Risk factors associated with Johne's disease test status in dairy herds in Ireland. *Veterinary Record* 168, 410.

Bech-Sàbat, G., López-Gatius, F., Santolaria, P., García-Ispierto, I., Pabón, M., Nogareda, C. *et al.* (2007) Progesterone supplementation during mid-gestation increases the risk of abortion in Neospora-infected dairy cows with high antibody titres. *Veterinary Parasitology* 145, 164–167.

Boelaert, F., Speybroeckb, N., de Kruifc, A., Aertsd, M., Burzykowskid, T., Molenberghsd, G. *et al.* (2005) Risk factors for bovine herpesvirus-1 seropositivity. *Preventive Veterinary Medicine* 69, 285–295.

Bolin, C.A. (2001) Clinical signs, diagnosis and prevention of leptospirosis in cattle. *Cattle Practice* 9, 267–273.

Brock, K.V., Redman, D.R., Vickers, M.L. and Irvine, N.E. (1991) Quantitation of bovine viral diarrhea virus in embryo transfer flush fluids collected from a persistently infected heifer. *Journal of Veterinary Diagnostic Investigation* 3, 99–100.

Carslake, D., Grant, W., Green, L.E., Cave, J.A., Greaves, J., Keeling, M.J. *et al.* (2011) Endemic cattle diseases: comparative epidemiology and governance. *Royal Society of London. Philosophical Transactions, Biological Sciences* 366, 1975–1986.

Daniels, M.J., Hutchings, M.R., Allcroft, D.J., McKendrick, I.J. and Greig, A. (2002) Risk factors for Johne's disease in Scotland – the results of a survey of farmers. *Veterinary Record* 150, 135–139.

Dhaliwal, G.S., Murray, R.D., Dobson, H. and Ellis, W.A. (1997) Effect of *Leptospira interrogans* serovar *hardjo* infection on progesterone concentrations in heifers. *Veterinary Record* 140, 19–20.

Drew, T.W., Yapp, F. and Paton, D.J. (1999) The detection of bovine viral diarrhoea virus in bulk milk samples by the use of a single-tube RT-PCR. *Veterinary Microbiology* 64, 145–154.

Dubey, J.P., Schares, G. and Ortega-Mora, L.M. (2007) Epidemiology and control of neosporosis and *Neospora caninum*. *Clinical Microbiology Reviews* 20, 323–367.

Ellis, W.A., Montgomery, J. and Cassells, J.A. (1985) Dihydrostreptomycin treatment of bovine carriers of *Leptospira interrogans* serovar *hardjo*. *Research in Veterinary Science* 39, 292–295.

Ellis, W.A., Thiermann, A.B., Montgomery, J., Handsaker. A., Winter, P.J. and Marshall, R.B. (1988) Restriction endonuclease analysis of *Leptospira interrogans* serovar *hardjo* isolates from cattle. *Research in Veterinary Science* 44, 375–379.

Ellis, J.A., Martin, K., Norman, G.R. and Haines, D.M. (1995) Comparison of detection methods for bovine viral diarrhea virus in bovine abortions and neonatal death. *Journal of Veterinary Diagnostic Investigation* 7(4), 433–436.

Fredriksen, B., Djonne, B., Sigurdardottir, O., Tharaldsen, J., Nyberg, O. and Jarp, J. (2004) Factors affecting the herd level of antibodies against *Mycobacterium avium* subspecies *paratuberculosis* in dairy cattle. *Veterinary Record* 154, 522–526.

Gerritsen, M.J., Koopmans, M.J. and Olyhoek, T. (1993) Effect of streptomycin treatment on the shedding of and the serologic responses to *Leptospira interrogans* serovar *hardjo* subtype *hardjobovis* in experimentally infected cows. *Veterinary Microbiology* 38, 129–138.

Green, L.E. and Medley, G.F. (2002) Mathematical modelling of the foot and mouth disease epidemic of 2001: strengths and weaknesses. *Research in Veterinary Science* 73, 201–205.

Greig, A., Stevenson, K., Perez, V., Pirie, A.A., Grant, J.M. and Sharp, J. (1997) Paratuberculosis in wild rabbits (*Oryctolagus cuniculus*). *Veterinary Record* 140, 141–143.

Greig, A., Stevenson, K., Henderson, D., Perez, V., Hughes, V., Pavlik, I. *et al.* (1999) Epidemiological study of paratuberculosis in wild rabbits in Scotland. *Journal of Clinical Microbiology* 37, 1746–1751.

Groenendaal, H., Nielen, M., Jalvingh, A.W., Horst, S.H., Galligan, D.T. and Hesselink, J.W. (2002) A simulation of Johne's disease control. *Preventive Veterinary Medicine* 54, 225–245.

Hage, J.J., Vellema, P., Schukken, Y.H., Barkema, H.W., Rijsewijk, F.A., van Oirschot, J.T. *et al.* (1997) Sheep do not have a major role in bovine herpesvirus 1 transmission. *Veterinary Microbiology* 57, 41–54.

Hathaway, S.C., Pritchard, D.G. and Little, T.W.A. (1984) Seroepidemiological studies of bovine Leptospira interrogans serovar hardjo infection. *Zentralblatt fur Bakteriologie, Mikrobiologie und Hygiene. Series A: Medical Microbiology, Infectious Diseases, Virology, Parasitology* 257(4), 526.

Hemphill, A. and Gottstein, B. (2000) A European perspective on *Neospora caninum. International Journal of Parasitology* 30, 877–924.

Houe, H. (1992) Serological analysis of a small herd sample to predict presence or absence of animals persistently infected with bovine viral diarrhoea virus (BVDV) in dairy herds. *Research in Veterinary Science* 53, 320–323.

Houe, H. (1999) Epidemiologic features and economic importance of bovine virus diarrhoea virus (BVDV) infections. *Veterinary Microbiology* 64(2/3), 89–107.

Innes, E.A., Wright, S.E., Maley, S., Rae, A., Schock, A., Kirvar, E. *et al.* (2001) Protection against vertical transmission in bovine neosporosis. *International Journal of Parasitology* 31, 1523–1534.

Kaashoek, M.J., Rijsewijk, F.A. and Oirschot, J.T. (1996) Persistence of antibodies against bovine herpesvirus 1 and virus reactivation two to three years after infection. *Veterinary Microbiology* 53, 103–110.

Kerkhofs, P., Renjifo, X., Toussaint, J.F., Letellier, C., Vanopdenbosch, E. and Welleman, S.G. (2003) Enhancement of the immune response and virological protection of calves against bovine herpesvirus type 1 with an inactivated gE-deleted vaccine. *Veterinary Record* 152, 681–686.

Kramps, J.A., Banks, M., Beer, M., Kerkhofs, P., Perrin, M., Wellenberg, G.J. *et al.* (2004) Evaluation of tests for antibodies against bovine herpesvirus 1 performed in national reference laboratories in Europe. *Veterinary Microbiology* 102, 169–181.

Lewis, F.I., Gunn, G.J., McKendrick, I.J. and Murray, F.M. (2009) Bayesian inference for within-herd prevalence of *Leptospira interrogans* serovar *Hardjo* using bulk milk antibody testing. *Biostatistics* 10, 719–728.

Lindberg, A., Groenendaal, H., Alenius, S. and Emanuelson, U. (2001) Validation of a test for dams carrying foetuses persistently infected with bovine viral-diarrhoea virus based on determination of antibody levels in late pregnancy. *Preventive Veterinary Medicine* 51, 199–214.

Lindsay, D.S., Dubey, J.P. and Duncan, R.B. (1999) Confirmation that the dog is a definitive host for *Neospora caninum. Veterinary Parasitology* 82, 327–333.

Lindsay, D.S., Ritter, D.M. and Brake, D. (2001) Oocyst excretion in dogs fed mouse brains containing tissue cysts of a cloned line of *Neospora caninum. Journal of Parasitology* 87, 909–911.

Lloyd, J.B., Whittington, R.J., Fitzgibbon, C. and Dobson, R. (2001) Presence of *Mycobacterium avium* subspecies *paratuberculosis* in suspensions of ovine trichostrongylid larvae produced in faecal cultures artificially contaminated with the bacterium. *Veterinary Record* 148, 261–263.

López-Gatius, F., Santolaria, P., Yániz, J.L., Garbayo, J.M. and Almería, S. (2005) The use of beef bull semen reduced the risk of abortion in Neospora-seropositive dairy cows. *Journal of Veterinary Medicine B: Infectious Diseases and Veterinary Public Health* 52, 88–92.

McGarry, J.W., Stockton, C.M., Williams, D.J. and Trees, A.J. (2003) Protracted shedding of oocysts of Neospora caninum by a naturally infected foxhound. *Journal of Parasitology* 89, 628–630.

McInnes, L.M., Irwin, P., Palmer, D.G. and Ryan, U.M. (2006) In vitro isolation and characterization of the first canine Neospora caninum isolate in Australia. *Veterinary Parasitology* 137, 355–363.

Munnoz-Zanzi, C.A., Thurmond, M.C., Johnson, W.O. and Hietala, S.K. (2002) Predicted ages of dairy calves when colostrum-derived bovine viral diarrhea virus antibodies would no longer offer protection against disease or interfere with vaccination. *Journal of the American Veterinary Medical Association* 221, 678–685.

Muylkens, B., Thiry, J. and Kirten, P. (2007) Bovine herpesvirus 1 infection and infectious bovine rhinotracheitis. *Veterinary Research* 38, 181–209.

Nielsen, S.S., and Ersbøll, A.K. (2006) Age at occurrence of Mycobacterium avium subsp. paratuberculosis in naturally infected dairy cows. *Journal of Dairy Science* 89, 4557-4566.

Nielsen, S.S. and Toft, N. (2006) Age-specific characteristics of ELISA and faecal culture for the purpose of specific testing for paratuberculosis. *Journal of Dairy Science* 89, 569–579.

Nielsen, S.S., Krogh, M.A. and Enevoldsen, C. (2009) Time to the occurrence of a decline in milk production in cows with various paratuberculosis antibody profiles. *Journal of Dairy Science* 92, 149–155.

Niskanen, R., Lindberg, A., Larsson, B. and Alenius, S. (2000) Lack of virus transmission from bovine viral diarrhoea infected calves to susceptible peers. *Acta Veterinaria Scandinavia* 41, 93–99.

Noakes, D.E., Parkinson, T.J. and England, G.C. (2009) *Veterinary Reproduction and Obstetrics*, 9th edn. W.B. Saunders, London, pp. 499–502.

Pritchard, G.C. (1999) Bulk milk antibody testing for Leptospira hardjo infection. *Cattle Practice* 7, 59–61.

Pritchard, G.C. (2001) Milk antibody testing in cattle. *In Practice* 23, 542–549.

Radostits, O.M. and Littlejohns, I.R. (1988) New concepts in the pathogenesis, diagnosis and control of diseases caused by the bovine viral diarrhea virus. *Canadian Veterinary Journal* 29, 513–528.

Roermund, H., Bakker, D., Willemsen, P. and de Jong, M. (2007) Horizontal transmission of paratuberculosis: A critical review and meta-analysis. *The Veterinary Journal* 179, 60–69.

Simon, A.J. (2004) A practical approach to the control and eradication of IBR using marker vaccines. *Cattle Practice* 12, 305–311.

Toft, N., Nielsen, S.S. and Jørgensen, E. (2005) Continuous-data diagnostic tests for paratuberculosis as a multi-stage disease. *Journal of Dairy Science* 88, 3923–3931.

Voges, H., Horner, G.W., Rowe, S. and Wellenberg, G.J. (1998) Persistent bovine pestivirus infection localized in the testes of an immunocompetent, non-viraemic bull. *Veterinary Microbiology* 61, 165–175.

Whittington, R. and Windsor, P. (2009) In utero infection of cattle with Mycobacterium avium subsp. *The Veterinary Journal* 179, 60–69.

Wittum, T.E., Grotelueschen, D.M., Brock, K.V., Kvasnicka, W.G., Floyd, J.G., Kelling, C.L. *et al.* (2001) Persistent bovine viral diarrhoea virus infection in US beef herds. *Preventive Veterinary Medicine* 49, 83–94.

# 8 Nutritional Management of Herd Health

**Alastair Hayton,[1] James Husband[2] and Richard Vecqueray[2]**
[1]*Synergy Farm Health, West Hill Barns, Evershot, Dorset DT2 0LD, UK;*
[2]*EBVC Ltd., Rural Enterprise Centre, Redhills, Penrith, Cumbria CA11 0DT, UK*

## Introduction: The Role of Nutrition in Dairy Herd Health and Production

The economics of milk production in recent decades has led to major changes in global milk industries: herds are increasing in size and yields are increasing per cow. The rate of genetic improvement has been rapid. Assuming milk of standard composition, improvements in genetic merit for milk yield have resulted in an increase of approximately 62 litres per lactation per year. In this context, the ration that cows are fed and the way in which the ration is fed are crucial to the efficient production of target milk yields and, depending on the requirements of the milk buyer, to target milk composition too. A diet should be formulated to meet the cow's dry matter intake (DMI), energy, protein, fibre, mineral and vitamin requirements according to recognized standards. Inappropriate nutritional management can strongly predispose cows to disease and poor reproductive performance, and thus nutritional requirements should be met without adversely affecting rumen function, reproductive performance, metabolic health, immune function or predisposition to disease. Therefore, nutrition plays a pivotal role in dairy herd health.

The nutritional challenges faced by dairy cows in early lactation are considerable.

The daily maintenance requirements depend on the size and breed of the animals, but a 700 kg Holstein has an energy requirement of approximately 80 MJ per day. Every litre of milk produced requires a further 5.5 MJ, so a cow producing 45 l of milk requires 325 MJ and is working at four times maintenance. Cows capable of producing 10,000 l in a lactation will often yield in excess of 45 l/day in the first month of lactation. If the likely DMI in the first month after calving and the energy density of typical feeds are considered, it is apparent that energy requirements cannot be met without the cow mobilizing some tissue stores. This results in negative energy balance (NEB). For example, if the cow cannot be persuaded to eat more than 21 kg DM of a ration with an energy density of 12.5 MJ/kg DM, then approximately 2 kg of body reserves (mainly fat, but muscle too) will be mobilized per day. If this degree of NEB carries on for 40–60 days then the total tissue loss will be approximately 80–100 kg, which represents the loss of approximately one body condition score (BCS). This, as will be discussed later in the chapter, is a level of loss that will jeopardize fertility, health and production, although in reality this degree of NEB is not uncommon in high-yielding cows.

Negative energy balance is a central and fundamental influence on cow health.

Attempts to minimize NEB in early lactation by increasing the proportion of high-energy feeds, such as cereals and exogenous fats, are often difficult. The main biological driver of body condition score (BCS) loss and NEB in dairy cows is BCS at calving rather than the composition of the fresh cow diet. A diet excessively high in starch and/or sugars can cause problems with ruminal acidosis in early-lactation cows, especially those that have had a poor transition from the dry to milking cow diets. Exogenous fats in early lactation can worsen NEB as these can drive milk production in excess of the extra energy provided, and certain fats such as the calcium soaps can depress DMI. Thus, the main challenge faced by the modern dairy cow producer is achieving high yields whilst minimizing NEB in early lactation, and this is a key focus in this chapter.

Production systems vary throughout the world, and low-input–low-output grass-based systems – and hybrids between low-input and high-input systems, which often show greater profitability in the face of low milk prices – are very common. The fundamentals of managing and monitoring grass-based systems are very different from high-input farms; in the former the focus tends to be on maintaining the quantity and quality of grass, while in the latter the focus is very much on monitoring cow performance and production. This diversity in feeding systems creates a challenge when reviewing and advising on nutritional health management, because the type of monitoring needed will be dependent to some extent on the system.

The purpose of this chapter is to provide a framework to approach dairy herd nutritional evaluation as a component of herd health, whatever the production system employed. We describe the key elements of monitoring and common areas where herd problems arise. We also discuss control strategies for important nutrition-related herd disease. While we address general principles of nutrition in relation to dairy herd health, most emphasis in this chapter will be placed on high-input systems.

## Background: Key Concepts

### The role of glucose in cow metabolism

High-yielding dairy cows have a huge and absolute requirement for glucose in early lactation for the production of milk lactose. The milk lactose concentration is relatively fixed compared with milk butter fat and protein, and since lactose is the determinant of the water content of milk (through osmolar effects) it is the driver for milk volume. Unlike other tissues (except the fetoplacental unit and the brain), the movement of glucose into the mammary gland is not under the influence of insulin. Hence, even at times of NEB, which is almost ubiquitous in early lactation, glucose is taken up by the mammary gland. Other tissues such as muscle, which require insulin for glucose uptake, will therefore use glucose as its primary energy source only at times of positive energy balance. Almost all ingested carbohydrates are fermented in the rumen to the three main volatile fatty acids (VFAs): acetic, butyric and propionic. Very little starch escapes ruminal degradation and so it follows that if glucose cannot be fed in the ration for direct use in the mammary gland for lactose production, then the vast majority has to be produced in the liver through gluconeogenesis.

An appropriate ration in early lactation has a relatively low quantity of cellulosic feed. This decreases the time required by the microbial population for degradation, increases rumen transit time and hence DMI. A delicate balancing act is required between rumen function and the availability of precursors for glucose synthesis. Too much fermentable energy can lead to ruminal acidosis, while too much structural carbohydrate limits glucose production and exacerbates NEB, thereby leading to excess fat mobilization and fatty infiltration in the liver ('fatty liver') and ketosis. This balance between energy and rumen function becomes more critical as yields increase, and makes the monitoring of responses to a ration, through cow signs and milk and blood parameters, of great importance.

## The pivotal role of the liver in adaptation to NEB

The liver has a pivotal role in adaptation to NEB. It is the main gluconeogenic organ and it also takes up a large proportion of the circulating non-esterified fatty acids (NEFAs) from the blood to process them into other forms of usable energy. The metabolic fates of NEFAs within the liver are regulated by several factors, including propionate metabolites, and are listed below.

**1.** Complete oxidation in the liver mitochondria to acetyl CoA (AcCoA) to be used in the Krebs cycle.
**2.** Partial oxidation to ketones (including beta-hydroxybutyrate (BHB)). When the cow is in NEB, liver glucose concentrations will be low and so will the supply of oxaloacetate (OAA) that is produced from rumen propionate (and hence is more plentiful when diets are rich in starch and sugars). OAA is required for the Krebs cycle and a deficit leads to the cycle slowing such that AcCoA, from complete oxidization of NEFAs, cannot be fed into the cycle to provide energy. Rather than full oxidation of NEFAs, the liver partially oxidizes these to ketone bodies which can be then used as energy sources in peripheral tissues. Ketone production does not result in as much net energy release as complete oxidation of FAs to AcCoA. Increasing concentrations of ketones may suppress DMI.
**3.** Re-esterification to triglycerides (TG), which remain in the liver parenchyma awaiting export as very low-density lipoproteins (VLDLs). VLDLs enter the circulation and are used by various tissues for energy, or by the mammary gland for the formation of milk fat.

Failure of the VLDL transport system will result in an increase in the TG content of the liver, which leads to a reduction in the functional capacity of the liver. Periparturient cows have a poor inherent capacity to produce VLDLs and, if the cow experiences intense fat mobilization and consequent high blood NEFA concentrations as a result of NEB, this can result in severe metabolic disruption.

Circulating concentrations of NEFAs and BHB can be used to measure the success of adaptation of the cow to NEB. NEFAs reflect the magnitude of mobilization of fat from storage, and BHB reflects the lack of ability of the liver to completely oxidize circulating fatty acids for use in the Krebs cycle. Monitoring of NEFA and BHB is described later in the chapter.

## Inappropriate metabolic responses of cows in NEB

Although cows have mechanisms for coping with NEB, recent research has shown that these adaptive mechanisms can function inappropriately and lead to excessive fat mobilization and an inability of the liver to cope with NEFAs. Adipose tissue should be considered a complex endocrinological organ as it excretes substances such as cytokines and leptin and behaves differently to a given stimulus depending on its metabolic history. 'Adipose sensitivity' is usually defined as an increase in the lipolytic response to a given stimulus. Certain factors affecting adipose sensitivity cannot be altered in a cow: examples include genetic influences and advancing gestation. Overfeeding during the dry period, however, especially when carried out over a long period (8 weeks is sufficient) results in excessive mobilization of adipose tissue after calving.

In recent years, two forms of ketosis, type I and type II have been distinguished. Type I is the 'traditional' ketosis which normally occurs as the cow approaches peak lactation (at 6–8 weeks) and is caused by glucose production being insufficient to meet demand. Type II occurs earlier, in the first week of lactation, and is believed to be related to insulin resistance resulting in excessive and poorly regulated lipolysis. This leads to raised blood NEFA concentration, which overwhelms the capacity of the liver mitochondria to take up NEFAs and convert them to ketones. The excess NEFAs, which cannot enter the mitochondria, are converted to TGs in the parenchyma. The failure of TG export out of the liver by VLDLs results in a pathological accumulation of TGs, usually termed 'fatty liver' disease. Type II ketosis is not always accompanied by high blood ketone concentrations; it can also result from the down-regulation of carnitine palmityl transferase 1 (CPT-1), which is the enzyme required for NEFA entry into the mitochondria.

Up to 50% of dairy cows have some degree of TG accumulation in the liver in the first 4 weeks of lactation. Severe fatty liver has been defined as when >10% of the fresh liver weight is TG, and moderate fatty liver when 5–10% is TG. Severe NEB and fatty infiltration are negatively correlated with health status and reproductive performance. It has been estimated from various studies worldwide over the last 30 years that 5–10% of cows acquire severe fatty liver after calving and 30–40% have moderate fatty liver.

The degree of NEB and the cow's ability to cope with it appears to be a major influence on cow health. There is growing evidence that failure to cope with NEB may be central to the aetiologies of several metabolic diseases in the immediate postcalving period. The interrelationships between diseases are not fully understood, but there may be a common causal pathway, possibly a profound disturbance of energy metabolism.

## Protein metabolism

Rumen microflora provide the cow with high-quality protein for digestion in the small intestine, provided they are supplied with rumen degradable protein (or non-protein nitrogen sources) and energy. Cows producing high yields (>30l) will require additional rumen bypass protein to meet their nutritional requirements. Cows producing low milk yields need virtually no bypass protein, and thus feeding expensive sources of bypass protein, such as soya and prairie meal, does not make economic sense.

Apart from the economic penalty of feeding high-protein diets, there is a potential fertility effect too. High-protein diets (>18% crude protein) tend to drive milk production but may be associated with a decrease in reproductive performance. Excess rumen degradable protein leads to the production of ammonia in the rumen, as the rumen microflora are unable to use all the supplied protein, and this ammonia passes to the liver where it is converted to urea. Excess urea can alter the uterine environment, making it less conducive to embryo survival. Some workers have observed reductions in conception rates with elevated blood urea concentrations but other studies, especially those looking at milk urea at the herd level, have failed to show any association. This is possibly because bulk milk urea comes from cows at different stages of lactation, only some of which will be at a stage where high-protein diets may have an adverse effect. It is worth noting that sudden elevations in bulk milk urea concentrations may represent a relative under-supply of fermentable energy so that the rumen microflora cannot use all the rumen degradable protein. The production of urea by the liver requires energy too, so high-protein diets can have important catabolic influences and worsen NEB, driving milk yields and the energetic cost of processing the ammonia.

There has been a move in the last 10 years, through the Feed into Milk (FiM) nutritional model, to limit the amount of rumen degradable protein fed and feed higher-energy density rations to drive yields, rather than rely on protein to drive production. Rather than feeding diets with a crude protein content of >18%, diets can be formulated at 16–17% with an energy density for high-yielding cows at >12 MJ/kg DM. The crude protein content can be decreased by maximizing microbial protein production by ensuring an adequate fermentable energy supply and feeding more bypass protein. This approach can be refined further, by not simply considering protein on the basis of its rumen degradation properties, but also by looking at its amino acid composition. Rations can be tailored so that they supply only sufficient protein sources or specific amino acids to meet the cow's specific amino acid requirements. Lysine and methionine are the two most common limiting amino acids, and these can be strategically supplemented. In this way, overall dietary crude protein even in high-yielding animals can be kept at 15–16%.

### Trace elements and vitamins

Six of the twenty-six trace minerals necessary for life have effects on health and productivity (Zn, Cu, Mn, I, Se, Co) and will be included in mineral supplements that are routinely fed to dairy cows in either total mixed rations (TMRs) or concentrate feeds. Trace elements and vitamins have diverse functions including involvement in many metabolic pathways, immune cell function, antioxidant effects, gene regulation and synthesis of enzymes and hormones. The effects of their deficiency are often neither pathognomonic nor clinically obvious and hence can be confused with other causes of disease that may be more likely to cause problems. The likelihood of suffering a herd deficiency will vary depending on the geographical area and soil type, but it is not known what proportion of dairy herds are underperforming due to trace element deficiencies. It is worth noting that supplementation is almost ubiquitous either through mineral supplements, dairy concentrate feeds or both, and thus deficiencies are probably not very common except perhaps in un-supplemented animals, such as pre-calving heifers at grass.

Inappropriate supplementation, however, is common and it is important to remember that an over-supply of most minerals can induce toxicity. This is especially the case with copper, where farmers supplementing by several routes (in feed, boluses and injectables), in the belief that it will improve fertility, have caused serious toxicity issues. Consequently it is important that trace element supplementation should be based on the best evidence available and not on anecdotal evidence.

## Monitoring of Nutritional Management, Including Herd Targets

While there are quantitative dietary guidelines to formulate a dairy cow ration by meeting nutritional requirements from estimated DMI, these guidelines are by no means foolproof. Uncertainty arises for a variety of reasons including innate variability in feedstuffs and their analyses, difficulties in quantifying the effect that different feed components have on rumen function, and variation in the mixing and feeding of the ration itself. Therefore the nutritional element of a dairy herd health programme is not based around the formulation of a ration, but rather on the evaluation of a wide set of cow and farm indicators to determine whether the current feeding practices are optimal. In this way, the veterinary surgeon (veterinarian) can work alongside and add value to the input of the ration formulator, to ensure that health and production are maximized and the farm's goals are achieved. For the purposes of this chapter, this process of evaluation will be subdivided into four key areas of monitoring: the records, the cow, metabolic markers, and feeds and feeding.

### Assessment of the records

#### Monitoring nutrition using milk recording information

The use of milk recording data for gauging the success or otherwise of any nutritional programme is not a precise science. There are numerous confounding factors and disparate research findings on the significance of individual parameters in relation to health and production. This means that drawing conclusions without further ancillary investigations may well be misleading. This is not to say that possible associations should not be examined, because the utilization of cheap, regular data is sensible practice. It should also be borne in mind that the percentages of fat and protein are frequently very significant contributors to the milk price a farmer receives, and therefore monitoring their trends is sensible practice, regardless of any further inferences that may be drawn with respect to nutrition.

MILK YIELD.    It is useful to monitor the level and variation in milk yield at the herd, group and cow level. Milk yield is influenced by frequency of milking, parity, days in milk, season of calving and feeding system, as well as by the quality of the nutrition. This can make fluctuations observed between time points or groups difficult to interpret. Consequently, when monitoring yield data it can be useful to use prediction data. Predictions of yield, based on previous lactation curves for that farm and month of calving – as well as, where applicable, previous lactations from the individual animal – allow these confounding factors to be controlled for, and to provide a benchmark from which to gauge performance. Prediction data can be unreliable on occasion, and care needs to be taken with such data, especially where (i) there has been a fundamental change to the management system; (ii) there is a high proportion of heifers within the group analysed (heifers provide the least accurate prediction as the effect of their own genetic base cannot be known); (iii) there are known issues with recording – some farms' data recording is consistently inaccurate; or (iv) 'factoring' – some farms opt not to record at consecutive morning and afternoon milkings but rather to record alternatively between morning and afternoons each month (thereby reducing costs). The 'missing' data are effectively estimated via the process of factoring. Unfortunately the predictions it creates can be unreliable, particularly in relation to butterfat. Consequently, knowledge of when and how recording is undertaken should be taken into account when commenting on the data.

Useful areas for monitoring milk yield on a monthly basis are now described.

• The average daily milk production per cow in the herd. As stated above, this will be influenced by a number of parameters, in particular the calving pattern; for a year-round calving pattern, the target will be to achieve the maximum possible level profile of daily production. Monitoring should be based on detecting differences between daily production and predicted performance, especially after changes to nutrition have been made. In a seasonal-calving herd, daily production should follow a lactation curve with a rise to a peak and then gradual decline as the herd moves away from the calving period. In this situation approximate targets for average daily production are easier to define, with the average peak target level reflecting the target lactation yield per cow for the herd. At peak production the target average daily production should be approximately the 305-day yield divided by 200 (e.g. a 30 l peak for 6000 l, 40 l for 8000 l, 50 l for 10,000 l and so on).

• Peak yield data (cows calved around 40–80 days). Given the level of production at which cows peak is highly correlated to overall lactation yield, and can also reflect on poor dry cow management, it is an important area to monitor. The relationship between peak yield and days post-calving, season of calving and parity are all useful parameters to monitor on a monthly basis. Very rapid rises to peak yield at 30–40 days, as opposed to slower rises at 50–60 days, are undesirable as they will result in larger negative energy deficits in the cows due to the slow rise to peak dry matter intakes at the start of lactation. The frequent consequence of this is poorer overall fertility and less overall milk produced (these cows often show very poor persistency after peak yield). Conversely, a failure to reach predicted yields at 30–40 days post-calving, in groups or individuals, is considered an indicator of potential transition period problems. Season may well have profound effects on peak yield, especially in systems where high-yielding cows are turned out to graze in the summer. In terms of parity, heifer performance should be evaluated with the expectation that they should peak within 25% of their herd-mates.

- Persistency of production. The decline from peak should be a maximum of 9% every month for multiparous cows and 6% every month for heifers. This decline will be heavily influenced by management – for example, frequency of milking and feeding system. Beyond ensuring that the cows are persisting as expected, the effects of month or season of calving and variation in parity, in particular the variation in performance between first lactation and multiparous animals, should be assessed. Poor performance in the heifers relative to the cows could suggest problems of excess competition for resources.

MILK CONSTITUENTS: ENERGY DEFICIT.    At the biochemical level, the quantities and proportions of the fats, proteins and lactose synthesized in the mammary gland at any point will depend on the relative amounts of available substrates and enzymes and the prevailing endocrine environment, which will partly be a function of the genotype of the animal.

Cows in early lactation in excessive NEB will be mobilizing high levels of body fat (as NEFAs), and these are sequestered and processed by the mammary epithelium, which results in elevated milk butterfat. At the same time, cows generally show a decrease in milk protein percentage, reflecting a shortage of glucose for milk protein synthesis in the udder.

As energy status is improved milk protein production increases. Along with increased glucose supply, this is thought to be for two main reasons: (i) the production of microbial protein increases in the rumen, and this can be incorporated into milk protein; and (ii) as more starch passes through the rumen (so-called 'bypass' starch) this helps to fulfil the energy requirements of the small intestine itself, which spares amino acids that can then be used for milk protein production. Protein synthesis is known to be modulated by endocrine signals as well as by substrate availability.

The basic premise of compositional monitoring strategies is that early-lactation animals in poor energy status will have lower milk protein and higher milk butterfat. Consequently, the monitoring of these processes via the individual yield and percentages of fat and protein and the ratio between them, at an individual and group level, should provide useful information on the adequacy of the diet in preventing excess NEB. Unfortunately, in many dairy systems, particularly those feeding high percentages of grass, butterfat percentages will be influenced by a large number of parameters independent of NEB, making the expected correlation with NEB unreliable. Consequently, such analyses should not be over-interpreted, or heavily relied upon to inform major decisions.

Some studies have established an association between milk constituent data and subsequent health/fertility and production, while others have failed to repeat such findings and/or concluded that the sensitivities and specificities of such techniques are not good enough to justify their use as a monitoring tool. As a consequence, if analysis of milk constituent data is suggestive of excessive NEB, this should not be seen as diagnostic in itself for assessing cow metabolic status, but as a potential warning indicator that there could be a problem and that further investigation is warranted. Similarly, simply because milk constituent data appear to be within target parameters, this should not preclude the possibility of the existence of nutrition-related problems.

A range of milk constituent analyses have been suggested to indicate energy balance. The analysis of monthly protein yield (kg) and protein percentage in relation to predicted yield and predicted percentage would be likely to produce the most reliable indicator, though as previously stated, care needs to be taken by ensuring that the predictive data are likely to be accurate. The principal target group to evaluate are the early-lactation animals. Performance of cows up to 50 days and 100 days post-calving should be considered. The number of days post-calving chosen for evaluation will partly be dependent on the time spent in fresh or high-yielding groups, and also on the number of animals that can contribute to the data set (very small numbers will reduce the chance of any trend being accurately highlighted).

There are no published levels of milk protein that clearly indicate when interference is needed, and judgement on this will partly be dependent on the quality of the data and the importance of protein to the income received by the farmer. The greater the likely accuracy of the prediction, the lower the required threshold for where poor performance should highlight the need for further investigation. In cases where data quality is good, more than 60% of cows below prediction for protein yield would be a reasonable point of concern, whereas with poor-quality data this cut-off may be extended to 75%. An alternative approach is to examine the mean weight of protein production for cows under 50 days in milk. This can be assessed on a rolling monthly basis to develop an understanding of what is normal for the herd. The expectation for cows yielding over 7000 l in one lactation is that the mean weight should be over 1 kg, and figures less than this raise concerns about inadequate energy supply.

Though not recommended by itself due to poor predictive capacity (often due to a large variability in fat production), the mean and median herd protein:fat ratio, in combination with the predicted protein yield, may provide limited additional evidence for the need for further investigation of energy status. Mean protein:fat ratios at a group level <0.75 for Holsteins and ~0.70 for the Channel Island breeds, in conjunction with poor protein yields, are considered an indicator of potential subclinical ketosis.

In systems where dietary consistency (uniform forages, fully housed, single TMR) mean that fluctuations in milk fat are less common, then the use of protein:fat ratios should be more reliable in terms of monitoring, and therefore greater significance can be given to the observation of low ratios as discussed above.

MILK CONSTITUENTS AND SUBACUTE RUMINAL ACIDOSIS.     Lowered milk fat is frequently cited as an indicator of subacute ruminal acidosis (SARA); however, fat percentages

may fall for other dietary reasons too, such as the introduction or increase in the supply of fats, particularly unsaturated fatty acids. Consequently, as with energy deficit, there is poor correlation between the presence or absence of SARA and milk fat percentage at the individual level. This is particularly the case in early-lactation cows when the fat percentage will be influenced by a variety of factors, including the degree of fat mobilization post-partum.

At the group or herd level, monitoring milk fat can be more appropriate particularly in mid-lactation (>100 days calved) cows. At this stage, a drop in fat production, particularly in association with feed changes, can be a useful indicator of a potential problem. Monitoring in mid-lactation should be based on average group fat percentages and yield of fat against prediction. As with protein, the threshold for interference will be dependent on the reliability of the predictive data and the importance of milk fat to income, but a minimum threshold of 60% below prediction for fat yield or fat percentage is a recommended cut-off for further investigation.

### Monitoring financial records

Feeding has a key effect on profitability and the analysis of financial indices related to nutrition, alongside nutritional evaluations related to cow health, is an essential component of a herd health programme. The example below is used to describe the use of feed-related indices. Since indices are calculated based on milk and commodity prices and the farm system involved, it is inappropriate to set target values for the indices described. In practice these should be monitored over time on a particular unit and, if available, useful comparisons can be made between farms with similar economic and management environments. As will be explored below, different parameters are particularly relevant to particular production systems and the following points are useful for the comparison and assessment of performance of different systems.

1. High-input systems have higher feed costs per litre but greater milk income per cow, because more 'marginal' litres are being chased that require relatively more feed per extra litre. For herds yielding >8000 l/cow/year, concentrate feed rates of 0.3–0.4 kg (corrected to 87% DM)/l are normal. When milk prices are high and concentrate feed prices relatively low, it becomes more worthwhile trying to pursue higher yields.

2. Low-input extensive systems, such as the New Zealand grazing systems, are not chasing more marginal, expensive litres. The aim is to minimize costs per litre produced, and this centres on maximizing grass usage. Hence margins over feed per litre will be high but, due to the lower production, margins over feed costs per cow will be relatively low.

EXAMPLE OF DERIVING FEED COSTS. Consider a UK herd of 200 cows with 160 cows in milk, averaging 200 days in milk and giving 30 l/cow/day (milk sold). The herd receives 25 pence per litre (ppl) for milk of the following

composition: 3.6% butterfat, 3.2% milk protein and 0.024% milk urea.

The 160 milking cows are fed the following ration on average through the month on a per-cow, per-day basis. The cost of feeding the dry cows can be included in these calculations, but for brevity they are excluded from the example shown in Table 8.1.

Thus the herd is fed 48 kg/day of a 43% DM ration, with 20.7 kg DMI, costing £3.54/cow/day or £2.72 if we consider only the purchased feeds element.

Dealing in DM terms allows a comparison between farms, since fresh weight intakes are very variable due to the DM variation of by-products and forages. For instance, in this example, the farm feeds molasses of 65% DM yet another farm may feed a distillery by-product of 48% DM. For this reason a 'dry matter correction' is made on the concentrate element of the diets to 87%. This allows comparison between farms using weights of concentrate that have some meaning to the farmer and can therefore be easily communicated. This farm feeds 9.9 kg

**Table 8.1.** Costs of feeding milking cows.

| Feed | Equation row | Dry matter (%) | Fresh weight (kg) | Dry matter intake (kg) | Fresh weight unit cost (£/t) | Cost/cow/day (£) |
|---|---|---|---|---|---|---|
| Column | | a | b | c | d | e |
| Equation | | | | a × b | | (b × d)/1000 |
| Grass silage | *i* | 30 | 36 | 10.8 | 22.8 | 0.82 |
| Concentrate pellets 20% | *ii* | 86 | 10 | 8.6 | 240 | 2.40 |
| Molasses | *iii* | 65 | 2 | 1.3 | 160 | 0.32 |
| Equation | | 100 × c*iv*/b*iv* | Sum (b*i*:b*iii*) | Sum (c*i*:c*iii*) | | Sum (e*i*:e*iii*) |
| Ration total | *iv* | 43 | 48 | 20.7 | | 3.54 |
| Equation | | | Sum (b*ii*:b*iii*) | Sum (c*ii*:c*iii*) | | Sum (e*ii*:e*iii*) |
| Conc. only total | *v* | | 12.0 | 9.9 | | 2.72 |
| Equation | | | c*v*/0.87 | | 1000 × e*v*/b*vi* | |
| Conc. 87% DM correction | *vi* | | 11.4 | | 239 | |

DM of concentrate per day, which is equivalent to 11.4 kg of DM corrected concentrate. Since the cost per day of this concentrate is known, this allows a cost per tonne to be calculated to allow a comparison of unit value (£239/t in this instance).

These indices are then further translated into other unit costs, as shown in Table 8.2.

It can be seen therefore that the ration costs 11.8 pence to produce 1 litre of milk, of which 9.1 pence/l is purchased or concentrate feed. This figure is much more accurate and easy to calculate than the 'all feeds' figure, which includes the forage component of the costs, and is the one predominantly quoted. However, where forage is purchased or expensive to produce, conclusions drawn by studying solely the concentrate costs, rather than the whole ration costs, can lead to spurious conclusions.

If any decisions are going to made on the basis of costs then it is important that they are placed in the context of the income against which they are set, the difference between the two being termed 'the margin over' the unit cost in question. The income, costs and margins for the example herd are shown in Tables 8.3, 8.4 and 8.5.

The unit of land area can also be considered by dividing the herd margin by the area of available land allocated to the dairy enterprise. This parameter is very relevant where costs are linked to high-value land prices or rental agreements.

Dry period policy, lactation persistency and herd fertility affect the percentage of

**Table 8.2.** Unit costs for milking cows.

| | Milk sold (l/cow/day) | Cost (£/cow/day) | Cost per litre (price/l) | Milk price (price/l) | Margin per litre (price/l) |
|---|---|---|---|---|---|
| Column | a | b | c | d | e |
| Equation | | | $100 \times b/a$ | | d–c |
| Milking cows (all feeds) | 30.0 | 3.54 | 11.8 | 25.0 | 13.2 |
| Milking cows (purchased feeds) | | 2.72 | 9.1 | | 15.9 |

**Table 8.3.** Income data for example herd.

| | Milk yield (l/cow/day) | Milk price (price/l) | Milk income (£/cow/day) | Days in month | Monthly milk income (£/cow) | Number of cows in milk | Monthly milk cheque (£/herd) |
|---|---|---|---|---|---|---|---|
| Column | a | b | c | d | e | f | g |
| Equation | | | (a × b)/100 | | c × d | | e × f |
| | 30 | 25 | 7.50 | 31 | 232.5 | 160 | 37,200 |

**Table 8.4.** Income costs for example herd.

| | Feed costs (all feeds; £/cow/day) | Days in month | Monthly feed costs (£/cow) | Number of cows in milk | Monthly feed costs (£/herd) |
|---|---|---|---|---|---|
| Column | a | b | c | d | e |
| Equation | | | a × b | | c × d |
| Milking cows (all feeds) | 3.54 | 31 | 109.76 | 160 | 17,562 |
| Milking cows (purchased feeds) | 2.72 | 31 | 84.32 | 160 | 13,491 |

the herd that is dry in any given time period. The influence of these factors is dramatic. If we consider the example herd, 20% of cows are dry (not milking). If this were improved with time so that only 10% of the herd were dry and other per-cow inputs and outputs remained the same, then the following margins would be achieved and the herd would generate another £3472.5 per month after all feed costs, as shown in Table 8.6.

However, none of the figures above can be interpreted in isolation; for example:

**1.** A high purchased feed cost per litre of milk may result in high-component milk, generating a high milk price and subsequently excellent margins.
**2.** An improving monthly margin over purchased feed per cow in the herd may run concurrently with a falling overall herd margin, as fewer cows are kept and milked.
**3.** There are significant costs associated with specific feeding systems, meaning that a high margin doesn't necessarily correlate with a large profit. For example, additional costs (beyond those accounted for in the forage cost of grazed grass) in a low-yielding, spring grazing system are relatively small.

In comparison a high-yielding, intensive, 365-day housed system fed a TMR would have extra costs associated with:

- concentrate storage;
- diesel for the feeding operation (tractor, mixer wagon, loader, for example);
- depreciation on feeding operation machinery;
- labour associated with feeding operation;
- slurry storage;
- slurry disposal;
- capital expenditure on housing facilities and investing in cow comfort; and
- additional labour units required per litre in attaining management standard to maintain a healthy, high-yielding herd and prevent losses.

Having considered financial efficiency, it is also important to consider physiological efficiency. Between-farm differences arise in the energy content of milk as a result of differing genetic, nutritional and management interactions. The biggest variation comes from varying butterfat percentages, and therefore milk is 'fat corrected' to allow meaningful physiological comparisons between farms. Four per cent is often used in the European context, whereas

**Table 8.5.** Income margins for example herd.

|  | Monthly income (£/herd) | Total monthly feed costs (£/herd) | Herd margins (£/herd) | Number of cows in herd | Margins per cow in herd (£/cow) |
|---|---|---|---|---|---|
| Column | a | b | c | d | e |
| Equation |  |  | a–b |  | c/d |
| Milking cows (all feeds) | 37,200 | 18,580 | 18,619.84 | 200 | 93.10 |
| Milking cows (purchased feeds) |  | 13,491 | 23,708.80 |  | 118.54 |

**Table 8.6.** Improved margins for example herd.

|  | Monthly income (£/herd) | Total monthly feed costs (£/herd) | Herd margins (£/herd) | Number of cows in herd | Margins per cow in herd (£/cow) |
|---|---|---|---|---|---|
| Column | a | b | c | d | e |
| Equation |  |  | a–b |  | c/d |
| Milking cows (all feeds) | 41,850 | 19,758 | 22,092.34 | 200 | 110.46 |
| Milking cows (purchased feeds) |  | 15,178 | 26,672.40 |  | 133.36 |

a 3.5% correction is more common in North America, as shown in Table 8.7.

In the example above the herd produces milk of 3.6% butterfat, 0.4% points below 4%. This represents an 'energy saving' of nearly 2 l of milk relative to producing milk of higher fat content. Once the standard 4% fat-corrected yield has been calculated, we can look at the efficiency with which it is produced to compare and assess differing farms. First, the DM-corrected concentrate weight per cow per day can be divided by this yield to calculate the 'feed rate' in kg/l. The feed rate for the herd in question is 0.4 kg/l of 4% FCM.

Feed rates rise when less milk is produced from forage. A figure is commonly quoted for this 'yield from forage' and is calculated on the blanket assumption that

all concentrate is 13 MJ/kg DM and therefore 0.45 kg of concentrate will produce 1 litre of milk. The calculation is fundamentally inaccurate but may be useful in communicating change to farmers, as shown in Table 8.8.

Finally, feed conversion efficiency should be considered. This is the amount of milk produced per 1 kg of dry matter consumed by the cow. Efficiency rises as yields rise, due to the dilution of maintenance requirements for the cow. It is calculated as shown in Table 8.9.

Increasing this efficiency figure is generally desirable, but the marginal cost per MJ of energy increases as yield rises, so margins must be monitored with the caveats given above.

**Table 8.7.** Fat correction data and milk yield.

| | Daily yield (l/cow/day) | Butterfat (%) | 4% FCM yield (l) | Concentrate fed (87% DM; kg/cow/day) | Feed rate (kg/l; 4% FCM) |
|---|---|---|---|---|---|
| Column | a | b | c | d | e |
| Equation | | | (0.4 × a) + (15 × a × b/100) | | d/c |
| Milking cows (all feeds) | 30.0 | 3.6 | 28.2 | 11.4 | 0.4 |

FCM, fat-corrected milk.

**Table 8.8.** Milk yield from concentrate and forage.

| | 4% FCM (l/cow/day) | Concentrate fed (87% DM; kg/cow/day) | Milk yield from concentrate (l/cow/day) | Milk yield from forage (l/cow/day) |
|---|---|---|---|---|
| Column | a | b | c | d |
| Equation | | | b/0.45 | a–c |
| Milking cows (all feeds) | 28.2 | 11.4 | 25.3 | 2.9 |

FCM, fat-corrected milk.

**Table 8.9.** Feed conversion efficiency.

| | 4% FCM (l/cow/day) | Dry matter intake (kg/cow/day) | Feed conversion efficiency (litres 4% FCM/kg DM) |
|---|---|---|---|
| Column | a | b | c |
| Equation | | | a/b |
| Milking cows (all feeds) | 28.20 | 20.7 | 1.36 |

FCM, fat-corrected milk.

## Monitoring disease and fertility parameters

Nutrition has the potential to influence the occurrence of many diseases (and general disease monitoring is dealt with in other chapters). Some diseases have stronger, more direct aetiological links with nutrition than others, and monitoring of these will provide more convincing direct evidence of nutritional mismanagement. Milk fever, displaced abomasum and retained placenta (see Chapter 4) are linked to nutrition, have clear clinical signs and should be recorded as they are useful nutritional monitors.

While metritis and endometritis are also considered to have a strong nutritional aetiology, they require veterinary expertise for accurate diagnosis and correct definition (see Chapter 4). Monitoring based on farmer-based diagnosis of these will need to be treated with caution, as this may be inaccurate. Furthermore, the incidences of these diseases are not solely influenced by nutritional status and other aetiologies, such as the level of dystocia, are relevant. Good records of other causal aetiologies and care in interpretation of the prevalence of these diseases is therefore required.

The frequency of examination of the records, and the decision as to when to take action in the face of an abnormal trend, will require careful thought. This is because it will depend on the incidence of the disease and the size of the susceptible population. For instance, retained placenta tends to be a more common condition than abomasal displacement, so trends may be more apparent over shorter time intervals. This will be the case particularly in larger herds that are seasonally calving with large 'at-risk' populations at certain times of the year. Thus, if 400 cows calve evenly over 3 months, more than 30 animals will be at risk of retained placenta every week of the calving season and hence monitoring of the weekly prevalence would be important.

As with the diseases discussed above, although many indicators of fertility status are strongly affected by nutrition, fertility parameters are also influenced by other management decisions and practices (see Chapter 4). For example, the time to first service and the apparent expression of oestrous activity are affected by nutrition, but they are probably more strongly influenced by the voluntary waiting period and the time allocated each day to the identification of cows in oestrus. There are further problems with fertility parameters: many suffer from being very historical and are only of use in retrospective analysis. Nutrition has a strong association with pregnancy rate, although it will be only one of many possible influences on this (see Chapter 4 for a detailed discussion).

Table 8.10 provides suggested guidance on the monitoring and proposed targets for

**Table 8.10.** Diseases to be monitored to evaluate nutritional influences on herd health.

| Disease or reproductive parameter | Achievable targets | Comments |
|---|---|---|
| Milk fever | <5% | Directly related to macro-mineral management in immediate pre-calving period and BCS (see later sections) |
| Retained placenta | <5% | Also need to record whether dystocia or |
| Endometritis[a] | <8,000l (<5–10%) 8,000–10,000l (<7.5–10%) >10,000l (<10–15%) | twins to establish whether there are non-nutritional influences |
| Displaced abomasum | Depends on yield <8,000l (0%) 8,000–10,000l (<2%) >10,000l (<3%) | Stage of lactation can provide important aetiological information (see later sections) |
| Pregnancy (conception rate) | NA | Pregnancy diagnosis must be performed |
| Fertility efficiency (see Chapter 4) | >20% | early and data examined regularly to avoid time lag |

BCS, body condition score. [a] Defined as purulent vulval discharge later than 21 days post-calving.

metabolic diseases. It should be noted that all targets are farm dependent and need to be determined by consultation with all parties involved on the farm to make them realistic and achievable.

### Monitoring nutrition: assessment of the cow

When monitoring nutritional status as part of a dairy herd health programme, individual cows provide useful information to inform decision making. Recording and evaluation of cow data is vital to understanding changes in a herd's nutritional status over time, and it is strongly recommended that the following assessments are made.

#### *Body condition scoring*

It is generally accepted that BCS is correlated to energy reserves, and therefore the management and monitoring of BCS (and changes in BCS) during the production cycle are central to the process of producing milk without predisposing the cow to excess mobilization of fat. While animals of high genetic merit produce more milk than those of lower merit – partly by increasing the mobilization of body reserves – it appears that cows have a genetically determined BCS target that they tend to achieve by the third month of lactation. Thus cows that are fatter than their BCS target show reduced feed intake and lose more condition after calving.

There are several different scoring methods described and utilized worldwide for BCS. However, for the purposes of this chapter the standard five-point scoring method (Edmonson *et al.*, 1989) has been used.

SYSTEMS AND TARGETS FOR SCORING. Monitoring systems either involve the monitoring of individual animals as they progress through the lactation or simply assessing the condition score of the cows at a given point in time and extrapolating BCS changes from this. This latter method is potentially unreliable, as it assumes that the current condition of any particular group is an accurate representation of the past condition of a group further on in the lactation cycle.

Ideally, all cows in any group should be scored but where individual group sizes become large (>100) then this will become onerous. Calculating a sample size that will provide sufficient confidence of obtaining a representative picture of that particular group is difficult – it will be affected by the variation of scores within the group. In practice, for a large group, a randomly chosen sample of 100 cows generally provides a good estimate of group BCS. An alternative approach is to set an acceptable level (prevalence) of low (or high) BCS cows and to estimate a sample size based on the principles described in Appendix 1.

The key groups to monitor are cows at drying off, calving, early lactation (during service and pregnancy diagnosis) and at mid-lactation (see Table 8.11). The latter group is often overlooked but is of great importance because this is the time when cow condition can be most easily influenced by dietary manipulation. This manipulation should be aimed at ensuring that cows reach the dry period at their target score (see below).

The key parameters to understand are (i) the mean score for the different stages of lactation and (ii) the percentage of cows outside (above and below) the target range. The target should be for 85% of cows to be

**Table 8.11.** Target body condition scores for dairy cows.

| Stage | Ideal score | Range (Holstein) | Range (Friesian) |
|---|---|---|---|
| Drying off | 3.00 | 2.5–3.0 | 3.00– 3.50 |
| Calving | 3.00 | 2.5–3.0 (heifers, 2.25–2.75) | 3.00– 3.50 (heifers, 2.75–3.25) |
| Early lactation | 2.50 | 2.0–2.5 | 2.50–3.00 |
| Mid-lactation | 2.75 | 2.0–2.5 | 2.50–3.00 |
| Late lactation | 3.00 | 2.5–3.0 | 2.75–3.25 |

within the target score range for that period of lactation.

A recent meta-analysis confirmed that modern dairy cows probably have lower BCS values than cows of 20 years ago and hence it can be argued that target BCS at drying off and calving is slightly less now than it was 20 years ago; for a modern, high-yielding Holstein cow the target condition score should be 2.5–3.0. In relation to the importance of understanding the percentage of outliers, researchers have examined the percentage of cows at less than target condition scores at given stages of lactation, and have concluded that herds with a higher percentage of 'faults' have a reduced reproductive performance, as defined by the percentage pregnant by 150 days in milk.

Table 8.12 demonstrates how to plot BCS in an example herd to derive these statistics, and provides an immediate picture of herd BCS. Dry cows should be scored in the early period and transition (<3 weeks to calving), and lactating cows must be divided into at least early, mid- and late groups (monitoring fresh cows is useful but not essential), so that the changes of score through lactation can be estimated. The example here demonstrates the need to understand the percentage of condition score faults as well as the mean score, because the mean scores in this herd are at target but there are too many cows scoring higher than the target score at any stage of lactation.

Monthly scoring will provide the most up-to-date information and thereby allow problems to be identified quickly, and should be considered the gold standard for frequency of monitoring. Not all farmers will wish to pursue such intensive monitoring, and so planning a targeted system of monitoring that coincides with higher-risk periods can be useful (e.g. at turnout to grass or three months prior to drying off, to allow dietary adjustment if cows appear to be destined to become over-fat at drying off).

### Rumen fill

Monitoring and scoring of rumen fill as a proxy indicator of DM intake is a useful procedure, and the protocol of scoring is shown in Table 8.13. Recent research suggests that this technique is valid for monitoring DMI, but that care needs to be taken with the method, and in particular the timing when scoring takes place. This is because cows will normally eat more during the day than at night and consequently rumen fill will be higher in the evening than in the morning. Therefore, when monitoring rumen fill and extrapolating these recordings to likely DMI, erroneous conclusions of changes of intake could be drawn from scoring at different times of day. For instance, monitoring in the morning would potentially lead to a conclusion that intakes appear low or dropping if compared with an evening result. The research suggests therefore that the technique should be used on a daily basis at the same time of day to determine changes of DMI in cows in early lactation. Suggested protocols for implementation of rumen fill scoring are outlined in Table 8.13.

MONITORING COW APPEARANCE AND RUMEN FILL IN THE DRY PERIOD. The aim for cows managed within late lactation and the early dry period is to have obvious cover over the transverse processes and overt ruminal distension. As a result, when viewed from behind, the cows should appear 'pear' shaped rather than an 'apple' shaped. Given the nature of their diet, faeces during this period should be stiffer than the early lactating cows and there should be a high degree of consistency between cows' faeces.

### Monitoring faeces

While monitoring the character of the faeces of individuals or groups of cows is a commonplace procedure on the farm, there is little scientific work on the relationship between the physical characteristics of faeces and inadequacies in the diet. Monitoring of faeces is based on observation of the appearance of the faeces and the observable level of variation within a group, and detection via washing and sieving of the faeces of (i) undigested and partially digested grain, (ii) long fibre particles (>1.25 cm) and (iii) the presence of mucin casts. When monitoring faeces,

**Table 8.12.** Example of condition scoring in a Holstein herd (targets set out in Table 8.11).

| Group | Days calved | Condition score ≤1.0 | 1.5 | 2.0 | 2.5 | 3.0 | 3.5 | 4.0 | ≥4.5 | Number scored | Mean score | Percentage of cows with BCS < target | Percentage of cows with BCS > target |
|---|---|---|---|---|---|---|---|---|---|---|---|---|---|
| Early dry | −60 to −21 | | 1 | 11 | 1111 | 1111 1111 | 11111 11111 | 1111 | | 30 | 3.1 | 10 | 47 |
| Transition | −21 to 0 | | | 11 1111 | 1111 | 1111 | 11 | 1 | | 14 | 2.8 | 14 | 21 |
| Fresh | <30 | | | 11111 1111111111 | 1111111111 | 1111 | | 1 | | 21 | 2.6 | 0 | 23 |
| Early | 30–100 | 1 | 1111 | 1111111 1111111 111111 | 1111111111 1111111 1111111 | 11111 1111 | 111 | 1 | | 63 | 2.4 | 6 | 22[a] |
| Mid- | 100–200 | | 11 | 1111111111 1111 | 1111111111 1111111 1111111 | 11111111 111111 11111 | 1111 | 11 | | 63 | 2.6 | 3 | 40 |
| Late | >200 | | | 1111111111 1111111111111111 | 11111111 1111111111111111 | 1111111 1111111 11111111 | 1111111 1111111 1111111 | 111111 111 | 1 | 75 | 3.1 | 12 | 41 |

[a] Cows scoring over target score in early lactation would not be considered a significant concern.

it should be borne in mind that faecal consistency will normally vary between cows and that some undigested material can be normal, especially in high-yielding cows where ruminal outflow levels are very high. The faeces of cows fed maize silage also tend to contain more undigested material than those fed grass or grass silage. Table 8.14 lists the observable abnormalities that can be detected and putative causes thought to generate such changes.

**Table 8.13.** Protocol for rumen fill scoring: cows should be monitored on level ground in the absence of obvious ruminal contractions, and performed while in their groups with access to feed (von Keyserlingk *et al.*, 2010, summarized from Zaaijer and Noordhuizen, 2003).

| | Appearance of paralumbar fossa | | | |
| Rumen fill score | Relationship to transverse lumbar processes | Relationship to last rib | Shape | Comment |
|---|---|---|---|---|
| 1 | Paralumbar fossa sinks in more than a hand's width below | Paralumbar fossa sinks in more than a hand's width | Empty rectangle | Cow highly likely to be ill |
| 2 | Paralumbar fossa sinks in less than a hand's width below | Paralumbar fossa sinks in more than a hand's width | Triangle | Not abnormal in the first few days post-partum, but otherwise abnormal and indicative of poor feed intake |
| 3 | Falls about a hand's width vertically down and then bulges out | Paralumbar fossa sinks in less than a hand's width behind the last rib | | Target early to mid-lactation cows |
| 4 | The skin arches out immediately below | Paralumbar fossa skin covers the area behind it | Fossa bulges out directly | Target late lactation |
| 5 | Transverse processes not visible | Last rib not visible | Rumen distended and almost obliterates fossa | Target dry cows |

**Table 8.14.** Presentation and potential causes of abnormal faeces (Kononoff *et al.*, 2012).

| Presentation of faeces | Possible reasons for abnormality |
|---|---|
| Large variation in consistency between cows on the same diet | Sorting of ration; poorly mixed ration; SARA |
| Excess undigested material | SARA; poor ruminal fermentation; large intestine fermentation |
| Undigested cereal grain particles | Failure to crack grain during harvesting; inadequate degradable protein; hard grains |
| Excessive looseness | Excess total and degradable protein; inadequate fermentable energy; low ADF/NDF; disease |
| Excessive firmness | Restricted water or protein intake |
| Presence of mucin casts | Extensive hind gut fermentation |
| Excessive faecal soiling | SARA |
| Foamy or bubbly | Lactic acidosis or excessive hindgut fermentation |

ADF, acid detergent fibre; NDF, neutral detergent fibre.

Suggested protocols for frequency of monitoring are listed in Table 8.15. The time required for rumen adaptation to dietary change means that any changes in faecal characteristics following dietary alteration will take in the region of 1 week. Any monitoring protocols will need to take this into account.

### Rumination (cudding)

Monitoring the frequency and proportion of animals that are ruminating while at rest is frequently cited as a good indicator of ruminal health. Despite this, there is little apparent scientific quantification of its true value. Rumination is correlated with saliva production, which is the primary buffering agent for the rumen, and thus an absence, or reduced quality, of rumination is inevitably undesirable. Standard maxims for herd assessment are that over 60% of cows resting should be ruminating at any point, that on average there should be 60 chews per cud and that cows should ruminate around once every minute. Recent work suggests that when monitoring rumination on a regular basis, utilizing a single time point is not accurate and that to develop an assessment of the overall percentage of cows ruminating, multiple observations within any day are required if accurate conclusions are to be drawn. Thus if an observation suggests that cows are not ruminating as frequently as desired, a minimum of a second observation that day is required to increase confidence that this is actually the case. Furthermore, while reductions in rumination can be indicative of an episode of SARA, this would not necessarily detect a herd with a chronic SARA situation with a prolonged but consistent low rumination rate.

The observation that cows are 'dropping their cud' while ruminating should be considered abnormal and noted. This is most commonly ascribed to be as a result of ruminal acidosis, though its presence should not be seen as pathognomonic for SARA.

### Subacute ruminal acidosis

Subacute ruminal acidosis can be defined as 'an intermittent fall of ruminal pH to non-physiological levels due to maladaptation of the ruminal environment in terms of ruminal microflora and ruminal mucosa', and is thought to occur when ruminal pH falls

**Table 8.15.** Suggested protocols for nutrition-related monitoring cows.

| Parameter | Critical groups to monitor[a] | Critical Times to monitor | Suggested interval between monitoring of dairy assessments (days) | Intervention(s) |
|---|---|---|---|---|
| Body condition scoring (BCS) | See section on BCS | NA[b] | 30 | See section on BCS |
| Rumen fill | Transition, early lactation and high-yielders[a] | After any diet/forage change | 1–7 | >25% outside target score for stage of lactation or where there is evidence of reduction in overall score |
| Faeces | Transition and early lactation | After any diet/forage change | 7 | >25% of faeces abnormal (see Table 8.14 for details) |
| Rumination | Early lactation | After any diet/forage change | 7 | >50% cows resting not ruminating; presence of cud balls |

[a]These groups are either at higher risk of problems occurring or should be monitored because faults at these stages will have greater impacts. [b] In seasonal calving herds, the start of the calving period and 3 months before drying off.

below 5.5 (clinical acidosis is considered to be seen below pH 5.2). Its significance in regard to cow health and productivity is probably dependent on the frequency and duration of the period during which ruminal pH remains below 5.5. High-producing dairy cows are considered to be at greater risk of SARA than their lower-yielding counterparts, as they will be fed rations with a higher concentrate:forage ratio and, most importantly, will have higher overall intakes (kilograms ingested) of readily fermentable carbohydrates. The mechanism of action is via either an excessive fermentation of sugars and starch or an inadequate buffering of the rumen, or a combination of both. This leads to a reduction in ruminal acidity below a pH of 6.0 at which optimal digestion can take place (due to depression of the ruminal microflora that aid cellulose digestion at these pH levels). Recent research suggests that cows appear to become more prone to SARA if they have been exposed previously and that the severity of further subsequent bouts becomes greater.

There are a number of indirect methods utilized to monitor SARA based on identifying the rather vague clinical signs associated with the disease, although none of these provide absolute evidence for the presence of the condition. Examples of such clinical signs include reduced or erratic feed intake, increased respiratory rate, diarrhoea possibly with greasy or foamy faeces and poor body and coat condition. The only reliable diagnostic test for SARA is based on a direct measurement of ruminal pH. This is normally performed through rumenocentesis, although even this test is limited because it provides only a snapshot of ruminal pH at any specific time. Consequently, the duration that the pH remains below 5.5 cannot be quantified unless repeated measurements are taken from an individual over a period of hours. A novel solution to this problem is via the use of indwelling ruminal boluses that monitor and relay the information on pH on a continuous basis, and the use of such monitors may become widespread in the next few years.

SELECTION OF COWS FOR RUMENOCENTESIS.    Given the epidemiological presentation, the main times during lactation to investigate cows

are around 2 weeks after calving and at peak yield, when maximum levels of food intake occur. The time of sampling during the day is important. For maximum sensitivity, where cows are receiving a concentrate feed sampling should occur approximately 3 h after this feed. In TMR herds it should occur 5–8 h after feed is delivered. If SARA is diagnosed at these time points then repeat sampling 2–3 h later could be considered, to ensure that the duration of the drop is a significant and not transient effect. Cows to be sampled should not be kept away from the feed for longer than 30 min.

The number of cows selected for rumenocentesis depends on the number in the group at risk, the prevalence at which a herd is deemed to have a problem and the certainty required to detect that prevalence (see Appendix 1 for details). It should be noted that given the defined time periods to investigate for SARA, there may be difficulties in selecting sufficient numbers of cows in the respective groups at risk. Furthermore, primiparous cows are more prone to low ruminal pH than multiparous cows and this should be considered when selecting which cows to sample. The number of heifers that should be represented within in any sampling group should be proportional to the number of heifers in the herd as a whole.

TECHNIQUE FOR RUMENOCENTESIS.    The sampling point for collection of the liquor is the ventral sac of the rumen and this is located at the level of the stifle joint, a hand's width caudal to the last rib (approximately 10–12 cm). Once the cow is adequately restrained, the insertion site should be aseptically prepared and a small amount of local anaesthetic introduced into the skin and muscle layers. A 10.0–12.5 cm, 16- or 18-gauge needle should be used for collection and this should be introduced quickly and decisively through the prepared site and into the rumen. A syringe can then be attached and the contents aspirated. Obstruction of the needle by particulate matter is not uncommon and this should be cleared by pushing air via the syringe through the needle (excessive suction should not be used as this is considered to produce inaccurate results). Samples should be tested via a calibrated pH meter as soon as possible after sampling.

DIAGNOSIS.     The diagnosis of SARA in a cow can be made if the pH measures <5.5. We recommend that an estimated herd prevalence of 10–15% of cows affected warrants further investigation of the diet (see Appendix 1).

There are other ancillary observations that can be performed on the ruminal liquor that can add useful information about ruminal heath status and have been reported to be correlated to SARA. These are (i) the gross appearance; normal ruminal liquor should look greenish and have an aromatic smell, whereas SARA samples tend to look yellow or whitish and often have a fetid, sour smell; and (ii) direct microscopy to visualize protozoa. Protozoa can be described as either large, medium or small. It has been reported that large protozoa are the first to disappear in digestive disorders, followed by medium then small; however, this is subject to variation and this observation cannot be considered a reliable indicator.

It should be noted that widespread rumenocentesis represents an invasive procedure and the welfare implications of this type of monitoring, on a herd basis, should be considered. Furthermore, it is increasingly recognized that ruminal pH tends to fluctuate over time in high-yielding cows, and the distinction between normal and abnormal is not absolutely clear. Decisions therefore as to the significance of any diagnosis should take into account the clinical picture and whether there is evidence that cow health and/or productivity appears to be adversely affected.

### Monitoring metabolic markers

*Non-esterified fatty acids and ketones*

Concentrations of NEFAs and BHB can be used as markers of NEB both at the individual cow and herd level. NEFAs are indicative of the degree of fat mobilization, and BHB the completeness of oxidization ('burning') of the mobilized fat in the liver (see section 'Background: key concepts').

The critical time to measure NEFA and/or BHB is during the transition from mid–late dry period to early lactation. The objectives of measuring these metabolic markers are:

1. To monitor, at herd level, the success of current management with the goal of early detection of problems or deviation from the management programme.
2. To identify individual cows at high risk of disease with the goal of intervening to prevent or mitigate clinical disease.

Unfortunately, no single test is perfect in terms of sensitivity and specificity and it is important to understand the performance of the tests to be able to understand when they are appropriate for one or both of these objectives. For example, if monitoring is aimed at finding individual cows with subclinical ketosis and the result of finding a 'positive' is that a cow receives treatment that requires withdrawal of milk from the bulk tank, then a test with poor specificity will result in more wasted milk than necessary.

Serum BHB is considered nearest to a 'gold standard' test for ketones, but urine and milk can also be used. There are test sticks which, when used at appropriate cut-off points, can be very cost effective in monitoring subclinical ketosis (SCK). In general, urine ketone tests are very cheap and are generally very sensitive (approaching 100%), and are hence good for ruling out SCK with a negative result. Milk ketone tests have a poorer sensitivity but are highly specific, and thus a positive result is likely to be a true positive. Due to the availability of relatively cheap human blood ketone tests, which can be used 'cow-side' and which have a sensitivity and specificity in excess of 90%, these are increasingly becoming the test of choice.

PRE-CALVING MONITORING OF NEB.     Significant associations have been found between NEB pre-partum, as reflected by elevated NEFA concentrations and the occurrence of displaced abomasum (DA). Most of the published work suggests that NEFA concentrations in excess of 0.6 mmol/l in the week prior to calving represent a significantly increased risk. However, NEFA concentrations rise as calving approaches and, if cows are sampled in a broader 2-week window prior to calving, target levels of <0.3 mmol/l are appropriate.

POST-CALVING INDICATORS OF NEB. The point at which a blood BHB concentration becomes abnormally high and puts an animal at increased risk of deleterious effects on health and fertility varies between research studies. The standard definition of SCK is that serum BHB exceeds 1.4 mmol/l, but recent work has suggested that values >1.03 mmol/l can have significant negative effects on health. A herd prevalence of SCK exceeding 20% in the first 2 weeks after calving has also been identified as representing an increased risk of fertility and metabolic disease, especially DA.

TESTING FOR TYPE I AND TYPE II KETOSIS. Testing strategies that concentrate on the first 2–3 weeks of lactation seem to be appropriate in most herds, bearing in mind the strong links between SCK, health and fertility. This is especially true in herds that are characterized by cows being too fat pre-calving and suffering from above-target left-sided DA (LDA) incidence. This early sampling window covers the peak incidence of fatty liver/type II ketosis, which stems from nutritional mismanagement during the dry period. However, in herds where dry cow management is adequate but where the nutritional demands of lactation are not met, type I ketosis may occur and this normally occurs 3–6 weeks after calving. Type I ketosis is more likely to be seen as disappointing yields and fertility, and occasionally LDA occurring later in late lactation (outside the first month). In such herds the lactating ration or low DMI is likely to be the main problem, rather than issues that started pre-calving as with type II ketosis.

Type II ketosis is associated with fatty infiltration of the liver and normally causes elevated NEFAs immediately post-calving, and elevated BHBs starting at day 5 post-calving. It is possible to have elevated NEFAs in very early lactation but normal BHBs, which means that testing for ketones alone may miss this population of animals and that NEFA testing is required.

LIVER DAMAGE AND FUNCTION. Increased concentrations of bile components are seen in cows with fatty liver. These and high concentrations of NEFAs, BHBs and cytokines are all cytotoxic and contribute to further liver damage. All liver enzymes increase, especially glutamate dehydrogenase (GDH), γ-glutamyl transferase (γGT) and aspartate aminotransferase (AST).

THE PRACTICALITIES OF TESTING

*Choice of cows.* Consistency is the key to being able to compare results on farms over time. Samples should be collected at approximately the same time of day to avoid confounding the results by diurnal or postprandial variations, and cows should be in the same 'window' relative to calving – ideally 2–10 days pre-calving and the first 2 weeks post-calving (avoiding the first 2 days). NEFA concentrations peak just before feeding. It is important not to choose cows that are 'oddities' but rather ones that seem to be 'normal' within the system. Cows for sampling should not be separated from their feed for several hours prior to testing.

*Sample handling.* Serum or plasma is acceptable for BHB and NEFA testing, but BHB levels will be falsely elevated by haemolysis. Samples should be collected from the tail vein or jugular vein and ideally chilled, separated within a few hours and then frozen or shipped chilled for receipt at the laboratory within 1–2 days. However, delays of up to 24 h for separation, and maintenance at room temperature for 24 h or refrigeration for <3 days do not substantially affect results. Cow-side tests are now available (such as the Optium Xceed meters (UK) and Precision Xtra meters (US)), which will eliminate errors associated with sample handling.

The number of samples required for group- or herd-level interpretation depends on the prevalence of affected animals that is judged important to detect, the certainty of detection that is desired, and the size of the group of interest (see Appendix 1). Fortunately, the latter criterion has a relatively small influence. We recommend that an estimated population prevalence of 10–15% warrants further investigations and, in practice, the minimum number of samples required is usually 9–12 to allow interpretation in most situations.

### Urea

An excess of rumen degradable protein results in an increased concentration of ruminal ammonia, which is absorbed through the ruminal wall and carried to the liver where it is converted to urea. Likewise, the catabolism of muscle protein for gluconeogenesis can also result in the production of ammonia, which is again converted to urea in the liver. Plasma urea is commonly used test to assess the efficiency of protein utilization. Urea moves passively from the blood into the milk, and hence there is a close and reliable relationship between the concentrations in milk and blood. Milk urea can therefore be used as a good, non-invasive substitute for plasma in testing for urea. Farmers commonly receive bulk milk urea concentrations on their milk quality reports.

INTERPRETATION OF UREA TESTS.     The concentration of urea in blood and milk reflects the balance of rumen available energy, and rumen available protein supplied to the ruminal flora. An increased urea concentration should probably be viewed as being more important for production and possibly fertility than a reduced urea concentration. An elevated urea concentration can suggest both an over-supply of rumen available protein and/or a lack of rumen available energy.

Both of these situations have an effect on the energy status of the animal. A lack of rumen available energy means that the rumen is not performing efficiently and an excess of rumen available protein, causing the conversion of excess ammonia into urea, requires ATP and hence incurs an energetic cost to the cow. A decreased urea concentration is more likely to reflect a lack of rumen available protein rather than an excess of rumen available energy (which can be difficult to achieve in high-yielding cows). Low urea can also occur in cows with reduced DMI in the previous 12–24 h. This can occur concomitantly with elevated serum BHB. A low urea concentration

in transition cows may be linked to those in NEB, perhaps reflecting a reduction in DMI or inability of the liver to convert ammonia efficiently to urea.

INDIVIDUAL TESTS.     Individual blood urea concentrations are routinely used in metabolic profiles, but can be difficult to interpret when considered in isolation. When blood BHBs are done at the same time, interpretation is more straightforward. As described above, a high urea with a high BHB should first suggest an under-supply of energy. The most appropriate action would normally be to increase DMI and energy supply and, secondly, to reconsider the level of protein supplementation if urea levels remain elevated. Unlike blood BHB, where high levels are known to have deleterious effects on production, disease and fertility, the upper threshold for blood urea where adverse effects occur is more difficult to elucidate (a normal value is generally considered to be 5–6 mmol/l). Individual milk tests are not often done but can be just as useful as blood tests. A 'normal' concentration is approximately 200–300 mg/l.

BULK MILK TESTS.     Bulk milk tests are a useful tool for overall monitoring of protein supply, but there has been a tendency for over-interpretation in the absence of clear scientific evidence to link high bulk milk urea levels to reduced fertility. It seems sensible not to be dogmatic about what are 'correct' bulk milk urea levels, but rather to use the readily available information provided by milk buyers to get an approximate idea of the protein and energy balance of the herd. Suggestions from the studies that have observed effects on fertility are to keep the milk urea values below 400–425 mg/l.

### Blood and urine macro-mineral monitoring for hypocalcaemia

Assaying blood calcium (Ca) concentrations can be useful in the first 36h after calving to demonstrate or monitor subclinical hypocalcaemia. Unfortunately, blood Ca concentrations will not yield any useful information as a *predictor* for hypocalcaemia, as it is under extremely tight homeostatic control, except in the immediate peri-parturient period. Surveys suggest that up to 25% of heifers can be subclinically hypocalcaemic (Ca <2 mmol/l) in this period, and this rises to over 50% in older animals. Herds with good hypocalcaemia control should experience a prevalence of subclinical hypocalcaemia in this time window of less than 20%.

Urine analysis (Table 8.16) can demonstrate the acid–base status of the cow and the reasons for that status. For instance, strong alkalosis is often associated with excess dietary K, which is shown as high urinary excretion of K. It is especially useful in predicting whether cows are sufficiently metabolically acidified to prevent hypocalcaemia or, on the other hand, too acidified (which causes excessive loss of Ca in the urine). (see later section "Nutritional control of hypocalcaemia").

### Monitoring trace elements

The trace element and vitamin status of dairy cows is often implicated in production problems but is rarely monitored consistently. Blood samples are sometimes used to investigate problems, but unless the choice of animals is consistent, sufficient numbers of animals are tested and the tests used are fully understood, it can be difficult to draw any conclusions.

METHODS FOR SCREENING TRACE ELEMENTS. Reference ranges differ at different points in the production cycle. In general, cows should not be sampled in the immediate peri-parturient period as the serum concentrates of many trace elements and vitamin precursors will fall during this time, this being partly due to normal sequestration

to colostrum. Sampling of 9–12 animals in the early dry period is useful to estimate herd status for the period of the production cycle that will be most affected by an inadequate status. Further sampling at 2 months into lactation can be useful too, as this coincides with the beginning of the peak service period and time of maximum production.

Monitoring should not be restricted to the cow, and mineral analysis of the forage components of the diet – particularly those derived from grass – can provide very useful information. This relates not only to the background supply of minerals (and their antagonists) to the cow but also to where they are to be fed, to the transition cow and the dietary cation–anion balance (DCAB) of the forage. It should be appreciated that any such analysis will provide only a snapshot of the mineral profile of the forage at that point, and as with dry matter content, the mineral profile is highly likely to alter between batches of forage.

It is recommended that dairy cow mineral and vitamin requirements are met by adhering to the independent Nutrition Research Center guidelines (freely available online at http://www.nap.edu/openbook. php?record_id=9825&page=1), but guidelines on the trace elements and vitamins most frequently encountered in dairy practice are provided in Table 8.17.

### Monitoring of nutrition: assessments of feeding

Whatever the complexity and precision of computer rationing software, successful

**Table 8.16.** Parameters used in pre-partum urine analysis.

| Urine parameter | Use |
| --- | --- |
| Potassium (K) | Demonstrates whether dietary K is excessive, the biggest driver for milk fever |
| Calcium (Ca) | Demonstrates Ca mobilization and evidence of acidification (rather than Ca intake) |
| | Prevention of excessive demineralization by adding more dietary Ca if the cow is excessively acidified |
| Magnesium (Mg) | Demonstrates adequacy of intake and uptake from the gut |
| Dissolved $CO_2$ | Related to blood bicarbonate concentration, hence acid–base status |
| pH | Demonstrates pre-calving acid–base status |

**Table 8.17.** Guidelines on trace elements and vitamins most frequently encountered in dairy practice.

| Trace element/vitamin | Uses/effects of suboptimal status | Requirements | Comments |
|---|---|---|---|
| Cu | Primary deficiency is rare; secondary deficiency – scour, coat colour changes, reduced reproductive function | Controversial – dietary levels >40 mg/kg DM can be toxic; depends on the presence of antagonists (Mo, S, Fe); certain pastures ('teart') in some geographical areas contain excess Mo; maize silage is low in antagonists | Diagnosis of secondary deficiency is difficult – caeruloplasmin:plasma Cu ratio may be a better indicator than plasma alone; liver biopsies (or abattoir sampling) and feed analysis can help; liver biopsies and liver enzymes may be worth monitoring to prevent over-supplementation |
| Se | Immune function; can cause retained fetal membranes (there are many other causes too); involved in iodine metabolism (conversion of T4 to T3) | 0.3 mg/kg DM | Blood tests normally assay glutathione peroxidase activity in erythrocytes and will be historical due to their long lifespan (~120 days); serum Se levels can be assayed too |
| I | Reduced fertility in both sexes; fetal death | 0.5 mg/kg DM should cover requirements even in the presence of goitrogens; supplementation levels often higher than requirements | Thyroxine (T4) and plasma inorganic iodine (PII) often assayed; T4 is an indicator of longer-term status but is affected by the metabolic status of the animal too; PII reflects recent intake; Se status affects I metabolism and should also be assayed; fetal thyroid required when investigating fetal death |
| Co | Required for vitamin $B_{12}$ production and gluconeogenesis; failure to grow, unthriftiness | 0.11–0.35 mg/kg DM | Deficiency unlikely in supplemented dairy cattle; liver vitamin $B_{12}$ content <0.1 mg/g wet weight is considered indicative of cobalt deficiency; abattoir sampling commonly used in NZ to monitor herd status; urinary methylmalonic acid (MMA) can be used |
| Zn | Involved in several reproductive and metabolic pathways; reduced horn quality and parakeratosis of skin | Affected by several antagonists including Cu and Ca; ~35 mg/kg DM, legal limit is 300 mg/kg DM | |

| | | | |
|---|---|---|---|
| Mn | Necessary for mucopoly-saccharide synthesis; growth abnormalities in neonates and ataxia reproductive failure | Requirements poorly defined; >22 mg/kg DM with toxicity at concentrations >1000 mg/kg DM; a cow producing 40 l/day requires 333 mg | |
| Vitamin A | B-carotene is the precursor of vitamin A and is required for rhodopsin (needed for night vision) and corpus luteum | Depends on background level, ~110 iu/kg DM | Abundant precursor (β-carotene) present in fresh grass; most likely time for deficiency is during the latter stages of the winter housing, especially when maize silage is the predominant forage source |
| Vitamin E | Antioxidant, often used as part of mastitis control strategy in dry period management | Depends on background level, ~20 iu/kg DM (500 iu/cow); transition diets often supplemented with 1000–1500 iu/cow | Abundant precursor (α-tocopherol) present in fresh grass; most likely time for deficiency is after winter housing |

feeding of cows will not be achieved if the cows and feed are not managed appropriately. The potential for error in formulation, preparation and delivery of feed and the subsequent intake of the ration by the cows is vast, and consequently cows often do not perform on a ration as predicted. Monitoring these related activities is an essential component of herd health management, as inadequacies in this area will limit milk yield and negatively impact on production and health. This is of particular concern during the transition and early postpartum period, where even relatively small effects on nutrition have been demonstrated to have important deleterious effects on health.

### The importance of normal cow behaviour

The most effective and welfare-friendly system of managing a cow is one that allows the cow to accomplish all her behavioural requirements without any form of hindrance. This constraint on behaviour can result from the physical environment, the time a cow has to perform certain behaviours or as a result of competition from other cows in the herd. In order to understand what to monitor to detect deviation from this requirement, it is important to understand what these behavioural requirements are.

FEEDING.    Cows are habitual creatures and divide their day up into distinct patterns of eating, drinking, resting and ruminating, each of which has individual time requirements. The total time taken to perform these behaviours, along with other minor behaviours, is considered to be around 21 h. If the management policy disrupts these requirements (e.g. excessive milking time), research suggests these will be an adverse effect on cow health and performance.

Cows, as herd animals, prefer to perform behaviours as a group, and thus the sight of one cow feeding will stimulate other cows to feed. If cows are prevented from acting in synchronicity, this trait will be diminished and the behaviour reduced. Cows are also hierarchical and this has two important consequences. Changes to a group structure will result in disruption to normal behaviours

(while the new hierarchy is established) and, in a situation where competition for resources exists, it will be the less dominant animals, typically heifers, that will suffer the greatest disruption to their behavioural needs.

Cows have peak feed intakes just after milking and after the delivery of fresh feed. Meal times are divided into approximately 30 min episodes and there are on average around 10 of these meals per day, though this number varies with parity, yield and days post-calving. Dry matter intake increases by approximately 1.5–2.5 kg/week during the first 3 weeks of lactation. Generally, older cows have a more rapid rate of increase in DMI during the first 5 weeks post-partum than primiparous cows. As lactation progresses, total daily eating time, meal frequency and meal duration are increased. If a cow is restricted from feeding for a prolonged period, then the lost time will be made up by increasing feed intake at the remaining meals, particularly at the initial meal, once that restriction is lifted. This is termed slug feeding and is considered undesirable because it results in reduced ruminal buffering and thus ruminal disruption, particularly if the ration is poorly mixed, prone to sorting or has a high proportion of concentrate.

DRINKING.    A cow's requirement for water is affected by the DM content of the diet, exercise level, food intake, milk yield, the environment and the quality of water. Cows will drink approximately 14 times per day, consuming approximately 13 ± 5 l/h, with a total time spent drinking of 30 min per day. As with feeding, cows prefer to drink together, and to alternate drinking with feeding and also to drink after being milked. More than a quarter of the daily fresh water intake is met during the 2 h after each milking, and almost 75% of the fresh water intake occurs during working hours (06.00–19.00 h). Even a small limitation in water intake, such as 0.5–1.0 kg/day, has been described as having negative impacts on DM intake. Water quality will affect palatability, and the presence of undesirable components, such as toxins, can be deleterious to the health of the cow. Cows tend to prefer to drink warm water (25°C versus 7°C), whatever the environmental temperature.

RESTING. A cow's desire to rest is very strong and is illustrated by the fact that, when cows are restricted from both the feed and resting space, they will make up for the lost time resting at the expense of feeding time rather than the other way round. Resting has been shown to take priority over feeding in a cow's time budget, with an additional 1.5 h/day standing time associated with a 45 min reduction in feeding time. Furthermore, since cows prefer to ruminate when resting, any impact on resting behaviour has the potential to impact on the quality and quantity of rumination and consequently on ruminal function. In particular, poor resting and ruminating is considered a risk factor for SARA. As a consequence, there appears to be a strong correlation between resting times and yield; this is based on the observation that the highest-yielding cows are those that rest the most, with each additional hour of rest promoting an extra 1.45 kg of milk per day. It is important to note that resting requirements are not only the preserve of the lactating cow but also the dry cow, with research indicating that transition cows that ruminate and rest for longer are more productive post-partum.

### Monitoring feeding: changes to cow groups

The three principal areas that need to be monitored, particularly within the peri-parturient period, in relation to grouping are (i) the impact of grouping on sub-dominant animals; (ii) the number of group changes an animal experiences; and (iii) the impact that group size will have on the cow's time budget.

The argument for separate grouping of heifers stems from two factors:

**1.** They are generally the smallest and most subordinate animals in a herd and therefore the most obvious group to be susceptible to the stress of group changes and bullying.
**2.** The differences in feed behaviour and intake between older and younger cows.

HEIFERS. There is a general perception and some evidence that heifers, if managed separately, perform better than if managed with other cows. The extent of the improvement observed will depend on the level of competition for resources they would otherwise experience. An observation of suboptimal heifer performance in relation to that of cows, particularly in terms of yield and fertility, could well indicate that there is excessive competition for resources in the herd generally. The poorer the heifer performance, the greater is the case for their being managed separately.

When evaluating competition for feed access, it is most germane to focus on the key areas of transition and early lactation, as restrictions in these areas will have the most profound impact (likewise, it is important to note that separate grouping does not need to occur for the whole lactation and could be restricted to one or both of these critical periods). Problems related to excessive competition for heifers will be compounded if they have not adapted to their post-partum environment. Therefore, cubicle training and introduction to the parlour and milking cow environment is an important desirable objective of maiden heifer management.

NUMBER OF GROUP CHANGES: TRANSITION AND CALVING. Management changes around calving time are critical to fresh cow health, with factors that compound the natural reduction in DM intake in this period being particularly relevant. It has been proposed that only around 30% of the variation in DMI may be explained by dietary and animal factors, suggesting that management factors account for 70% of the variation. Changes to group structure will result in a period of altered behaviour while cows redefine the new hierarchy of the group, and this disruption will last for 48 h. Group changes are therefore considered to have a significantly negative impact on DMI, with an increased number of group changes resulting in more social perturbation and a greater effect on DMI. Consequently, the method and frequency with which group changes are performed needs to be managed and monitored carefully. Ideally, group changes within a herd should occur no more frequently than once per week, are better performed as a batch than as an individual, and performed in the evening rather than in the morning.

It should be borne in mind that the freshly calved cow will often be weak and tired and therefore susceptible to competition. Management of such cows should ensure that they are not placed in an environment that will expose them to the risk of excess competition and bullying. A further significant observation in this area is that cows that spend a prolonged period in a maternity pen (3–5 days as opposed to 1–2 days) are at a higher risk of lowered productivity, culling, increased body fat mobilization, displaced abomasum and ketosis. Therefore it is recommended that, provided the cow is in a physiologically suitable state, that she should be moved from the calving pen within the first 24 h.

TIME BUDGETS AND MILKING.      Given the requirement for cows to have 21 h to perform their daily behaviour requirements, it is important that groups are managed in such a way that total milking time (including time in the pre- and post-milking yards) does not exceed 3 h per day.

*Monitoring feeding: competition for resources*

FEED SPACE REQUIREMENTS.      Stocking density at the feed face, particularly in the transition period, has been linked to compromised cow health and reduced productivity and fertility. Increasing feed space reduces aggressive interactions between cows and results in increased feed activity, particularly for subordinate cows. A further problem with a reduced feed space is that dominant cows may attempt to 'sort' (preferentially eat different components of the ration), resulting in less dominant animals not only eating less but also eating a poorer ration.

Suitable feed space allocation is considered to be 0.75 m per cow (for a Holstein-Friesian). However, in the transition period, feed space allocation should be 20% higher for both fenceline feeding systems and headlocks. Therefore it is recommended that cows are stocked at 80% of normal capacity (i.e. to provide ten headlocks to eight cows or, in feedline systems, a feed-space of 0.9 m per cow).

FEED FACE DESIGN.      Cows are reported to eat for longer and produce more saliva when they eat in a natural grazing position with their head 10–15 cm above their foot height. Raised feed troughs above 45 cm will result in dominant cows controlling more of the feed face, thereby reducing the effective feed area. Cows will spend less time at a head-to-head feeder than at a fenceline design, and this can be reflected in reduced intake. Post and rail designs appear to be more accommodating for cows to feed at, as compared with headlocks, resulting in increases in feeding time and less inactive standing at the feed area, although lower hierarchical cows may be displaced less often in headlock designs. Therefore, if feed space is limited, headlocks may be useful in reducing competition and consequently displacement of a cow's lower status in the hierarchy. The physical condition of the trough surface also needs to be assessed – cows are likely to eat more when presented with a smooth floor (e.g. plastic or tile-lined) than with a rough surface.

WATER PROVISION.      There should be at least two water troughs per housed group and these should be located away from direct sunlight and dead ends of passageways and close to the feed and lying area of the cows. There should be adequate space for cows to move freely around the troughs – failure to provide this will result in dominant cows inhibiting access to the trough. Troughs should be located in the loafing area post-milking because cows drink 50–60% of their total intake post-milking, with a linear trough space per cow exiting the parlour of 0.3–0.6m. Total linear space for water provision should be 10 cm per cow in the herd. Water pressure should be sufficient to avoid cows waiting for a drink. Deep troughs should be avoided (no deeper than 30 cm) to reduce water stagnation and aid cleaning.

Water quality will also impact on intake. The prime anti-quality factors known to affect dairy cattle and the interference levels associated with these are (i) total dissolved solids >7000 ppm; (ii) sulfur/sulfates >200 ppm;

(iii) nitrates >130 ppm; and (iv) iron >0.3 ppm. Further information on this subject can be found at http://www.das.psu.edu/research-extension/dairy/nutrition/pdf/water.pdf. A subjective initial assessment however is more practical – simply ask whether you would be willing to drink from the trough. When assessing the adequacy of water supply, look for confrontations at the trough, particularly after milking – if they are observed, increased availability is required.

### Monitoring feeding: the cow's environment

A variety of aspects of the cow's environment are important to optimize nutrition and production. Excellent cow comfort and ventilation are important areas and are discussed in other chapters. Some additional aspects of the cow's environment are highlighted below.

HEAT STRESS. A primary consequence of heat stress is a drop in feed intake, and heat stress has the capacity to severely reduce a cow's health and productivity. Monitoring for heat stress is based on measuring both temperature and humidity and then comparing these with the temperature and humidity index (THI). When humidity levels are <30%, cows can generally handle temperatures up to 32°C without a drop in production; however, when humidity levels increase to 80% or higher, a drop in production may be observed at temperatures as low as 21–23°C. The problem is exaggerated if temperatures remain high at night so that cows cannot cool down.

Housing can significantly affect the environmental temperature that cows experience. Increases in the region of 10°C between housed cattle and the outside environmental temperature are not uncommon, particularly in poorly designed, under-ventilated buildings. Consequently even relatively mild external temperatures at high humidity could be significant where cattle are housed. Monitoring of both the internal and external humidity and temperature can allow an understanding of this dynamic, and consequently an understanding of what external environmental conditions should

prompt further management methods to reduce the effect of heat stress on the cows. Further information on this subject can be found at http://www.das.psu.edu/research-extension/dairy/pdf/heatstress.pdf.

PHOTOPERIOD. Photoperiod is defined as the duration of light to which an animal is exposed within a 24 h period. It is defined in day length: a long day length is considered to be 16–18 h of continuous exposure to light, while a short day length is <12 h. There are a variety of published papers suggesting that milk production increases with increased day length relative to cows under natural photoperiod day lengths, with a typical response to artificially increasing the day length being ~2 l/cow/day (further information on the requirements to create this environment can currently be found at http://www.livestocktrail.uiuc.edu/photoperiod/).

### Monitoring feeding: food management

FOOD PREPARATION. The ration fed can be completely different from that formulated if mistakes are made in its preparation and presentation. The two main sources of variation, when estimating DM intakes, are human error and variation in forage dry matter. The following are common examples of why divergence from a formulated diet occurs and should be assessed.

1. Farmer 'interpretation' of the supplied ration formulation to account for issues of supply and rounding (e.g. a nutritionist may work to three decimal places of a single kilogram, while farmers often work to 25 kg units for bagged products and 50 kg units for forages and straights).
2. Communication errors between the operator responsible for feeding and the farmer:

- The operator responsible is not aware of the protocols and procedures for mixing such as the order of addition, time for mixing and maximum and minimum loads.
- Diet sheets/protocols do not provide for changes in DM of forage and changes in group size.

**3.** Practical considerations in using the feeding equipment:

- Difficulties are encountered in cutting silage blocks to required weights or dropping straights from a loader bucket into the mixer wagon (i.e. driver-dependent errors).
- Weigh scales are inaccurate or not clearly visible.
- There are worn or broken parts in the mixer wagon.
- Straights were not mixed prior to loading (this can reduce time and increase accuracy).

**4.** Dry matter variation for by-products and forages can be marked, and these are therefore frequently very different from what was estimated for rationing (the monitoring of DM is discussed later).

To account for the human component there is no substitute for good verbal communication between *all* parties involved in the feeding operation, and the first stage in monitoring should involve speaking to the person who actually feeds the cows to find out what is truly being fed. A more quantitative analysis of feeding accuracy can be gained by:

**1.** Comparing the expected level of feed used, be this straights or forage, with the actual amount fed. This is frequently the issue that indicates a possible problem.
**2.** Assessing that a uniform mix is distributed among all the cows. This should be undertaken regularly, at least weekly, and can be assessed at its simplest by identifying whether the proportion of an easily identifiable straight is the same at various sites in the feed trough.
**3.** A more accurate method of assessment can be performed by identifying whether the relative proportions of particle sizes on the Penn State separator trays are the same at various sites along the feed trough.
**4.** Intermittent sampling of the TMR for DM and analysis using near-infrared spectroscopy (NIRS) or wet chemistry (DM, crude protein, NDF, macro-minerals) and comparison of the results with the formulated ration.

The frequency with which the latter two methods are employed will depend on the size of the unit (cost of error higher), the performance of the cows and whether concerns have been raised by other aspects of monitoring.

DISCRIMINATION (SORTING) OF THE DIET. If cows are able to discriminate and select different ration components ('sorting'), this can result in the consumption of a very inconsistent ration. Sorting is thought to contribute to ruminal dysfunction such as SARA and variation in performance due to cows eating 'unbalanced' diets. However, a recent study of sorting found that, despite large differences in particle size and some chewing and ruminating differences, no changes in ruminal fermentation, milk production or milk components were found. Typically, long particles are selected against, resulting in some meals having much greater grain content than intended. Cow sorting can lead to multiple 'rations' being consumed by animals apparently fed the same ration. To minimize sorting, the aim should be for the forage particle size to be mostly between 0.9 and 2.7 cm.

SIGNS OF SORTING.

- presence of fibre being left over in a mix (usually >10 cm);
- 'holes' eaten into the TMR in the trough;
- variation in faecal consistency and composition; and
- a large variation in the proportions of particle size on the Penn State separator trays between freshly delivered feed and feed in the trough left 12 h later.

FEED DELIVERY. Cows are habitual and therefore benefit from being fed at a consistent time each day. Feeding twice daily does provide the advantage of a reduction in wasted feed, as cows can be fed more accurately. There is evidence that providing the delivery of fresh feed a few hours after the time cows return from the parlour may be beneficial in terms of intake, since this avoids the overlap of the two greatest stimuli to feed, namely milking and the provision of fresh feed.

Prior to a fresh allocation of feed, the feed trough should be cleaned out to remove spoiled feed. Cows should have access to the trough for at least 21 h each day. To maximize intake and provide for true ad lib feeding there should be a target of 5%, and certainly no less than 2%, feed remaining in the trough prior to the delivery of fresh feed. If this is not the case, it is likely that cows are not consuming the formulated diet and this should prompt investigation into the reasons – for example, the DM content of the forages should be checked.

Despite the fact that presentation of feed is recognized as a strong stimulus to feed, there is little evidence to show that providing fresh feed more than once per day increases DMI, provided the feed remains stable (a function of the environmental conditions and inherent stability of the feed). Pushing up feed can encourage cows to eat more, but principally will be of benefit only where they cannot reach the feed or where there is relatively little feed left, as cows do not like licking feed directly off the floor surface, particularly if that surface is rough.

UNDERTAKING REGULAR FEEDING EVALUATIONS. The frequency with which the parameters pertaining to the monitoring of feeding are assessed will be highly dependent on the size of the farm and the system of management. Common sense should dictate the necessity for monitoring a particular area, and thus if cow numbers are constant within a group there is no point in measuring the adequacy of the physical facilities, as this will remain constant. Table 8.18 summarizes the areas discussed above that should be measured, and provides recommended measures of how often this should occur and in which groups.

### Monitoring feeding: forages

The forage component of the diet is not only the most significant but also the most variable part of a dairy cow's diet and regular evaluations of forage, whether grazed or conserved, are consequently very important.

### Monitoring grazed grass

While it is unlikely that a herd health advisor will always be directly involved in the monitoring of grazing, understanding the principles and practices governing this area is very useful when working with farms where grazed grass is a significant proportion of the diet. Failure to manage grazing correctly will increase the risk of a shortfall in supply and potentially jeopardize the future quality and productivity of the sward, with consequent deleterious impacts on the nutrition of the herd.

MONITORING THE QUANTITY AND QUALITY OF GRAZING. Monitoring the quantity and quality of grazing on a weekly basis throughout the year is vital in determining both short- and long-term decisions on the manipulation of grazing management, to ensure that there is sufficient feed available to maximize DMI and that the sward's quality and productivity is maintained. The best method of assessment of quantity is from the estimation of the kilograms of DM within a sward, termed the 'field cover', with a score range from 1 to 5 reflecting a change from 1500 kg/DM grass/ha (the post-grazing target) to 3500 kg/DM grass/ha, respectively (a rise of 500 kg/DM grass/ha per point). Although it is possible with experience to develop reasonable visual estimations of likely cover, the use of a rising plate meter or new scanning technology provides more accurate data, which are very useful when calculating growth rates accurately.

An understanding of quality can be made by basic assessment of the species of plant and appearance of the swards. Open swards (no plant material), high levels of weed species, large areas of rejected grazing, low levels of clover and an overt amount of dead or dying leaf matter are all indicators of reduced quality and are all easily observed when walking the pastures. The focus should be on developing a sward where the energy content is consistently at or above 11.5 ME/kg DM by ensuring it contains a high level of live leaf and ryegrass species. Monitoring the ratio of live to dead leaf in the sward provides a good

**Table 8.18.** Recommended measures and frequencies for monitoring aspects of feed management.

| | Frequency of monitoring | Comments |
|---|---|---|
| **Grouping policy** | | |
| Maximum group size | Every 6 months – dependent on calving pattern and herd size | |
| Average duration in group | | |
| Moved as individuals or in batches | Annual | |
| Heifers trained to cubicles | Annual | |
| **Feeding trough management** | | |
| Liner trough space or no. headlocks per cow | | Essential for transition cows |
| Floor height of trough | | |
| Neck rail height | | |
| Fenceline/head-to-head? | Assuming no changes to farm facilities, only needs measuring once | |
| Troughs clean? (Y/N) | Daily | |
| Feed distributed along length of face? (Y/N) | Daily | |
| **Water trough management** | | |
| Water trough space | | |
| No. troughs per group | | |
| Depth of troughs | | |
| Maximum distance from cubicles | Assuming no changes to farm facilities, only needs measuring once | |
| Restricted space around troughs? (Y/N) | | |
| Trough in loafing area and linear space offered? | | |
| Troughs clean? (Y/N) | Weekly | |
| Water temperature | Every 3 months | |
| **Housing** | | |
| No. rows cubicles in house | Assuming no changes to farm facilities, only needs measuring once | |
| Width of feeding alley | | |
| Cow comfort assessment | Monthly | Staff should be trained to recognize this |
| **Feed preparation** | | |
| Parlour feeders calibrated | Monthly | |
| Staff trained in feed preparation? (Y/N) | Annual or after staff change | |
| Straights mixed prior to loading? (Y/N) | As required | |

| | | |
|---|---|---|
| Diet sheets available with forage DM increments and animal numbers? | - | |
| Scales visible and calibrated? (Y/N) | Monthly | |
| Mix delivered with uniform consistency? | Daily | Staff should be trained to recognize this |
| Evidence of sorting? | Daily | |
| Time spent away from feed for milking, feeding, scraping, etc. | Every 6 months – dependent on calving pattern and herd size | |
| Feeding frequency | | |
| Feed pushed up/frequency | Annual | Staff should be trained to recognize this |
| Feed left before new feed delivered (%) | Daily | |
| Physical nature of feed | | |
| Abnormal odour?(Y/N) | Daily | Staff should be trained to recognize this |
| Evidence of mould? (Y/N) | Daily | |
| Evidence of heating? (Y/N) | Daily | |
| Forages | | |
| Chopped length of forages | Monthly | |
| How often is DM of forages checked? | Monthly | |
| How often are feed analyses done? | Monthly | |

understanding of the D-value (organic matter digestibility) of the grazing with a target for this value to be always greater than 65%.

MONITORING GRASS GROWTH.    Monitoring sward cover every week will allow the plotting and calculation of the level of growth that occurs on individual pastures. This is usful when calculating rotation length and in the monitoring of the grazing wedge (see below). It will also allow the assessment of average farm cover, which is the farm cover divided by the hectares available for grazing. The average cover provides a very effective way of planning forage supply throughout the year, and budgeting sward availability. As an example, the following targets are recommended in the UK for average farm cover (courtesy of the DairyCo grass + programme; Table 8.19).

A further refinement to monitoring growth is to monitor the number of leaves on a number of rye grass tillers, because rye grass tillers support only three green leaves; if the plant becomes sufficiently mature to have four leaves, the fourth leaf at the bottom of the tiller will be dead. This is obviously undesirable as it will reduce the plant's nutritional quality and will also lead to reduced productivity, as leaf death and decay have already commenced. Conversely, if a tiller is re-grazed before the emergence of the second leaf, this severely reduces the vigour of the plant and subsequent regrowth. Consequently, monitoring the emergence of these leaves allows the best pre- and post-graze points to be established, and can help determine whether the correct rotation lengths have been established.

SETTING THE DM INTAKE FROM GRAZING.    The decision about the targeted level of DMI for cows is fundamental to successful productivity and to the health of the cow. Unfortunately, monitoring DMI from grazing is very difficult but some level of estimation can be made from the reduction in the sward's cover following a period of grazing and, where an extra feed (buffer) is fed, subtracting this quantity from the overall value for

**Table 8.19.** Proposed UK average farm cover targets.

| Month[a] | Target cover (average) | Comments |
|---|---|---|
| Turnout | At least 1900–2000 kg DM/ha | Fields of 2500 kg DM/ha or more (grade 3) should be grazed first |
| Late April | 1800 kg DM/ha | Average farm cover is likely to fall after turnout until 'magic day', when grass growth matches grazing demand, usually around 1 May |
| May–August | 2500–3000 kg DM/ha | Fields should be grazed when they reach 2800 kg DM/ha; the highest covers are eaten first and the remainder should be cut for silage or topped if grass growth is ahead |
| Early September | 2500–3000kg DM/ha | Fields to be grazed should carry a cover of 3500 kg DM/ha (grade 5); as this will be the penultimate grazing, fields that may become waterlogged should be grazed first; fields should be grazed well down to 1500 kg DM/ha (grade 1) |
| Late September | 2500–3000 kg DM/ha | Fields should be grazed at no more than 3500 kg DM/ha; pre-grazing covers of >3500 kg DM/ha should be avoided to encourage autumn/winter tillering and the production of thick swards the following season |
| October–late November | 1900–2000 kg DM/ha | Grazing should be terminated when average farm cover drops to 2000 kg DM/ha; any paddocks grazed from mid-October should not be re-grazed |

[a] Throughout the season, swards should be grazed to a field cover of 1500 kg DM/ha (grade 1) and a height of 4–5 cm.

expected DMI. Understanding the processes that govern the setting of the target DMI for a group or herd is vital, as this will allow an understanding of whether such targets are realistic in relation to both animal factors (such as the target yield) or the genetic base of the herd and the pasture conditions.

The maximum DMI from grazing is considered to be 17–18 kg of grass under optimal grazing and sward conditions. The following factors need to be considered when determining the actual DMI selected.

SWARD QUANTITY.    If the average farm cover is falling below target and additional grazing area is not available, the introduction of increased levels of nutritional supplementation will be required to avoid future shortfalls in grazing.

SWARD CHARACTERISTICS.    As DM falls in a sward, a greater fresh weight of grass will need to be eaten to maintain the same level of DMI. For instance, a fall in sward DM from 20 to 15% means that cows need to consume an additional 25 kg of fresh sward to maintain the same daily DMI. In practice, the lower the sward DM, the more likely it is that cows will be unable to achieve target DMI because they run out of grazing time. The daily amount of fresh weight of grass that a cow can eat is subject to debate and, though there are instances of cows reportedly eating considerably more than this, a figure of 80 kg fresh weight is a reasonable maximum target. Similarly, as the D-value of the herbage decreases below 68%, this will result in decreased intake. A frequently quoted figure for D-value in regard to DMI is that a 1% fall in dry matter digestibility (DMD) is estimated to result in a fall in daily DM intake of 0.6 kg DM. Thus, as D-values decrease through the summer, so will intake of grass.

Sward mass, height and uniformity are also important variables that can significantly affect pasture intake, with the higher and thicker the sward the greater the intake. Herbage intake can be maximized by offering a good-quality, tall, dense sward. High-yielding cows need leafy swards with an average field cover of 2800–3000 kg DM/ha. These should be removed from the allocated field when grass reaches a height of 6–8 cm.

YIELD.    Supplementation is necessary where there is likely to be a shortfall in DMI as a result of inadequate quantity or quality (low D-value or DM content), and also where grazing will not meet the dietary requirements of high-yielding cows (usually defined as those producing >25 l). This is due either to a direct shortfall in supply and/or dietary imbalance. These imbalances result from inadequate levels of undegradable protein, starch and fibre and excess degradable protein. The consequence of supplementation of the cow's grass DMI will to a large extent depend on (i) the quantity of grass available: if grazing is in short supply, supplementation will have little effect and vice versa for high levels of grass availability; (ii) the nature of the supplement: in general forages have high substitution rates (the reduction in grazing intake from grass silage supplementation when adequate grazing is available has been shown to be almost 0.9 kg DM for every 1.0 kg DM fed), whereas concentrates will substitute to a lesser extent (0.4 kg DM for every 1.0 kg DM fed).

As the nutrient quality of well-managed swards is usually higher (higher energy and crude protein and lower fibre content) than the same plant material harvested as silage or hay, unnecessary substitution is undesirable and will result in reduced productivity of the animal and reduced quality of the sward, as well as increased feed costs.

GENETIC BASE OF THE HERD.    While the advantages of optimizing the potential DMI from grazing are obvious, if over-optimistic intakes are predicted this will result in reduced nutrient intakes. When assessing the level of risk can be taken, the genetic base of the herd needs to be considered primarily and, to a lesser extent, the average yield, number of days in milk and the proportion of heifers in the herd. Cows with a high genetic merit for milk production are far more prone to metabolic disturbance if their DMI is compromised, particularly in early lactation. Heifers are less able to achieve high DMI from grazing than their multiparous counterparts.

Thus more conservative estimates for DMI need to be made when dealing with these cows than with Friesian or Channel Island breeds, which will tend to respond to inadequacies of intake by simply reducing yield rather than developing metabolic complications. It should also be borne in mind, when grazing high-yielding cows, that on average Holsteins will achieve 20% greater DMI when presented with a TMR than by grazing alone, and it is reasonable on this basis to question whether high-yielding, early-lactation cows should be expected to graze at all.

MONITORING GRAZING SUPPLY: THE GRAZING WEDGE. The best way to calculate, plot and monitor the status of the grazing supply is via the use of a grazing wedge. This technique employs the use of a target line to allow a very easy means of predicting shortfalls or surpluses in grass supply (see Fig. 8.1). The key to the creation of a wedge is to understand the target for the pre-grazing cover. This can be set by using targets for the time of the year, as discussed above, or

can be derived from the following parameters: rotation (round) length, DM intake/cow, number of cows and current grazing area, and is calculated by the following equation.

Pre-grazing cover = (DMI × no. of cows)/
(grazing area/rotation length)
+1450 kg DM/ha (post-grazing target).

Thus, for example, in a 270-cow herd grazing 55 ha where the rotation length is 21 days and the expected DMI is 14 kg, the pre-grazing target is

$$(14 \times 270)/(55/21) + 1450$$
$$= 2893 \text{ kg DM/ha}.$$

The target line is derived by understanding the required growth figure, which in turn is calculated by

Daily growth required (kg DM/ha)
= (no. of cows × DMI)/grazing area.

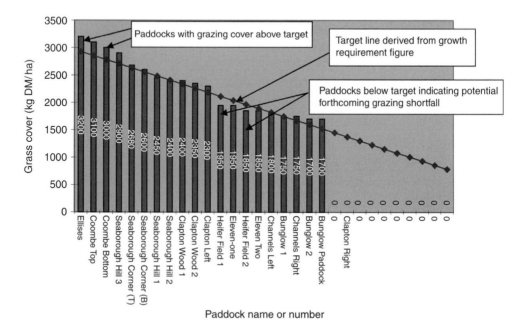

**Fig. 8.1.** Example of a grazing wedge. The columns indicate the grass cover of individual paddocks. Where a column exceeds the target line there is a potential surplus to be removed as silage; conversely, paddocks below the line show a potential forthcoming deficit in grazing supply. Observation of these patterns allows management decisions to be taken before the issues materialize and cause problems.

Thus in our same example the target would be

Daily growth required
$$= (270 \times 14)/55 = 68 \text{ kg DM/ha}$$

The measurements taken from the examination of the covers to determine the growth rate (see above) can then be used to create the columns on the wedge and thereby allow decisions on potential forthcoming shortfalls or surpluses of grazing to be taken (Fig. 8.1).

### Monitoring conserved forages

FORAGE INTAKES.    When assessing on-farm forages it is important to establish how much the cows are currently eating, because intakes are frequently overestimated. When grass is involved this has to be estimated too, but in housed cows forage intake can usually be established fairly accurately. If care is taken in obtaining correct DM and allowing for wastage, the results can be very enlightening and frequently explain problems of poor milk yield, cow health and milk quality. Common average forage intakes for herds are between 10.0 and 12.5 kg DM, depending on forage types and palatability.

CALCULATION OF FORAGE RESERVES.    Monitoring the amount of conserved forage and the rate of consumption is critical to ensure that there are sufficient reserves to last until new forages become available. Having to purchase silage or by-product forage 'extenders' is financially undesirable and, occasionally, logistically difficult. Basic calculations can therefore be made to provide estimates of rates of progression through the clamp:

**1.** Take approximate measurements of the length, width and height of the silage clamp to give an approximate volume (e.g. 30 × 10 × 3 m = 900 m³).
**2.** Work out the fresh-weight density of the whole clamp. The fresh-weight density of silage is approximately 600 kg/m³, with wet, long-chopped and poorly compacted silage being lower (~500 kg/m³) and fine-chopped,

well compacted silage being higher (700 kg/m³) (e.g. 900 m³ × 600 kg/m³ = 540,000 kg).
**3.** Estimate how long the clamp will last at the current feed rate using the amount of silage fed per head via the ration. It is advisable to allow 10–15% for wastage in collecting and feeding (e.g. 200 cows being fed 15 kg/head/day = [540,000 × 0.85]/[200 × 15] = 153 days).

A slightly less accurate method can be employed in herds with ad lib access to feed or poor diet records by estimating the number of metres removed from the face of the clamp over a set time period, and projecting forwards (e.g. a herd with a 30 m clamp losing 2 m off the face per week will last 15 weeks).

FORAGE QUALITY.    Variability in feed quality changes the balance of nutrients and may change feed stability and palatability. Early lactation cows naturally have limitations on DMI, and high quality forages provide a high level of nutrients from the feed. While silage analysis is an invaluable tool in predicting the nutrient and fermentative quality of what usually forms the main component of the diet, it cannot be overemphasized that it remains only a guide to the likely feeding value. Farmers will often obtain just one analysis for a particular clamp for its entire feeding period. Dependency on a single report to ensure the ongoing health and productivity of animals will result in erroneous conclusions, as there will be large variation within and between clamps of forages in relation to their physical and chemical characteristics.

Samples should be taken from the silage face in a 'W' pattern and then mixed thoroughly on a clean surface before sending ~300 g to a laboratory for analysis. The analysis from NIRS is based on a prediction rather than a direct measurement and, consequently, results should be interpreted with caution. At present, since laboratories use a wide variety of techniques, there are no agreed NIRS calculations for nutritive values, for whole-crop or leguminous silage or for organic bi-crop energy. Therefore, if whole-crop cereal or lucerne silage is intended to form a significant part of the diet, it would seem prudent to use primary (wet chemistry) analytic methods to assess quality. Aspects of feed quality to monitor are DM content, chemical analysis results, physical characteristics, palatability, stability, mould and appearance.

DM CONTENT.    The monitoring of forage DM on a regular basis is extremely important as this will vary considerably within a clamp, and failure to correct for this will lead to errors in feeding. The exact frequency that is adopted will be dependent on the farmer, observations of unexpected variation in performance and intake of the cows and on changes in the appearance and characteristics of the clamp. However, as a minimum, this monitoring should occur monthly, assuming there are no changes between clamps during this time. Samples need not be sent to a laboratory – analysis can be performed using an oven DM calculation. This can be undertaken using either microwave ovens, low-temperature heated ovens, Koster™ forage DM testers (similar to a large, inverted hair dryer) or adapted food dehydrators.

PHYSICAL CHARACTERISTICS

*Assessment of forages using the Penn State separator.*   The Penn State separator comprises a series of three sieves of declining aperture size and thickness that allow the ration to be fractionated into varying particle sizes. It works on the principle that increasing fibre level and forage particle size have been shown effectively to increase chewing activity and to increase saliva flow, ruminal pH, acetate:propionate ratios and milk fat levels. Conversely, excessive amounts of long, coarse forage may also limit intake and digestibility, ultimately affecting the energy balance of the animal. The Penn State separator helps determine whether the right balance of particle size has been achieved (Table 8.20). Detailed instructions on the practical use of the Penn State separator can be found at http://www.das.psu.edu/research-extension/dairy/nutrition/pdf/evaluating-particle-size-of-forages.pdf/. In temperate conditions, with wetter rations (typically 40–45% DM) the fine particles tend to stick to the wetter forage and confound the results. Another problem is that grass silage tends to weave together and does not necessarily fall through the top sieve despite smaller particle sizes – it therefore needs to be carefully teased apart. To overcome these factors it is best to dry the TMR or the forages to a standard DM before using the separator, and this does detract from its on-farm usefulness.

*TMR physical characteristics: 'openness'.*   This is very subjective, but useful; healthy rations are generally 'open', i.e. they spring open when squeezed. This reflects their effective fibre content and must be a function of rigidity or 'scratch', and also reflects the ration's DM percentage. Rations <40% DM and with inadequate long fibre tend to squash slightly rather than spring open.

*Secondary fermentation.*   This is the process in which feed begins to ferment again after it is removed from storage, and is usually the

**Table 8.20.** US targets for the Penn State separator.

| Screen | Corn silage | Haylage (lucerne) | TMR[a] |
|---|---|---|---|
| Upper sieve (% of total) | 3–8 | 10–20 | 2–8 |
| Middle sieve (% of total) | 45–65 | 45–75 | 30–50 |
| Lower sieve (% of total) | 30–40 | 20–30 | 30–50 |
| Bottom pan (% of total) | <5 | <5 | <20 |

[a] When assessing rations where concentrate is fed outside the total mixed ration (TMR), it should be remembered that parlour cake will sit in the bottom tray (<1.18 mm) since it is very finely ground. These are US targets, and the proportion allocated to the upper sieves (specifically the 'middle sieve') will need to be greater where consistently higher butterfat is required.

result of incomplete fermentation when the feed was initially put into storage. Fermented or wet feeds are more likely to be unstable and undergo secondary fermentation. In the heat of summer it will occur much more quickly than in the cold of winter. Since cows prefer not to eat feed that is hot and fermenting again, harvesting and storage protocols should be reviewed to prevent this from happening.

Aerobic spoilage occurs where

- There is oxygen.
- There is a plentiful carbohydrate source.
- There is a higher pH (this tends to occur in drier crops).
- There is a heavy inoculation of yeasts and moulds.

Simple assessments of secondary fermentation can involve examining the clamp or TMR to detect heating and mould formation. More involved assessments can be made via laboratory analysis of mould and mycotoxin load and physical measurements of the temperature of the feed.

## Key Concepts in Formulation

To review ration formulation and make recommendations as part of a herd health programme, it is recommended that the herd health advisor either undertakes specialized training in diet formulation or works closely with a credible nutritionist. There are numerous computer software systems and models available, and the differences between these lie in their energy and protein calculations and in the feed databases upon which they draw to make these calculations. Comparison of energy values and metabolizable protein values between systems and models is therefore possible, but difficult in practice, since they are subject to hundreds of variables including default cow weights, yields, milk components, environmental factors (temperature, humidity), activity measures and varying fractional feed degradability. Even differing software programs running the same formulation/rationing model may well give significantly differing outputs.

Therefore, we recommend the following approach when reviewing nutrition as part of a herd health programme.

**1.** Investigate cow responses to the offered ration as described in the earlier sections in terms of output (milk yield and constituents), body condition, faecal consistency and metabolic response.
**2.** Place these observations in the context of the metabolic disease history.
**3.** Build a picture of financial and physiological performance and evaluate this over time.
**4.** Evaluate environmental and management factors that may be impacting on the above responses to the formulated diet.
**5.** Audit, by DM testing, NIRS and wet chemistry, the ration and its component feedstuffs in terms of its nutrient content.
**6.** Note the previously described caveats; enter the ration actually eaten by the cows in a computer model as precisely as possible.

Having built a picture of the whole farm feeding system, alterations can be made to the formulated ration guided by these findings. A summary of guidelines for manipulating the major macro-nutrients applicable to the numerous formulation models is given in Table 8.21.

## Control of Major Nutrition-related Disease

It has been reported in epidemiological studies that dystocia, milk fever, retained placenta, metritis, ketosis, displaced abomasum, fatty liver and lameness are interrelated. Indeed, some authors position all these diseases together as the 'peri-parturient disease complex'. The relationship between these diseases is not fully understood, but there may be a common causality, possibly a profound disturbance of energy metabolism. While the prevention of conditions associated with reproduction and lameness is considered in other chapters, we set out below the important aspects of preventing specific nutrition-related diseases: hypocalcaemia,

**Table 8.21.** Summary guidelines for checking macro-nutrients in a ration formulation.

| Nutrient parameter | Minimum value and circumstances where this may be seen | Maximum value and circumstances where this may be seen | Typical (UK) values and caveats |
|---|---|---|---|
| DMI (kg) | 18.0<br>1. Poor forage quality. This is characterized by poor fermentation, showing high non-lactic, VFA levels, ammonia levels or ash content. Heavy faecal contamination prior to cropping is typical, as is the presence of yeasts and moulds. Field weed contamination favours such fermentation. Low digestibility affecting intake occurs when weeds are present or old varieties or poor species are used. Later harvest dates raise NDF content, which reduces intake.<br>2. Poor bunk management practice (e.g. restricted access).<br>3. Small cows of low genetic merit eat less.<br>4. High incidence of herd disease (e.g. lameness) | 26.0<br>1. Excellent forage quality, characterized by low VFA and ammonia levels, high digestibility, zero weed contamination and no spoilage. No faecal contamination prior to cropping.<br>2. Excellent bunk management practice, including access and presentation.<br>3. Large cows of high genetic merit eat more.<br>4. Relatively low 'days in milk' for the group. | 21.5<br>For a 7000–8000-l herd, the average figure would represent a feed conversion efficiency of ~1.31 4% FCM/kg DM. |
| fNDF (% ration DM) | 18.0<br>1. Slowly digestible, longer-chop length forages (e.g. straw).<br>2. TMR feeding.<br>3. Good bunk management practices.<br>4. Good concentrate characteristics, such as having particle size >1.18 mm (e.g. coarse brewer's grains or dried sugarbeet pulp pellets, or using slowly digested ingredients such as cracked maize grain or caustic treated wheat). Use of whole cottonseed allows this lower limit to be broken if all other factors above apply. | 26.0<br>1. Rapidly digestible, short-chop length forages such as spring grass, low-NDF grass silage (44%), short-chop/low-NDF maize silage or the use of brown, mid-rib maize varieties.<br>2. Component feeding allows concentrate slugs and requires a greater fibre 'safety net'.<br>3. Poor bunk management practices.<br>4. Poor concentrate characteristics, such as fine grinding and using rapidly digested products (e.g. milled wheat or confectionery). | 23.0<br>fNDF negatively correlates to DMI (the lower the fNDF the higher the intake until acidosis effects take over). When modelling fNDF values, always account for the substitution effect where component feeding is taking place. |

| | | | |
|---|---|---|---|
| CP (% ration DM) | 15.0<br>1. High DMI<br>2. Excellent amino acid profile of supplemented protein, a balance of lysine and methionine.<br>3. High-quality, slowly degraded protein sources.<br>4. Low levels of background soluble nitrogen from forages.<br>5. High levels of slowly degraded carbohydrate supplied to generate high microbial protein yields. | 18.5<br>1. Lower DMI<br>2. High levels of dietary soluble protein and nitrogen:<br>• common in grass-based or grass silage-based diets; and<br>• poor supplemental protein quality. | 17.5<br>Despite recent research demonstrating the effectiveness of low-protein diets, it is not uncommon to find 18.5–19.5% CP diets formulated routinely – we recommend these are avoided. |
| Starch (% ration DM) | 12%<br>1. Wet diets with a high background forage acid loading, such as 20% DM grass silage that has undergone extensive lactic fermentation.<br>2. Low dietary and physically effective NDF typically found where the concentrate presented is compounded or finely milled.<br>3. Presence of rapidly digested starch or sugar sources (e.g. ground wheat, biscuit meal or molasses).<br>4. Component feeding. | 26%<br>1. Dry diets.<br>2. Low background forage acid loading.<br>3. High dietary and physically effective NDF from all components.<br>4. Well-presented TMR will little sorting.<br>5. Slowly digested starch sources; typically, most starch derived from forage maize grain that is very mature and coarsely processed. | 14%<br>Starch levels vary hugely by geography. Where maize feeding is more common, starch levels will frequently reach 18%. |
| Oil (% ration DM) | 3.0<br>1. Poor energy density for high levels of milk production where intake is limiting.<br>2. Potentially limiting precursors for reproductive steroid hormone production.<br>3. Maintains low cost/kg of DM. | 6.0<br>1. May restrict DMI at or above this level, since high levels of calcium soap-protected fat in certain dietary contexts are unpalatable or where free oil affects rumen fibre digestion.<br>2. Unsaturated oil increases CLA production due to either high dietary supply or low ruminal pH (or both).<br>3. High butterfat % may be seen where fat is saturated C:16 (palm oil). | 5.0<br>This is a typical inclusion in diets for higher-yielding animals; however, the inclusion of 5% oil (if all unprotected and free in the rumen) would produce serious fibre digestion effects in many instances. |

DMI, dry matter intake; fNDF, forage neutral detergent fibre; CP, crude protein; VFA, volatile fatty acid; FCM, fat-corrected milk; TMR, total mixed ration; CLA, conjugated linoleic acid.

fatty liver, ketosis, displaced abomasum and subacute ruminal acidosis.

## Nutritional control of hypocalcaemia

Although the aetiology of hypocalcaemia (milk fever) relates more to the macro-mineral composition of the transition ration than to aberrations in energy metabolism, hypocalcaemia can affect peri-parturient energy status through depression of DMI. Calcium (Ca) is also involved in the release of insulin. The aetiology of hypocalcaemia is reasonably well understood and it can be thought of as a 'gateway disease' for other diseases, so prevention is a high priority in herd health management.

The main method of control previously was dietary Ca restriction in the 2 weeks prior to calving, to improve the activation of homeostatic Ca mechanisms. If Ca can be restricted sufficiently (<30g/day in a typical Holstein-Friesian cow) this method is effective, but the practical problem is that background dietary Ca levels are too high to be able to achieve this.

Since the start of the new millennium, the control of hypocalcaemia has moved towards managing the dietary cation–anion balance (DCAB) in the transition ration. The DCAB value of a ration or an individual feedstuff is calculated from the relative concentrations of sodium (Na) and potassium (K), the strong cations, relative to sulfur (present as $SO_4$) and chloride (Cl), the strong anions, and is measured in milliequivalents/kg DM (meq/kg DM). High-DCAB rations induce a metabolic alkalosis which decreases the efficiency of binding of parathyroid hormone (PTH) to its receptor, and this reduces the activation of vitamin D3. The role of vitamin D3 is to increase Ca release from bone stores and increase Ca uptake from the gut.

Cows are usually metabolically alkalotic (urinary pH in lactating cows is >8.0), due to the high K content of grass-based forages; the only situation where strong metabolic alkalosis is a clinical problem is in the period prior to calving. The primary aim of the DCAB method of hypocalcaemia control is to reduce metabolic alkalosis. It is also important to ensure adequate magnesium (Mg) status, as this is involved in the production, release and binding of PTH to its receptors.

### *The partial and full DCAB approaches*

The partial DCAB approach is the most commonly used method of hypocalcaemia control, and is based on selecting forages with low DCAB values (K concentration is the most important determinant of this) and ensuring an adequate Mg status. The full DCAB approach involves the addition of anionic salts such as ammonium chloride, magnesium sulfate, calcium sulfate (gypsum) and calcium chloride, which have strongly negative DCAB values (an excess of Cl and S over Na and K to induce a mild metabolic acidosis as shown by urinary pH values of 6.0–7.0). The full DCAB approach has considerable practical disadvantages and can worsen metabolic disease if not managed correctly, as the anionic salts required are unpalatable. The partial DCAB approach is usually the recommended default for overall metabolic health, but occasionally a well-managed full DCAB approach can be very effective for hypocalcaemia control and may not depress intakes sufficiently to precipitate excess fat mobilization. Table 8.22 highlights the differences between these two approaches. A practical approach to reducing the risk of peri-parturient hypocalcaemia using the DCAB control method is summarized below.

- Reduce K intake so that overall K in the diet is <2% DM (target, 1.3–1.5%). This usually centres on choosing grass-based forages with the lowest DCAB values (K concentrations >2% should be avoided) for use in transition diets or partially/totally replacing these with reliably low DCAB forages such as straw, maize silage or whole crop cereals. (There may be marked variation in the DCAB of different silage cuts and across different clamps, but multiple silage analyses

**Table 8.22.** Comparison of partial and full DCAB rations for the control of hypocalcaemia.

|  | Partial DCAB | Full DCAB |
|---|---|---|
| Basis of approach | Reduce forage DCAB base and add 50–100 g $MgCl_2$ to attain a Mg concentration of 0.4% DM | Reduce forage DCAB base and add sufficient anionic salts to attain urine pH of 6.0–7.0 |
| Calcium requirement | Not normally manipulated, and typically 0.5–0.6 % DM | Increased to 1.2% DM to compensate for urinary losses associated with acidification |
| DCAB range | –50 to +100 meq/kg DM | –100 to –150 meq/kg DM |
| Urine pH | 7.8–8.1 | 6.0–7.0 |
| Monitoring | Urine pH is not helpful at high pH values; periodic forage DCAB sampling | Regular urine pH sampling essential |
| Comments | Can be very effective and simple if theory is understood | Anionic salts are unpalatable and can depress DMI severely; this should not be used on farms where urine monitoring will not be done regularly |

DCAB, dietary cation–anion balance.

will help to identify the lower DCAB forages to be selected).

- Balance the diet using relatively low-DCAB feedstuffs such as cereals, rapeseed meal and straw.
- Magnesium supplementation via feed or water troughs should be considered (aim for 0.4% DM). Magnesium chloride has the dual benefit of lowering DCAB and providing magnesium. However, it is unpalatable and care should be taken in hot weather when cows are thirsty, as strong solutions can prevent cows drinking.
- Managing dry cows out at grass is difficult due to the relatively high potassium content and lack of control of their diet; cows should be removed from pasture prior to calving. Changing the DCAB has rapid effects on Ca metabolism, and high-risk cows can be removed from grass for the last few days prior to calving. Practically, it is often better to manage cows away from grass for the last 3 weeks of the dry period, to avoid any ration and group changes too close to calving.
- If transition cows have to be kept at grass, they should be tightly stocked with sward height <7 cm and, ideally,

only on later-season grass. However, care is required with mastitis prevention (see Chapter 2).

- To formulate low-DCAB forages for transition cows:
  - Use a small acreage and plant a long-lived grass; avoid clover leys.
  - Use moderate to heavy nitrogen fertilization (14–18 kg/ha at harvest).
  - Avoid fertilization with manure or potash.
  - Harvest grass twice a year (June and September), but avoid harvesting autumn 'flushes'.
- Over-supply of phosphorus to counter hypophosphataemia problems is counterproductive, as it reduces the activation of Vitamin D by inhibiting renal 1-α-hydroxylase. The principles that apply to the control of hypocalcaemia also apply to the control of hypophosphataemia.

*Targeted calcium supplementation*

It is possible to target high-risk cows and supplement them with Ca around calving. The most appropriate preparations for rapid Ca uptake, which are appropriate for the treatment of stage 1 (cow still standing but hyperaesthetic and staggering) hypocalcaemia, contain rapidly absorbable Ca. The most commonly employed salt is calcium chloride. This targeted approach can work well, but it is still important to try to control the DCAB of the pre-calving ration as this will reduce the likelihood of relapse and there will also be fewer high-risk cows requiring supplementation. Blood Ca concentrations are normally depressed only in the immediate calving period, with maximum risk approximately 6–12h pre-calving to 36h post-calving. This is because PTH secretion increases very rapidly in response to depressed blood Ca, but production of activated vitamin D3 takes approximately 36h. The most appropriate period for supplementation is therefore from 12h pre- to 24h post-calving. Most commercial preparations will contain approximately 40–50g of Ca, and a review of different methodologies suggests that the most successful prevention strategy is four doses over this time period. In practice, one dose 12h pre-calving followed by another post-calving should suffice. It is worth noting that if a cow does not calve within 12h of her pre-calving dose, then a further dose will probably be required.

### Nutritional control of fatty liver and ketosis

Fatty liver and type II ketosis are caused by excessive fat mobilization in the immediate peri-parturient period. Adipose tissue is often regarded simply as a means to store energy, but it is effectively the largest endocrine organ with a 'metabolic memory' of nutritional status. Excess body condition score (BCS) and overfeeding in the far-off dry period both increase the risk of fatty liver occurring, by increasing the level of fat mobilization precipitated by the metabolic demands of lactation.

When appraising management practices and cows in the face of a problem it is important to appreciate that assessing the average cow is useful, but perhaps more important are the deviations from this average. Variation in BCS across a group is especially important and will result principally from variations in individual cow mobility,

genetics and calving interval. However, there will be other less obvious variations that need to be considered too, and these arise from the quality of labour and the consistency of feeding practices. Forage quality, cow comfort, seasonal variations in feeding (e.g. proportion of maize silage in the ration) and numbers of cows calving all have to be considered.

### BCS management

Fundamental control of fatty liver and type II ketosis depends on maintaining appropriate herd BCS. The target BCS at various stages of the production cycle has been described earlier in this chapter. If monitoring reveals that these targets are being missed, the nutritional management needs to be altered. The most common cause of excess BCS in late lactation is feeding a single group on TMR that is too energy dense for lower-yielding, late-lactation cows. Cows with a greatly extended calving interval are particularly susceptible, and improving fertility is an important medium-term aim. Reduction of the energy density of the ration of the diet (for all cows or just those with high BCS) in late lactation can be considered – for example, by decreasing the amount of maize silage or concentrate feeds – but this strategy is not as straightforward as it sounds. Lower-yielding animals that are placed on lower-energy density diets often readjust their yield downwards and can still be over-supplied with energy relative to production. The best strategy is probably to focus on the reproductive performance of the herd and, if a single TMR system is required, then culling cows with inappropriate genetics may be necessary.

### Appropriate dry cow feeding: early dry period (drying off to three weeks prior to calving)

It is possible to increase the risk of fatty liver by overfeeding cows in the far-off dry period. This can occur even in the absence of grossly excessive BCS (>3.5). Farms where very high-quality forages are produced may be particularly susceptible to overfeeding. The energy requirements at this stage are low and can be satisfied by 5–7 kg of straw, with the remainder of intake provided by grass silage of low digestibility. When feeding a high straw inclusion in the transition ration it is important to acclimatize cows to this type of ration in the early dry period. The starch content of maize silage is too high, and neither maize silage nor concentrate feeds should normally be fed in the early dry period. Exercise can be useful especially in over-fat cows required to lose some condition; very bare pasture with straw provided in racks is ideal.

### Appropriate dry cow feeding: transition` period (3 weeks prior to calving)

There is a natural drop in DMI as parturition approaches, and one of the main aims of transition cow feeding is to minimize this drop by providing a palatable, well-balanced ration that is constantly available and fed from adequate, clean trough space. Exercise again may be beneficial and feeding cows outside, provided there is very little grass growth to cause complications with excess K intake, is possible. However, in practice this is difficult to achieve and cows are often more easily managed when housed. As discussed in the earlier section on cow behaviour, group changes should be kept to a minimum for the last 3 weeks prior to calving.

### Single-group dry cow management

Single-group dry cow management can have advantages – it minimizes stressful group changes, eliminates the risk of a cow moving to the transition group too late and reduces the number of rations that need to be fed and monitored. However, managing cows throughout the dry period as one group can be a high-risk strategy for fatty liver if cows receive a ration with an inappropriately high energy density. Even with an average dry period length of 45–60 days, there is the potential for cows with an excessive calving interval to have a considerably longer dry period than this. Overfeeding is much more common and likely to cause problems than underfeeding, and to reduce the chances of overfeeding on this system

the ration should be 'diluted' with straw. The inclusion of 5 kg of short, pre-chopped straw throughout the dry period can work extremely well to increase rumen size and prevent overfeeding.

### Management of the post-parturient cow

Recommended management practices for maximizing DMI in the post-parturient cow can be summarized as.

- Provide warm drinking water immediately after calving and place it next to the calf so that the cow doesn't have to move.
- In the calving pen, provide a highly palatable lactating ration that the cow can eat (urea and some fats can depress intake). Monitor how much of the ration is eaten.
- Leave the cow with the calf for no longer than 24–48 h.
- Consider a high-comfort fresh cow group, especially if the cow accommodation is lacking in loafing and feed space or floor surfaces are slippery. Keep cows in this group for 3–4 weeks if possible.
- Keep ad lib fresh feed available at all times.
- Assign one individual to monitor the demeanour and feed intake of the fresh cows. Consider other forms of monitoring such as rectal temperature.

## Nutritional control of displaced abomasum

Displaced abomasum (DA) is often regarded as a wholly nutritional disease, but the complicated multifactorial aetiology of the condition means that nutritional management will probably only provide part of the answer. Social stresses and other factors that cause reduced DMI need to be considered, as do management factors that render endotoxaemia more likely.

The recorded statistical associations between fatty liver/ketosis and DA do not indicate causation but do suggest that some of the aetiological pathways and predisposing factors for these peri-parturient diseases may be shared. Hence, the same factors that apply to the control of fatty liver/ketosis mentioned above probably also apply to the prevention of DA.

Displaced abomasum occurring in the first week post-calving are very likely to be related to fatty liver/type II ketosis, and may also be due to a lack of an adequate rumen fibre mat. It is impossible accurately to quantify what an adequacy of dietary fibre intake is, although the provision of adequate chopped straw, as highlighted in earlier sections, will provide sufficient fibre. Round bales and haylage can also be useful to increase long, palatable fibre inclusion, but the DCAB should be considered and also the means of incorporation in the ration, to ensure even intake across the group.

Displaced abomasum occurring later in lactation can be related to type I ketosis. Higher-yielding cows at grass may be particularly susceptible if weather conditions are poor, grass quality or quantity are inadequate or if buffer feeding is lacking. In the face of an outbreak of DA at grass, it is worth considering housing the early-lactation cows either completely or just at night until weather conditions or grass supply and quality improve. Buffer feeds should be more energy based (maize silage, molasses, mollassed sugarbeet) than protein based to balance the high protein content of grass, but the buffer ration should not predispose to acidosis. Finally, care should be taken in ensuring these cows are well within the safe limits of their likely DMI from grass (see section on monitoring of grazing).

## Nutritional control of subacute ruminal acidosis

The two fundamental causes of SARA are a failure of ruminal buffering and an excessive level of starch and sugars. These factors are frequently linked because increasing the proportion of fibre is highly likely to reduce the proportion of non-fibrous carbohydrate. While control has frequently centred on the levels of physically effective fibre and total

fibre in the diet, the overall DMI and physical and degradability characteristics of the non-fibrous carbohydrate (NFC) component are equally important in the occurrence of SARA. The factors that govern decisions on the type and quantities of fibre and NFC components of the diet when formulating are briefly discussed in the section on monitoring.

### Failure of buffering

Failure of rumen buffering will primarily result from factors that reduce the level of chewing that a cow undertakes (thus reducing the level of bicarbonate-rich saliva secreted per bolus of food). This can occur either at the initial intake of the food or later if there is a reduced level of rumination. A further factor to consider is that certain feeds have their own natural compounds (buffers) that help reduce the fall in ruminal pH. The main reasons for failure of buffering are:

- Inadequate long fibre (also see section on monitoring of the formulation): adequate long fibre must be present to form the fibre mat that floats on top of the liquid ruminal contents. The mat performs a vital role in rumen function by physically trapping food particles and allowing their controlled breakdown by the microbial flora associated with the mat. Lack of an adequate fibre mat allows undigested food particles to pass out of the rumen. Central to this issue is the chop length of silage. Short chop lengths of grass silage will allow for greater compaction and fermentation in the clamp and consequently a more stable feed, but long chop lengths provide a better buffering capacity.

- Sorting of long fibre (discussed in earlier sections): this is reported to be minimized when the highest proportion possible of particles is between 9 and 27 mm.

- Slug feeding (discussed in earlier sections): the feeding of relatively large quantities of highly fermentable foodstuffs does not facilitate good rumen buffering.

- Low-DM forages: wet forages require less chewing and will tend to have a higher acidic load.
- Excessive mixing of a TMR diet: if a diet is over-mixed in the TMR mixer wagon, long fibre will become less effective.
- Poor cow comfort (discussed in earlier sections): comfortable conditions that promote long lying time will also enhance rumination time.
- Silages with very low pH contents; this occurs more commonly than expected, and underlines the importance of consistently re-analysing feed values in silage clamps.
- Presence of mycotoxins: recent work has demonstrated that the presence of mycotoxins can alter the metabolism of lactic acid, allowing it to build up and cause acidosis.

### Excess fermentable energy

Feeding excess proportions of NFC relative to the fibre component, particularly where these are highly fermentable and/or where cows have a high DMI, will increase the risk of SARA. The common causes and risk factors for this are:

- The requirement to achieve high energy densities in the feed for high-yielding cows.
- Parlour feeding: despite the investment and cost of using mixer wagons, farms do not necessarily practise a complete TMR diet. Commonly, a level of production is expected from the TMR and then individual cows are fed additional concentrates using in- or out of-parlour feeding. This tends to provide greater control over feed rate and thus diet cost. The consequences of this are that cows, particularly those fed in the parlour, receive large slugs of concentrate, often around 4 kg at one time. This can be a significant factor for the induction of SARA. Cows in early lactation are at the greatest risk because these animals have not yet reached their maximum voluntary feed intake and consequently there is less forage to buffer the slugs of concentrate.

Cows in early lactation should receive a minimal proportion of in-parlour feed until their yield reaches the level provided by the TMR. The objective during the post-calving period is to maximize DMI rather than keep up with the daily energy requirements of the cow. Ensuring that protein levels of rations are kept low (~16%) in early lactation may help prevent cow yields rising too rapidly, and consequently reduce the potential for a negative energy gap.

- Poor transition cow management: specifically, this involves either a failure of rumen adaptation to the lactation ration (due to a poor transition cow diet) or the feeding of inappropriately high levels of concentrate too quickly and too soon post-calving, or a combination of the two. The general theory that the introduction of concentrates in the late dry period is important in stimulating ruminal papillary development is questionable. Recent research suggests that the type of diet fed during this period has little effect on papillary development, the rapid increase in size post-calving being a normal physiological response.
- Feeds containing high levels of soluble starches and sugars and/or an excess of finely ground feed particles (see previous sections on monitoring with the Penn State separator and monitoring the formulation).
- Grazing: SARA is not limited to concentrate feeding. Grazing, particularly in the spring, will provide all the key conditions to induce SARA in terms of low DM, high rapidly fermentable carbohydrates and low fibre content, and consequently SARA is thought to be common in grazed cattle.
- Reduced voluntary food intake (VFI): if VFI is poor – for example, due to poor palatability of the forages or heat stress – then diets will need to have an increase in their energy density (relative to a higher feed intake) to match a particular yield. This may also occur if the DM content of the forage is overestimated such that the proportion of the forage in the ration is lower than expected.

*Additives to control SARA*

A further method of correction or control, useful where it is difficult in practice to correct the issues discussed above, is the use of a variety of additives to control SARA. These are principally yeasts (e.g. *Saccharomyces cerevisiae*), bacteria (e.g. strains of *Enterococcus* spp.), alkaline agents (e.g. magnesium oxide) and buffers (e.g. sodium bicarbonate), all of which have been shown in trials to have some benefit in modifying ruminal pH. Further products such as acarbose, a commercially available α-amylase and glucosidase inhibitor, are also being trialled and may also become commercially available.

## Summary

Nutrient intake is closely linked to the health of dairy cows and it is therefore important that nutrition is a key component of a herd health programme. This chapter has detailed how to incorporate nutrition into herd health management through the careful monitoring of records, cows, feeds and feeding management. Although it is useful for the herd health advisor to work closely with the nutritionist responsible for ration formulation, it should be recognized that problems related to feeding are more commonly associated with management of feeds and feeding rather than diet formulation. Therefore the role of the herd health advisor is critical in ensuring that nutritional management is dealt with in a holistic manner and included alongside other areas related to cow health.

## Acknowledgements

We would like to thank Tom Overton and Tom Chamberlain for their invaluable thoughts and comments on the content of this chapter.

## References and Further Reading

Agnew, R.E., Yan, T. and Gordon, F.J. (2002) Nutrition of the high genetic merit dairy cow – energy metabolism studies. *Recent Developments in Ruminant Nutrition* 4, 255–282.

Albright, J.L. (1993) Feeding behaviour of dairy cattle. *Journal of Dairy Science* 76, 485–498.

Bach, A (2011) Causes, prevention and control of rumen acidosis. The Dutch Bovine Conference. February 10, Utrecht, The Netherlands.

Bach, A., Iglesias, C. and Busto, I. (2006) A computerized system for monitoring feeding behavior and individual feed intake of dairy cattle in loose-housed conditions. *Journal of Dairy Science* 87, 358 (Abstr.).

Bach, A., Iglesias, C., Devant, M. and Ra'fols, N. (2006) Performance and feeding behavior of primiparous cows loose housed alone or together with multiparous cows. *Journal of Dairy Science* 89, 337–342.

Bach, A., Valls, N., Solans, A. and Torrent, T. (2008) Associations between non-dietary factors and dairy herd performance. *Journal of Dairy Science* 91(8), 3259–3267.

Batchelder, T.L. (2000) The impact of head gates and overcrowding on production and behaviour patterns of lactating dairy cows. In: *Proceedings of the 2000 Dairy Housing and Equipment Systems: Managing and planning for profitability*, pp. 325–330.

Beauchemin, K.A. (1991) Ingestion and mastication of feed by dairy cattle. *Veterinary Clinics of North America: Food Animal Practice* 7(2), 439–463.

Bede, D.K. (2005) The most essential nutrient: Water. In: *Proceedings of the 7th Western Dairy Management Conference*, p. 13.

Behnke, K.C. (2005) Mixing and uniformity issues in ruminant diets. In: *Proceedings of the Penn State Dairy Cattle Nutrition Workshop*, pp. 39–45.

Bertics, S.J., Grummer, R.R., Cadorniga-Valino, C. and Stoddard, E.E. (1992) Effect of prepartum dry matter intake on liver triglyceride concentration and early lactation. *Journal of Dairy Science* 75, 1914–1923.

Bobe, G., Young, J.W. and Beitz, D.C. (2004) Invited review: Pathology, etiology, prevention, and treatment of fatty liver in dairy cows. *Journal of Dairy Science* 87(10), 3105–3124.

Bolinger, D.J., Albright, J.L., Morrow-Tesch, J., Kenyon, S.J. and Cunningham, M.D. (1997) The effects of restraint using self-locking stanchions on dairy cows in relation to behaviour, feed intake, physiological parameters, health, and milk yield. *Journal of Dairy Science* 80, 2411–2417.

Brand, A., Noorhuizen, J.P.T.M. and Schukken, Y.H. (2001) *Herd Health and Production Management in Dairy Practice.* Wageningen Press, Wageningen, The Netherlands.

Brouk, M.J., Smith, J.F. and Harner, J.P. (2003) Effect of feedline barrier on feed intake and milk production of dairy cattle. In: *Proceedings of the Fifth International Dairy Housing Conference*, pp. 192–195.

Burgos, S.A., Dai, M. and Cant, J.P. (2010) Nutrient availability and lactogenic hormones regulate mammary protein synthesis through the mammalian target of rapamycin signalling pathway. *Journal of Dairy Science* 93, 153–161.

Butler, W.R., Claman, J.J. and Beam, S.W. (1996) Plasma and milk urea nitrogen in relation to conception rate in lactating dairy cattle. *Journal of Animal Science* 74, 858–865.

Cameron, R.E.B, Dyk, P.B., Herdt, T.H., Keneene, J.B., Milller, R., Bucholtz, H.F. *et al.* (1998) Dry cow diet, management and energy balance as risk factors for DAs in high-producing dairy herds. *Journal of Dairy Science* 81, 132–139.

Caraviello, D.Z. and Weigel, K.A. (2006) Analysis of reproductive performance of lactating cows on large dairy farms using machine learning algorithms. *Journal of Dairy Science* 89, 4703–4722.

Cardot, V., Le Roux, Y. and Jurjanz, S. (2008) Drinking behavior of lactating dairy cows and prediction of their water intake. *Journal of Dairy Science* 91(6), 2257–2264.

Cook, N. (2007) Pen moves and facility designs to maximise transition cow health and productivity. In: *Proceedings of the 8th Western Dairy Management Conference*, pp. 161–171.

Cook, N. (2008) Time budgets for dairy cows: How does cow comfort influence health, reproduction and productivity? In: *Proceedings of the 2008 Penn State Dairy Cattle Nutrition Conference*, pp. 53–60.

Cook, N.B., Nordlund, K.V. and Oetzel, G.R. (2004) Solving fresh cow problems: The importance of cow behavior. In: *Proceedings of the 8th Dairy Symposium of the Ontario Large Herd Operators*, pp. 248–255.

Cooper, R. (2011) An assessment of milk compositional indicators as a predictor for subclinical and clinical ketosis in UK dairy cattle. Dissertation submitted as part of the requirements in the examination for the RCVS Diploma in Cattle Health and Production, RCVS Library, London.

Correa, M.T., Curtis, C.R., Erb, H.N., Scarlett, J.M. and Smith, R.D. (1990) Ecological analysis of risk factors for postpartum disorders of Holstein-Friesian cows from thirty-two New York farms. *Journal of Dairy Science* 73, 1515.

Cottrill, B., Biggadike, H.J., Collins, C. and Laven, R.A. (2002) Relationship between milk urea concentration and fertility of dairy cows. *Veterinary Record* 151, 413–416.

Coulon, J. and Rémond, B. (1991) Variations in milk output and milk protein content in response to the level of energy supply to the dairy cow: A review. *Livestock Production Science* 29, 31–47.

Coulon, J.B., Doreau, M., Rémond, B. and Journet, M. (1987) Development of feeding activities in dairy cows at the start of lactation and relation to the quantities of feed ingested. *Reproduction and Nutritional Development* 27, 67–75.

Curtis, C.R., Erb, H.N., Sniffen, C.J., Smith, R.D. and Kronfeld, D.S. (1985) Path analysis of dry period nutrition, postpartum metabolic and reproductive disorders, and mastitis in Holstein cows. *Journal of Dairy Science* 68, 2347–2360.

Dado, R.G. and Allen, M.S. (1994) Variation in and relationships among feeding, chewing and drinking variables for lactating dairy cows. *Journal of Dairy Science* 77, 132–144.

Dahl, G.E. (2002) Lighting the way to optimal performance. In: *Proceedings of the AABP 35th Annual Convention*, pp. 92–95.

DeVries, T.J. and von Keyserlingk, M.A. (2005) Time of feed delivery affects the feeding and lying patterns of dairy cows. *Journal of Dairy Science* 88(2), 625–631.

DeVries, T.J., von Keyserlingk, M.A. and Beauchemin, K.A. (2003a) Diurnal feeding pattern of lactating dairy cows. *Journal of Dairy Science* 86, 4079–4082.

DeVries, T.J., von Keyserlingk, M.A. and Beauchemin, K.A. (2003b) Measuring the feeding behavior of lactating dairy cows in early to peak lactation. *Journal of Dairy Science* 86(10), 3354–3361.

DeVries, T.J., von Keyserlingk, M.A. and Weary, D.M. (2004) Effect of feeding space on the inter-cow distance, aggression, and feeding behaviour of free-stall housed lactating dairy cows. *Journal of Dairy Science* 87(5), 1432–1438.

DeVries, T.J., Beauchemin, K.A., Dohme, F. and Schwartzkopf-Genswin, K.S. (2009) Repeated ruminal acidosis challenges in lactating cows at high and low risk for developing acidosis: Feeding, ruminating and lying behavior. *Journal of Dairy Science* 92, 5067–5078.

Dickson, D.P., Barr, G.R., Johnson, L.P. and Wieckert, D.A. (1970) Social dominance and temperament of Holstein cows. *Journal of Dairy Science* 53, 904–909.

Dohme, F., DeVries, T.J. and Beauchemin, K.A. (2008) Repeated ruminal acidosis challenges in lactating dairy cows at high and low risk for developing acidosis: Ruminal pH. *Journal of Dairy Science* 91(9), 3554–3567.

Duffield, T.F. and Bagg, J. (2002) Herd level indicators for the prediction of high risk dairy herds for subclinical ketosis. In: *Proceedings of the 2002 AABP Convention.*

Duffield, T.F., Kelton, D.F., Leslie, K.E., Lissemore, K.D and Lumsden, J.H. (1997) Use of test day milk fat and milk protein to detect subclinical ketosis in dairy cattle in Ontario. *Canadian Veterinary Journal* 38(11), 713–718.

Duffield T.F., Lissemore, K.D., McBride, B.W. and Leslie. K.E. (2009) Impact of hyperketonemia in early lactation dairy cows on health and production. *Journal of Dairy Science* 92, 571–580.

Edmonson, A.J., Lean, I.J., Weaver, L.D., Farver, T. and Webster, G. (1989) A body condition scoring chart for Holstein dairy cows. *Journal of Dairy Science* 72(1), 68–78.

Enemark, J.M.D. (2008) The monitoring, prevention and treatment of sub-acute ruminal acidosis (SARA): A review. *The Veterinary Journal* 176, 32–43.

Enemark, J.M., Jorgensen, R.J. and Kristensen, J.B. (2004) An evaluation of parameters for the detection of subclinical rumen acidosis in dairy herds. *Veterinary Research Communications* 28(8), 687–709.

Ferguson, J.D., Calligan, D.T., Blanchar, T. and Reeves, M. (1993) Serum urea nitrogen and conception rate: the usefulness of test information. *Journal of Dairy Science* 76, 3742–3746.

Froetschner, J.R. (2005) Mixing, a detailed look at the factors that influence mix uniformity. In: *Proceedings of the Penn State Dairy Cattle Nutrition Workshop,* pp. 19–28.

Gábor, G., Tóth, F., Ozsvári, L., Abonyi-Tóth, Z. and Sasser, R. (2008) Factors influencing pregnancy rate and late embryonic loss in dairy cattle. *Reproduction in Domestic Animals* 43(1), 53–58.

Garnsworthy, P.C. (2007) Body condition score in dairy cows: targets for production and fertility. In: Garnworthy, P.C. and Wiseman, J. (eds) *Recent Advances in Animal Nutrition.* Nottingham University Press, Nottingham, UK, pp. 61–86.

Garnsworthy, P.C. and Topps, J.H. (1982) The effect of body condition of dairy cows at calving on their food intake and performance when given complete diets. *Animal Production* 35, 113–119.

Garret, E., Pereira, F., Nordland, M.N., Armentano, K.V., Goodger, W.J. and Oetzel, G.R. (1999) Diagnostic methods for the detection of subacute ruminal acidosis in dairy cows. *Journal of Dairy Science* 82, 1170–1178.

Geishauser, T., Leslie, K., Duffield, T. and Edge, V. (1998) An evaluation of protein/fat ratio in first DHI test milk for prediction of subsequent displaced abomasum in dairy cows. *Canadian Journal of Veterinary Research* 62, 144–147.

Grant, R.J. (1993) Water quality and requirements for dairy cattle. Nebguide. G 93-1138-A. Cooperative Extension Institute of Agriculture and Natural Resources, University of Nebraska, Lincoln, Nebraska.

Grant, R.J. (2007a) Effect of stocking density on cow comfort, health and productivity. In: *Proceedings of the 2007 Cornell Nutrition Conference for Feed Manufacturers.*

Grant, R.J. (2007b) Taking advantage of natural behaviour improves dairy cow performance. In: *Proceedings of the 8th Western Dairy Management Conference,* pp. 225–236.

Grant, R.J. (2009) Stocking density and time budgets. In: *Proceedings of the Western Dairy Management Conference,* pp. 7–17.

Grant, R.J. and Albright, J.L. (1995) Feeding behaviour and management factors during the transition period in dairy cattle. *Journal of Animal Science* 73, 2791–2803.

Grant, R.J. and Albright, J.L. (1997) Dry matter intake as affected by cow grouping and behaviour. In: *Proceedings of the 58th Minnesota Nutritional Conference, University of Minnesota,* pp. 93–103.

Green, M.J., Husband, J., Vecqueray, R. and Green, L. (2008) Variability in feed components of animal diets: Implications for animal performance and decision-making. In: *Recent Advances in Ruminant Nutrition,* presented at the Nottingham Feed Conference, 2007.

Grummer, R. (2008) Nutritional and management strategies for the prevention of fatty liver in dairy cattle. *The Veterinary Journal* 176, 10–20.

Herdt, T. (2000) Ruminant adaptation to negative energy balance. *Veterinary Clinics of North America* 16(2), 215–231.

Heuer, C., Schukken, Y.H. and Dobbelaar, P. (1999) Postpartum body condition score and results from the first test day milk as predictors of disease, fertility, yield, and culling in commercial dairy herds. *Journal of Dairy Science* 82, 295–304.

Holtenius, P. and Holtenius, K. (1996) New aspects of ketone bodies in energy metabolism of dairy cows: A review. *Journal of Veterinary Medicine A* 43, 579.

Hooijer, L., Rehage, G.A. and Noordhuizen, J.P.T.M. (2004) Rumenocentesis (rumen puncture): a viable instrument in herd health diagnosis. *Deutsche Tierarztliche Wochenschrift* 111, 458–462.

Huzzey, J.M., DeVries, I.T., Valois, P. and von Keyserlingk, M.A.G. (2006) Stocking density and feed barrier design affect the feeding and social behavior of dairy cattle. *Journal of Dairy Science* 89, 126–133.

Kertz, A.F., Reutzel, L.F. and Thomas, G.R. (1991) Dry matter intake from parturition to mid-lactation. *Journal of Dairy Science* 74, 2290–2295.

Keunen, J.E., Plaizier, J.C., Kyriazakis, L., Duffield, T.F., Widowski, T.M., Lindinger, M.I. *et al.* (2002) Effects of a subacute ruminal acidosis model on the diet selection of dairy cows. *Journal of Dairy Science* 85(12), 3304–3313.

Keunen, J.E., Plaizier, J.C., Kyriazakis, L., Duffield, T.F., Widowski, T.M., Lindinger, M.I. *et al.* (2003) Short communication: effects of a subacute ruminal acidosis on free-choice intake of sodium bicarbonate in lactating dairy cows. *Journal of Dairy Science* 86, 954–957.

Klein, J.L. (2004) Prevalence of subacute ruminal acidosis in Dutch dairy herds – a field study. Inaugural dissertation. Zur Erlangung des Grades eines Doktors der Veterinärmedizin (Dr. med. vet.) durch die Tierärztliche Hochschule, Hannover, Germany.

Kondo, S. and Hurnik, J.F. (1990) Stabilization of social hierarchy in dairy cows. *Applied Animal Behavioral Science* 27, 287–297.

Konggaard, S.P. and Krohn, C.C. (1978) Performance of first-calf heifers in two different grouping systems. *Reports of the National Institute of Animal Science, Copenhagen, Denmark.*

Kononoff, P., Heinrichs, J. and Gabriella, V. Using manure evaluation to enhance dairy cattle nutrition (www.das.psu.edu/teamdairy/).

Kristula, M., Reeves, M., Redlus, H. and Uhlinger, C. (1995) A preliminary investigation of the association between the first postpartum milk fat test and first insemination pregnancy rates. *Preventive Veterinary Medicine* 23, 95–100.

LeBlanc, S., Leslie, K. and Duffield, T. (2005) Metabolic predictors of displaced abomasum in dairy cattle. *Journal of Dairy Science* 88(1), 159–170.

Leonardi, C. and Armentano, L.E. (2003) Effect of quantity, quality, and length of alfalfa hay on selective consumption by dairy cows. *Journal of Dairy Science* 86, 557–564.

Littledike, E.T., Witzel, S. and Whipp, S.C. (1968) Insulin: evidence for inhibition of release in spontaneous hypocalcemia. *Proceedings of the Society of Experimental Biology and Medicine* 129(1), 135–139.

Loeffler, S.H., deVries, M.J. and Schukken, Y.H. (1999) The effects of time of disease occurrence, milk yield and body condition on fertility in dairy cows. *Journal of Dairy Science* 82, 2589–2604.

Madouasse, A., Huxley, J., Browne, W., Bradley, A., Dryden, I. and Green, M. (2010) Use of individual cow milk recording data at the start of lactation to predict the calving to conception interval. *Journal of Dairy Science* 93, 4677–4690.

Markusfeld, O. (1987) Periparturient traits in seven high dairy herds. Incidence rates, association with parity, and interrelationships among traits. *Journal of Dairy Science* 70, 158.

Martinez, M.J.T. (2004) The use of milk quality components as predictors of fertility performance in the commercial dairy cow. D Phil thesis, Veterinary Epidemiology and Economics Research Unit, School of Agriculture, Policy and Development, University of Reading, UK.

Matzke, W.C. (2003) Behaviour of large groups of lactating dairy cattle housed in a free stall barn. MS thesis, University of Nebraska, Lincoln, Nebraska.

Maulfair, D.D., Zanton, G.I., Fustini, M. and Heinrichs, A.J. (2010) Effect of feed sorting on chewing behavior, production, and rumen fermentation in lactating dairy cows. *Journal of Dairy Science* 93(10), 4791–4803.

MDC (DairyCo) Grass+. Grassland Management Improvement Scheme. CD-ROM. Milk Development Council. Author Harland J.I., Contributors; Fox, C., Bailey, A., Bax, J., Brandon, S., Browne, I., Harland, J., Lane, G., Mayne, S., Simpson, R.

Metz, J.H. (1975) Time patterns of feeding and rumination in domestic cattle. Communications of the Agricultural University of Wageningen, The Netherlands.

Murphy, M.R. (1992) Water metabolism of dairy cattle. *Journal of Dairy Science* 75, 326–333.

Murphy, M.R., Davis, C.L. and McCoy, G.C. (1983) Factors affecting water consumption by Holstein cows in early lactation. *Journal of Dairy Science* 66, 35–38.

Nordlund, K.V. (2010) Creating the physical environment for transition cow success. In: *Proceedings of the 2010 Penn State Dairy Cattle Nutrition Workshop*, pp. 47–52.

Nordlund, K.V., Cook, N. and Oetzel, G. (2006) Comingling dairy cows: pen moves, stocking density and health. In: *Proceedings of the 2006 Annual Convention of the American Association of Bovine Practitioners*.

NRC (2001) *Nutrient Requirements of Dairy Cattle, 7th revised edn*. National Academic Press, Washington, DC.

Oetzel, G.R. (2004) Monitoring and testing dairy herds for metabolic disease. *Veterinary Clinics of North America: Food Animal Practice* 20, 651–674.

Ospina, P.A., Nydam, D.V., Stokol, T. and Overton, T.R. (2010) Associations of elevated nonesterified fatty acids and β-hydroxybutyrate concentrations with early lactation reproductive performance and milk production in transition dairy cattle in the northeastern United States. *Journal of Dairy Science* 93, 1596–1603.

Patton, J., Kenny, D.D., McNamara, S., Mee, J.F., O'Mara, F.P.O., Diskin, M.G. *et al.* (2007) Relationships among milk production, energy balance, plasma analytes, and reproduction in Holstein-Friesian cows. *Journal of Dairy Science* 90, 649–658.

Peeler, E.J., Otte, M.J. and Esslemont, R.J. (1994) Inter-relationships of periparturient diseases in dairy cows. *Veterinary Record* 134, 129–132.

Phelps, A. (1992) Vastly superior first lactations when heifers fed separately. *Feedstuffs* 11, 11–13.

Podpecan, O., Mrkun, J. and Zrimsek, P. (2008) Diagnostic evaluation of fat to protein ratio in prolonged calving to conception interval using receiver operating characteristic analyses. *Reproduction in Domestic Animals* 43, 249–254.

Rook, A.J., Huckle, C.A. and Penning, P.D. (1994) Effects of sward height and concentrate supplementation on the ingestive behaviour of spring-calving dairy cows grazing grass clover swards. *Applied Animal Behaviour Science*. 40:101–112.

Rukkwamsuk, T., Wensing, T. and Geelen, M.J.H. (1998) Effect of overfeeding during the dry period on regulation of adipose tissue metabolism in dairy cows during the periparturient period. *Journal of Dairy Science* 81, 2904–2911.

Samarutel, J., Ling, K., Waldmann, A., Jaakson, H., Kaart, T. and Leesmae, A. (2008) Field trial on progesterone cycles, metabolic profiles, body condition score and their relation to fertility in Estonian Holstein dairy cows. *Reproduction in Domestic Animals* 43, 457–463.

Shaver, R.D. (1997). Nutritional risk factors in the etiology of left displaced abomasum in dairy cows: a review. *Journal of Dairy Science* 80, 2449–2453.

Stokol, T. and Nydam, D.V. (2005). Effect of anticoagulant and storage conditions on bovine nonesterified fatty acid and β-hydroxybutyrate concentrations in blood. *Journal of Dairy Science* 88, 3139–3144.

Thilsing-Hansen, T., Jørgensen, R.J. and S. Østergaar, S. (2002) Milk fever control principles: A review. *Acta Veterinaria Scandinavica* 43, 1–19.

von Keyserlingk, M. and DeVries, T. (2004) Designing better environments for cows to feed. *Advances in Dairy Technology* 16, 65.

von Keyserlingk, M.A.G., Weary, D.M., Veira, D.M. and Heuwieser, W. (2010) Technical note: Evaluation of a scoring system for rumen fill in dairy cows. *Journal of Dairy Science* 93(8), 3635–3640.

Wiltbank, M.C., Weigel, K.A. and Caraviello, D.Z. (2007) Recent studies on nutritional factors affecting reproductive efficiency in U.S. dairy herds. In: *University of Nottingham Feed Conference*, 2007.

Windig, J.J., Beerda, B. and Veerkamp, R.F. (2008) Relationship between milk progesterone profiles and genetic merit for milk production, milking frequency, and feeding regimen in dairy cattle. *Journal of Dairy Science* 91, 2874–2884.

# 9 Dairy Farming, Food Security and Environmental Issues

Jonathan Statham,[1] Martin Green,[2] Jon Huxley[2] and Sian Statham[1]
[1]Bishopton Veterinary Group, Mill Farm, Studley Road, Ripon, North Yorkshire HG4 2QR, UK; [2]School of Veterinary Medicine and Science, University of Nottingham, Sutton Bonington Campus, Leicestershire LE12 5RD, UK

## Introduction

Looking after the world in which we live and caring for our natural environment are becoming increasingly important to society. It is now widely accepted that dairy farming influences this environment and, in some areas, this raises cause for concern. It is clear that we can minimize the negative environmental effects of dairy farming by increasing the efficiency of production and modifying farming practices and management. In this respect, there is a role for the herd health advisor: to consider the environmental aspects of dairy farming when conducting herd health, and to work with farm staff to limit negative impacts. In this chapter we outline areas in which dairy farming can interact with the environment and discuss ways in which adverse effects can be limited.

## Background: Food Security, Energy Security and Climate Change

Livestock activities have a significant impact on virtually all aspects of the environment, including air and climate change, land and soil, water and biodiversity (Steinfeld *et al.*, 2006). Together with the combustion of fossil fuels for energy generation and land-use changes (which destroy organic carbon in soil), the livestock sector is considered one of the top three most important influences on the environment, both at local and global levels. Greenhouse gas (GHG) emissions, notably carbon dioxide, methane and nitrous oxide specifically from the dairy cattle sector, have been assessed using a 'life cycle' approach that focuses on the entire dairy food chain (FAO, 2010). The environmental impacts of dairy farming may be direct – for example, through grazing and production of methane via the ruminal fermentation of grass, or indirect, such as the expansion of soybean production for intensive dairy feeds, replacing forests in South America.

By the end of the 20th century, governments and policy makers around the world faced three key issues: (i) renewed worries about energy security; (ii) commitment to economic development, including the creation and sustainability of jobs, particularly in agriculture in the developing world; and (iii) the need to mitigate global climate change and achieve lower GHG emissions (Nuffield Council Report, 2011). The issue of world 'food security' (Beddington, 2011) has to be balanced with these global needs of energy security, improving the livelihoods of human populations (especially those dependent on agriculture) and ecological intensification and sustainability of natural resources (Bonnet *et al.*, 2011).

We summarize below the important issues surrounding food security, energy security and climate change in the context of dairy farming, and the provision of a herd health programme.

## Food security

Food security as a concept is more than food self-sufficiency. Since the World Food Summit of 1996, food security has been defined at individual, household, national, regional and global levels as 'being achieved when all people, at all times, have physical and economic access to sufficient, safe and nutritious food to meet their dietary needs and food preferences for an active and healthy life'. Importantly, there is a wide contrast in food security between countries throughout the world (Maplecroft, 2011).

The world's population is forecast to reach 9 billion by 2050, and the challenge for agriculture is to feed this population while at the same time preserving the earth's resources and ecological structures. The global growth in demand for food products requires a significant shift away from purely 'production at all costs' agricultural practices to balanced, ecological methods of intensification. Food security is not, however, limited solely to the quantitative aspects of food supply. If food security exists only when there is reliable access to safe and nutritious food that meets dietary needs and food preferences for an active and healthy life, then livestock farming offers an excellent contribution by providing energy and protein with a high nutritional value and micronutrients. It may also support the income of those engaged in the production, processing and marketing chains at national and international levels, and ultimately to a country's gross domestic product (GDP) (Bonnet *et al.*, 2011). The global sustainability of

food and farming is discussed in detail by Beddington and others (2011) in *The Future of Food and Farming*.

Dairy farming specifically offers a contribution to global food security through the provision of high-quality protein sources, calcium and essential fatty acids from dairy products, together with beef as a by-product from cull cows and beef crossed calves for the beef industry.

The veterinary sector is essential as one of the guarantors of the stability and development of global food security through the activities it deploys at each stage in the system: production at farm level and processing, distribution and marketing at national and international levels.

### Food security: key concepts

The literature on food security identifies three areas that are applicable to products of animal origin: availability of food, access to food and effective and safe utilization of food (Bonnet *et al.*, 2011). A fourth dimension of sustainability is now applicable in the environmental context (see Table 9.1).

### Veterinary activities and their impact on food security

In a food security context, 'veterinary services' have a role in organizing a technical and regulatory environment in which health risks can be identified and controlled, in order to limit their impact on livestock production sectors and humans. Veterinary services consequently contribute to food security, economic development and human health protection. Veterinary activities are deployed at each stage in the food system: production at farm level, processing, distribution and marketing at the local and national level or for export. This demands a wide range of organizational, legislative and technical competencies across both the public and private sectors. The focus of this book is on veterinary activities at farm level and the role of herd health management in optimizing productivity through minimizing poor health and reproductive inefficiency. However, it is important to remember veterinary services that occur beyond this and that play an important role in food security; these are summarized in Box 9.1 below.

New food security challenges are emerging. Globally, veterinary services must continue to acknowledge the desire for diets and food systems that are sustainable from an environmental, societal and territorial perspective. The International Office of Epizootics (OIE) offers the 'OIE Pathway', a procedure designed to sustainably improve a country's veterinary services, using the OIE tool for the evaluation of performance of veterinary services (OIE PVS Tool). These evaluation methods aim to reflect the major

**Table 9.1.** Components of food security (after Bonnet *et al.*, 2011).

| | |
|---|---|
| Availability | Domestic production together with international trade to acquire, through imports or food aid, a sufficient volume to supplement domestic products. Availability also involves the acquisition of foreign currency, through export of high-value products with which to purchase other food commodities |
| Access | The physical and financial capacity of households to provide themselves with food:<br>• Physical access: concerns the distance from the producer to the consumer and the stability of supply cycles. Generally, consumers are dependent on local producers or on distribution and marketing channels for unprocessed and processed food products. There may be direct supply (farm-gate sales or markets) or supply systems involving a complex arrangement of operators. There may be an indirect contribution of livestock to physical access to food, for example in transport of products to the local market<br>• Financial access: concerns access to a range of products at prices compatible with income and purchasing power |
| Utilization | The quantity and quality of products, socio-cultural preferences and consumption patterns. This encompasses undernourishment of persons whose energy and caloric intake is insufficient for them to lead an active life (~925 million people worldwide) and malnutrition, characterized by inadequate intake of energy, protein (and specific amino acids) and micronutrients (vitamins, minerals), giving rise to delayed growth and intellectual development and ill health. In developed countries, it also relates to diseases associated with excessive food intake and obesity |
| Sustainability | The capacity for sustainably maintaining agricultural production (including animal production), national and international trade, storage and supply that will meet demand over the long term. It involves the development and sustainable manage-ment of natural resources used in animal production, and productivity margins that are feasible under various scenarios and capable of contending with new societal and consumer requirements |

---

**Box 9.1.** An outline of veterinary activities in food security.

**1.** Epidemiological surveillance at the national level and at borders.
**2.** Emergency or routine disease diagnosis.
**3.** Sanitary interventions to control or eradicate endemic, exotic or emerging diseases.

Two mechanisms are essential if a system is to be effective:
• animal identification to ensure the traceability of animals and animal products throughout the production chain and to control animal movements at the national level, including animals for export (quarantine); and
• veterinary diagnostic laboratories operating under a reliable quality control system for the tests they perform.

worldwide impact of veterinary services on food security.

### Food security: political influences

Maplecroft's global map of food security (Maplecroft, 2011) shows that the developed world is at low risk of food insecurity when compared with the risks experienced by, for example, much of the African continent. However, the stability of the global food market and the ability to purchase food with generated wealth are critical to preserving food security in many developed countries. Political instability represents a threat to this status quo and may result from global pressures on food and other scarce resources.

Global food security will remain dynamic. The effects of climate change may mean that countries that are currently primary food producers and exporters may, through necessity, become importers. This will require the generation of wealth by alternative means to support the purchase of food.

In terms of milk production, the FAO predicted that milk production is set to double from 580 to 1043 million tonnes in the period 1999–2050 (Steinfeld *et al.*, 2006). Where will this additional production come from? While scope exists for an increase in milk production worldwide, the key challenge is to meet this increasing demand for dairy products using farming methods that are environmentally sustainable.

## Energy security

Total world energy consumption has been predicted to increase by 49% between 2007 and 2035, mainly attributed to increased demand in developing countries. Almost one third of total world energy consumption comprises fuel for transport, i.e. cars, aviation and shipping. The need for energy security has been expressed as one of the principal priorities for governments in the 21st century.

Energy security has been defined as 'The uninterrupted physical availability of energy products on the market, at a price which is affordable for all consumers (private and industrial)' (European Commission, 2000). Many threats to energy security exist; some disrupt the provision of energy to consumers and businesses (e.g. through limited availability of fuel), while others affect the price of energy (e.g. price spikes as a result of political tensions).

With rising demand, biofuels have been considered as one solution to energy security, by increasing the diversity of supply choices. These can provide a new source of income for farmers as well as being a renewable source of fuel, and may lead to reduced greenhouse gas (GHG) emissions when compared with fossil fuels. The USA is the world's largest producer of biofuels. A major motivation for biofuels production was economic – to use surplus agricultural production. However, concerns over energy security following the oil crisis in the early 1970s also played an important role. Production of biofuels might also be an attractive prospect in developing countries, where a large proportion of the population is engaged in agriculture and where biofuels might provide a local energy source in energy-deprived areas.

The two principal biofuels are (i) bioethanol (to blend with petrol) made from, for example, corn, wheat or sugar cane; and (ii) biodiesel (to blend with diesel) made from palm oil or rapeseed oil.

Biofuel production has increased very rapidly. Between 1998 and 2009, the production of biodiesel in the European Union (EU) increased more than tenfold (European Biodiesel Board, 2009). Worldwide, it is expected that by 2030 biofuels will account for 7% of road transport fuel (International Energy Agency, 2007).

### Controversies over energy security versus food security

Problems with large-scale production of biofuels have begun to emerge. Concerns have been raised over threats to food security and food prices because of the competition of biofuels with food production, and this has led to political unrest.

For example, in the UK, the onset of bioethanol production from wheat was one of the factors that caused the commodity price to more than double (from £80/t to around £180/t in 2011), with a consequent rise in dairy feed input costs. Biofuel production also results in both direct land use change (dLUC) and indirect land use change (iLUC). Some reports suggest that the production of corn-based bioethanol overall produces more GHG emissions than fossil fuels; other studies cite far more favourable results (Renewable Fuels Association, 2010). Fierce debate continues over the consequences of biofuel production for food security and the environment. Biofuels do appear to be one contributing factor to changing food prices, but the scale of effects is both complex and uncertain to model (Renewable Fuels Agency, 2008). Other factors, such as high energy prices and the weak dollar, are also significant – blaming food price spikes on biofuel production alone is too simplistic. None the less, there is clearly the potential for serious effects on food security as biofuel production increases.

*Energy security solutions sparing food supply: second generation biofuels*

Concerns over the use of potential food sources for biofuels has prompted diverse research into more efficient sources of biomass and more efficient production and conversion techniques. The goals are to provide biomass sources/feedstocks that

- do not compete with food production;
- have a high energy yield with low inputs of water, land and fertilizer;
- do not negatively affect the environment or local populations; and
- can be produced in sufficient quantities to allow economically viable biofuel production.

Among the most promising candidates so far are those biofuels made from waste products and energy crops using full lignocellulosic conversion and, more speculatively, biofuels made from algae. These are termed 'second generation' biofuels.

*Anaerobic digestion: an alternative energy source*

Anaerobic bacterial digestion (AD) processes plant biomass into methane gas for heating and power. Suitable plant biomass includes solid waste, manure, crop residues, compost, food waste and paper. Crops can be grown specifically for use in AD. The UK produces over 100 million tonnes of organic material 'feedstock' that is suitable for treatment by AD, including 90–100 million t of agricultural by-products like manure and slurry. Digesting 1 t of food waste can generate about 300 kWh of energy. Cereals and rape meal can be used as AD feedstocks, giving high methane yields, but since these are expensive commodities they are generally not grown solely for digestion. The yield of methane from a particular product will vary according to

- dry matter content;
- storage time (prolonged storage may result in poorer yields because breakdown may have commenced);
- length of time in the digester;
- the type of AD plant and the conditions in the digester; and
- the purity of the feedstock.

Methane can be combusted to produce heat alone (when burned, 1 m$^3$ of methane produces around 2.5 kWh of heat) or can be used in electricity generation, or a combination of both. While coal- and gas-fired power stations have an efficiency of around 34 and 55%, respectively, combined heat and power (CHP) plants can achieve overall efficiencies in excess of 70% at the point of use.

## Environmental Issues: Significance for the Dairy Industry

New food security challenges are taking shape, in particular relating to sustainability of the environment and natural resources. The livestock industry accounts for ~40% of global GDP, employs 1.3 billion people (including 1 billion of the worlds' poor), supplies approximately one third of global protein intake and is a potential solution for malnutrition as well as a potential cause of obesity (Steinfeld *et al.*, 2006). Global milk production is projected to double from 580 to 1043 million t and global production of meat to more than double from 229 to 465 million t between 1999 and 2050. The environmental impact per unit of livestock production must halve in this time period just to remain standing still (Steinfeld *et al.*, 2006).

## Impacts of dairy farming on the atmosphere and climate change

'Warming of the climate system is unequivocal, as is now evident from observations of increases in global average air and ocean temperatures, widespread melting of snow and ice and rising global average sea levels' (Intergovernmental Panel on Climate Change, 2007). Global warming is one of the greatest challenges to have faced mankind. The best estimates from six possible GHG emission scenarios predict an increase in temperature of between 1.8 and 4.0°C by 2090–2099 compared with the period 1980–1999. Similarly, sea levels are predicted to rise between 0.18 and 0.59 m over the same period (Intergovernmental Panel on Climate Change, 2007). The United Nations Framework Convention on Climate Change was developed at the Rio de Janeiro Earth Summit in 1992 in an attempt to limit the impact of global warming. Initially its contents were non-binding, although the treaty allowed for the development of mandatory requirements in the future. The Kyoto Protocol came into force in 2005, and nearly 200 countries have now signed up to the agreement. Just over 40 of these signatories (including the EU, Australia, Canada, Japan, New Zealand, the Russian Federation and the USA) have committed to reducing their emissions of GHG. At the end of 2008, the UK government passed the Climate Change

Act, a long-term and legally binding framework to tackle climate change. The Act commits the UK to reduce GHG emissions by at least 34% by 2020 and 80% by 2050 compared with 1990 levels.

Dairy farming and other ruminant agriculture makes a significant contribution to GHG emissions, and therefore will have an obligation to reduce emissions in line with national and international agreements. A failure to reduce emissions would require larger cuts to be made in other areas, a situation that is unlikely to be acceptable to governments and those industries involved. Dairy farming results in the production of three of the four principal gases with global warming potential (GWP) – carbon dioxide, methane and nitrous oxide. While overall, carbon dioxide is the most important GHG, methane and nitrous oxide make significant contributions. Carbon dioxide 'equivalents' are used to standardize the GWP of different gases: methane and nitrous oxide have 23 and 296 times the GWP of carbon dioxide, respectively.

The most significant sources of GHG from dairy farming are methane produced during enteric fermentation – which is released into the atmosphere when animals eructate – and the methane and nitrous oxide released from mineral fertilizers and manure (both when stored and spread). Emissions are also generated from fuel and electricity produced from fossil fuel sources used for equipment on the farm, during the production and transport of resources required for dairy farming, and in the milk and dairy supply chain. The Food and Agriculture Organization (FAO) of the United Nations has recently published a full life cycle assessment of GHG emissions from the worldwide dairy sector (Steinfeld *et al.*, 2006). The report encompasses the entire life cycle of dairy products, including the production and transportation of resources, transportation of milk, processing and distribution and includes all animals linked to milk production (e.g. milking cows, replacements and surplus calves reared for beef). The report's overall conclusions are striking and provide an excellent summary of the dairy sector's contribution to GHG emissions:

- Methane contributes most to the global warming impact of milk (~52% of the GHG emissions from both developing and developed countries). Nitrous oxide emissions account for 27 and 38% of GHG emissions in developed and developing countries, respectively, while $CO_2$ emissions account for a higher share of emissions in developed countries (21%) compared with developing countries (10%).
- In 2007, the dairy sector emitted 1969 million t of $CO_2$ equivalent emissions (± 26%), of which 1328 million t were attributed to milk, 151 million t to meat from culled animals and 490 million t to meat from fattened calves.
- The global dairy sector contributes 4.0% to the total global man-made GHG emissions.
- The average global emissions from milk production, processing and transport are estimated at 2.4 kg of $CO_2$ equivalent emissions per 1 kg of FPCM (fat- and protein-corrected milk) at the farm gate.
- Average regional emissions (per 1 kg of FPCM at the farm gate) range from 1.3 to 7.5 kg of $CO_2$ equivalent emissions (± 26%). The highest emissions were found in the developing regions, with the average for sub-Saharan Africa, South Asia, and North Africa and the Near East recording 7.5, 4.6 and 3.7 kg of $CO_2$ equivalent emissions, respectively. Industrialized regions such as Europe and North America had the lowest emissions per 1 kg of FPCM.
- The level of GHG emissions, per 1 kg of FPCM, is higher in grazing systems than in mixed systems. Grassland systems contribute about 2.72 kg of $CO_2$ equivalent emissions per 1 kg of FPCM compared with mixed systems, which on average contribute 1.78 kg.
- Along the entire dairy food chain, 'cradle-to-farm gate' emissions (i.e. from young calf to adult milking cow on the farm) contribute the highest proportion of emissions (93% on average). In industrialized countries, the relative contribution ranges between 78 and 83% (i.e. ~20% of emissions occur after the milk

has left the farm), while in developing regions this figure ranges between 90 and 99% of total emissions.

Dairy farmers have already started to act to reduce their GHG emissions, and they will undoubtedly have to play their part in reducing emissions over the coming decades. Recent data from the UK suggest that dairy businesses in the top 25% of performance (measured by cost of production) produce milk with a carbon footprint of well over 300 g of $CO_2$ less per litre than farms in the bottom 25% (DairyCo Roadmap, 2010). A failure to act will lead to increasing pressure from government and consumers and, ultimately, the imposition of mandatory targets and sanctions to ensure that reduction targets are met. There is scope to reduce emissions in a range of areas; many are possible now and others are likely to become viable options in the future. It is important to remember that while sudden and large changes requiring significant financial investments are possible, for most individual units these are unnecessary as long as farms continue to make small changes leading to year-on-year reductions in emissions.

A discussion of methods to reduce GHG emissions and the role of herd health is provided later in the chapter. However, the impacts of various management strategies on methane emissions has recently been evaluated (Chadwick et al., 2007). The following changes were reported to have the most significant impact on emissions.

- an increase in milk yield per cow (by 30% in the modelled scenario), coupled with a reduction in dairy cow numbers – to maintain a constant level of production (24% reduction in emissions);
- a high fat diet (14% reduction);
- increased heat detection rate (7% reduction);
- a high starch diet (5% reduction); and
- the provision of high-quality forage (3% reduction).

It is likely that a variety of other methods are also useful in reducing GHG emissions, in particular the improvement of cow health and reproduction. These areas are considered in detail later in the chapter.

## Impacts of dairy farming on water

Water is vital for life and dairy farming has the potential to pollute this vital resource, which is becoming increasingly scarce in many parts of the world. Groundwater is water held beneath the surface in soil and in porous rock formations; larger deposits of porous rock containing water are termed aquifers. Surface water is any water collected above ground in water courses, ponds, lakes, wetlands and oceans. Both surface and groundwater have the potential to become contaminated. Pollution can be caused by either a single catastrophic accident or event ('point source', e.g. slurry discharging into a river) or it can be the cumulative result of agricultural activity over a prolonged period of time ('diffuse pollution'). A range of different pollutants can contaminate water from dairy farms: nitrogen and phosphorus are probably the most high profile, but a range of others can be important in certain circumstances.

### Nitrogen

About 60% of the nitrates in English rivers come from agriculture (DEFRA, 2009). Both chemical fertilizers and organic animal waste (slurry and manure) can cause nitrate pollution. Nitrates are soluble – if they are not taken up rapidly by grass and other crops they are leached out of the soil. Leaching primarily occurs when the concentrations of nitrate are high and when the water containing it moves below the root zone. It is particularly a problem during periods and in areas of heavy rainfall and on lighter soil types. Sandy soils are more prone to leaching as they cannot hold as much water, and rain passes through them. In some heavy clay soils leaching is not a significant issue because water is retained. Once leached, nitrates are either carried into water courses or continue down into groundwater through porous rocks.

There are two principal dangers of elevated levels of nitrates in water: (i) nitrates in drinking water pose a risk to human health; and (ii) they can lead to the eutrophication of surface water (see below). High levels of nitrates in drinking water represent one of the possible causes of methaemoglobinaemia. Methaemoglobin is the oxidized form of haemoglobin, has a strong affinity for oxygen and therefore high levels reduce the blood's ability to oxygenate body tissues. Children under 6 months of age are particularly vulnerable and can develop the potentially fatal 'blue baby syndrome' as a result. Three-quarters of Europeans obtain their water supply from groundwater, and water companies invest large amounts of money ensuring that the levels of nitrate in drinking water are below safe and legal limits.

Eutrophication is the enrichment of water with nitrogen and phosphorus. It causes the rapid and excessive growth of plants and algae, altering the fragile equilibrium present in the ecosystem. This can lead to a range of consequences including the death of other species (e.g. fish and other plants) resulting in a loss of biodiversity, overgrowth of some types of plant that can obstruct watercourses used for navigation and recreation, and the growth of toxic algal blooms that can be poisonous to fish, animals and man.

### Phosphorus

Phosphorus is a component of both chemical fertilizers and organic animal waste; however, unlike nitrogen, phosphorus is largely insoluble and not prone to leaching. Phosphorus generally causes contamination when particles of soil enter water courses as a result of soil erosion. Soil erosion occurs through a combination of erosion by weathering – particularly rain and wind – and the impact of agriculture itself, e.g. tillage, poaching and erosion by agricultural machinery. Excessive levels of phosphorus in water can lead to eutrophication. In European freshwater systems, phosphorus is usually the rate-limiting nutrient and the main cause of eutrophication. In sea water, nitrogen is usually rate limiting.

*Control of nitrate and phosphorus pollution*

Within Europe, the Nitrate Directive (1991) aims to protect water quality by promoting and legislating for good farming practices to prevent the pollution of surface and groundwater with nitrates of agricultural origin. The directive is interpreted and implemented at the national level and has five steps: (i) identification of polluted or threatened waters; (ii) designation of nitrate-vulnerable zones (NVZs); (iii) establishment of codes of good agricultural practice; (iv) establishment of compulsory action programmes to be implemented by farmers within NVZs; and (v) national monitoring and reporting every four years. Farms outside NVZs are encouraged to comply with the codes of good agricultural practice. For farms within NVZs the codes become mandatory, and there are additional requirements around the application of both chemical and organic fertilizers. These regulations can be particularly challenging for dairy farmers, as they specify the capacity of slurry storage vessels, designated periods when slurry cannot be spread on land and limit the amount that can be applied, and restrict the application of fertilizer in high-risk areas (e.g. sloping ground, land close to water courses). Within Europe, phosphorus pollution is less stringently controlled than nitrogen pollution, although other parts of the world are subject to stringent control measures (e.g. Florida, USA).

*Slurry, manure and other organic materials*

In addition to the risk posed by nitrates and phosphorus, slurry, manure, silage effluent and other organic materials such as milk and animal carcasses can cause substantial damage if they escape into water courses from dairy farms. Environmental microorganisms that break down organic matter can deplete water oxygen levels, with catastrophic consequences for other life and in some circumstances killing everything else present. The polluting strength of organic materials is measured in terms of biochemical oxygen demand (BOD). The BOD of raw

sewage is 200–300 mg/l; slurry from cattle farms has a BOD of 10,000–20,000 mg/l and even dirty farm water (yard run-off and washing water) has a BOD of 1000–5000 mg/l. Worse still, silage effluent has a BOD of 30,000 mg/l and milk 140,000 mg/l (DEFRA, 2009). Thus even small quantities of such contaminants can have devastating consequences for the environment local to the spill. Control of such forms of pollution is now much more highly regulated by many local authorities.

*Farm chemicals*

Agrichemicals such as veterinary medicines, dairy chemicals, disinfectants, pesticides, herbicides and fuels are all commonly used on dairy farms and all have the potential to cause huge damage to the environment if they escape into water courses. The use and disposal of all these chemicals is highly regulated in most countries to minimize the risks of either accidental or negligent pollution.

*Poaching and soil erosion*

The banks of water courses, ponds, lakes and canals inevitably become poached and eroded over time if animals have direct access to them. In addition to being unsightly, the damage reduces water quality by adding silt and faecal contamination, and has the potential to increase phosphorus levels.

## Impacts of dairy farming on biodiversity and local ecology

'Biological diversity means the variability among living organisms from all sources including, inter alia, terrestrial, marine and other aquatic ecosystems and the ecological complexes of which they are part; this includes diversity within species, between species and of ecosystems' (United Nations, 1992). Biodiversity describes the quantity of variation in life forms (plants, animals and microorganisms) in an environment or ecosystem. There is growing concern that man's activities are causing a decline in biodiversity (termed the 'Holocene extinction'), particularly through habitat destruction. Human activities have caused extinction rates to increase to 1000 times their natural level (UK Biodiversity Partnership, 2007). In addition to our moral responsibilities and the income and enjoyment we gain from diverse and vibrant habitats, there is a fear that the ecosystems that sustain human life may collapse if the rate of extinction continues.

To address this concern, the international Convention on Biological Diversity was signed by leaders from over 150 countries at the 1992 Rio de Janeiro Earth Summit and is dedicated to promoting sustainable development worldwide. The convention has three main aims: (i) the conservation of biological diversity; (ii) the sustainable use of its components; and (iii) the fair and equitable sharing of the benefits from the use of genetic resources (Convention on Biological Diversity, 2011). In 2010 a revised and updated Strategic Plan for Biodiversity for the 2010–2011 period was adopted. The convention requires all parties to create a National Biodiversity Strategy and Action Plan to implement the convention at the national level and to ensure that the strategy is adopted by all those sectors whose activities impact on biodiversity (Convention on Biological Diversity, 2011).

Agriculture is one of these sectors; by their very nature, all agricultural monocultures inevitably have a huge impact on biodiversity as almost by definition the farmer is trying selectively to exclude the growth of other plants and pests. This is particularly true of 'industrial' agriculture, which has undergone a rapid expansion in many parts of the world since the end of World War II. Over that period the increasing size and mechanization of dairy farms has had a significant impact on the local ecology and biodiversity. Hedgerows were removed to create larger fields and heath-, moor- and marshlands were drained and improved to create uniform pastures for grazing. Developments in plant science, herbicides, pesticides and fertilizers created near-perfect monocultures of forage crops and cereals for feed. The problems continue in many parts of the world where ancient and complex ecosystems (e.g. the rainforests of South America) are being removed to make way for intensive agriculture, including dairy farming.

While modern agricultural systems are responsible, it certainly does not mean to say that farmers are to blame. Initially the impacts on biodiversity were not clear and its importance not fully understood, and in many parts of the world farmers were simply responding to the demands of the populace to produce more and cheaper produce for a rapidly expanding and increasingly affluent population. The Convention on Biological Diversity (2011) is dedicated to 'promoting sustainable development around the world'. Continuing improvements in agricultural outputs and efficiency are vital if we are to meet the requirement predicted by the FAO over the coming decades: 'By 2050 the world's population will reach 9.2 billion, 34 percent higher than today … In order to feed this larger, more urban and richer population, food production must increase by 70 percent' (FAO, 2008).

The impacts of agriculture, including dairy farming, on biodiversity and local ecology are now well recognized, and many countries are addressing the challenges created by modern farming techniques. This does not mean turning back the clock or reverting to outdated, inefficient practices, but it does mean that dairy farming must be undertaken with an understanding of the countryside and the complex ecosystems and environments it contains. Replanting hedgerows and trees; creating small areas of specific habitats for previously common or endangered species; delaying or changing the timing of agricultural practices to allow the completion of lifecycles; leaving margins around watercourses, woodlands, hedgerows and other habitats to limit the impacts of agriculture and protect delicate ecosystems; providing roosting and breeding sites and boxes for birds in agricultural buildings; avoiding the use of fertilizers, herbicides and pesticides on small areas of land; and the identification and protection of particularly important habitats and sites, are just some examples of practices that improve biodiversity and which are now undertaken alongside dairy farming and other agricultural systems.

## Promoting and enforcing environment protection

The environmental challenges facing dairy farming and agriculture more generally are demanding. Schemes to promote and enforce environmental protection are vital if national and international goals are to be met over the coming decades. Two examples of such schemes are the EU Single Payment Scheme and the UK Environmental Management Scheme, and these are briefly outlined below.

### EU Single Payment Scheme

In 2003 the European Commission reformed the Common Agricultural Policy (CAP) and removed the link between subsidy payments and the level of production ('decoupling'). A system of single payments was introduced to guarantee farmers a more stable income providing they meet certain obligations under 'Cross Compliance' standards. These standards relate to public, animal and plant health, the environment and animal welfare and the maintenance of land in good agricultural and environmental condition. The standards are laid out in two strands: 'Standards of Good Agricultural and Environmental Conditions (GAECs)' and 'Statutory Management Requirements (SMRs)'. Farmers who fail to meet these requirements can have some or all of their single payment withheld.

### UK Environmental Management Scheme

In many parts of the world, farmers are encouraged to participate in schemes designed to protect the environment. For example, the Environmental Stewardship Scheme run by Natural England on behalf of DEFRA in England is divided into a range of different schemes and levels. Its primary objectives are to conserve wildlife and biodiversity, maintain and enhance landscape quality and character, protect the historic environment, protect natural resources and promote public access and understanding of the countryside. Approximately 70% of England's farmland is currently covered by this or previous schemes.

## Reducing the Impact of Dairy Farming on the Environment

As described above, there are a wide variety of ways in which dairy farming can have a damaging effect on the environment and these need to be considered and addressed where possible. A fundamental aspect of managing dairy herd health is that decisions are made within the context of other interrelated aspects of dairy farming, one of which should be environmental citizenship. The environmental impact of dairy farming represents an opportunity for involvement for the herd health advisor; the advisor is an ideal coordinator of this process, with an overview of animal health/welfare, food production and environmental management. Therefore, a useful role of the herd health advisor is to form a cohesive farm policy that balances animal health/welfare, economic and environmental considerations.

An individual farm can take steps to reduce its impact on the environment, and these should be tailored to local circumstances. Examples of practical measures to reduce the environmental impact of dairy farming are outlined in Table 9.2.

### The influence of increased efficiency and improved health and reproduction

### Health and reproduction

For all dairy systems, improved efficiency of milk production helps to reduce the negative environmental effects of dairy farming. For example, for any particular system, if fewer cows (and replacements) are required and there are fewer 'lost' litres of milk, then the environmental impacts per litre of milk sold or per animal on the unit will be reduced. 'Lost' milk here includes milk that does not enter the food chain following animal treatment or a

**Table 9.2.** Examples of methods to reduce the environmental impact of dairy farming (after Green et al., 2011).

| Area | Suggested methods for improvement |
|------|-----------------------------------|
| Soil | Aerate if compacted. Use soil analysis for precise evaluation of the additives required. Improve swards with minimal soil disturbance (reduces $N_2O$ losses) – e.g. use oversowing and direct drilling |
| Water | Reduce dietary protein as much as possible to reduce nitrogen excretion (the use of essential oils and specific amino acids may decrease overall crude protein requirement). High-yielding dairy cows can be sustained on rations <17.5% crude protein (dry matter basis). Adhere to Nitrogen Vulnerable Zone regulations if applicable. Excess dietary phosphorus will be excreted in urine and faeces and is a potential cause of eutrophication. Therefore check dietary content so that mineral specifications are not excessive for phosphorus |
| Manure/slurry | Compact manure and cover slurry stores or manure heaps to reduce ammonia and $N_2O$ levels. Slurry application: $N_2O$ emissions are lower if spread in spring compared with autumn/winter. Match nutrient content of slurry/manure to crop requirements while allowing for ground type and local fertilizer rules. Direct injection of slurry reduces ammonia and $N_2O$ compared with surface spreading. Consider anaerobic digestion to capture and utilize methane, which can be used as an energy source on the farm |
| Nitrogen (N) | Effective N utilization requires an understanding of soil and crop requirements and matching this with fertilizer rates. Maximizing use of organic manures can reduce $N_2O$, ammonia and nitrate losses. Feed cows so as not to provide excess N in diet |
| Cow health and fertility | Optimizing efficiency of production; fewer cows and less waste milk reduce the environmental impact per litre sold. This provides a major role for the herd health advisor (see later sections for details) |
| Cow diets | Effective use of feed improves performance and reduces inputs and waste per litre of milk produced: high dry matter intakes, high-quality forage, high sugar forage, use of clover, addition of specific oils or other feed additives to reduce methane emissions are current areas of research |
| Housing | More frequent slurry removal reduces ammonia emissions. Bolder and longer-term strategies could include scavenging greenhouse gases from negatively ventilated, sealed buildings. Collected gases could be used as an energy source on the farm |
| Genetics | In future, it may be possible to select for 'low-emission' animals by making use of the relatively large between-animal variations that exists in emission characteristics |
| Energy consumption/$CO_2$ emissions | Make energy-saving changes to lighting, machinery, dairy equipment (e.g. plate coolers, heat recovery units), reduce delivery numbers (increase storage capacity), use local feeds or by-products where possible. Consider 'carbon storage' – e.g. conversion of cultivated land to permanent pasture or woodland. Consider production of energy from renewable or home-produced sources |

reduction in yield that occurs following clinical or subclinical disease or poor reproductive performance. This highlights the central importance of herd health in terms of the environment, and is a fundamental reason why the management of herd health, described throughout this book, is so important. Clinical mastitis illustrates this point:

**1.** Milk is discarded because of antimicrobial usage and the associated withdrawal periods.
**2.** Milk yield is reduced for the remainder of lactation as a consequence of compromised mammary gland function.
**3.** There is an increased risk of culling and requirement for extra replacement heifers.

Thus a reduction in GHG and use of non-renewable resources and chemicals, per litre of saleable milk, is an inevitable consequence of improved health and fertility, because fewer cows at a given level of production are required to produce the same quantity of milk.

The effects of fertility on GHG emissions have been evaluated using a model linking changes in fertility to herd structure, number of replacements, milk yield, nutrient requirements and gas emissions (Garnsworthy, 2004). Fertility has a major effect on the number of heifer replacements required to maintain herd size for a given milk quota or number of cows. Restoring fertility to 1995 levels was predicted to reduce methane emissions by 10–11% and ammonia emissions by about 9%. Improving submission rate from 50 to 70% produced improvements in fertility that could reduce emissions of methane by up to 24% and of ammonia by about 14% (Garnsworthy, 2004). Thus improved submission rate alone represents a realistic, achievable route to improve herd profitability, while at the same time reducing the environmental impact of dairy farming (see Chapter 5).

A holistic herd health programme that incorporates many of the areas detailed in this book is likely to have a significant effect on reducing the environmental impact of milk production. Improving health and fertility to reduce the environmental impact of dairying has the substantial advantage that it is also beneficial for cow welfare and farm financial returns; in this respect it is a potential 'win–win' situation. This is an area in which the herd health advisor can and should take a leading role.

### Dietary formulation to optimize carbohydrate utilization

Dietary manipulation is an interesting area and one that demonstrates some of the difficulties and anomalies that exist when considering the environment. Feeding more starch and less fibre to a dairy cow will mean that relatively more propionate and relatively less acetate and butyrate are produced in the rumen, and this leads to reduced methane production. As reviewed by Moss *et al.* (2000), the carbohydrate source within a diet will influence the methane-producing capabilities of the food consumed. A herd producing 8000 litres per annum, that has a relatively high starch content in the diet, will have a lower methane production per litre (assuming an equivalent feed rate) than a herd producing the same milk with a lower dietary starch content and higher digestible fibre. The work of Lana *et al.* (1998) supports this theory by confirming that low ruminal pH regulates methane production.

However, high starch-based diets have the potential to cause ruminal acidosis and subsequent deleterious effects on cow health and welfare. This is an example of a potential conflict between environmental and cow considerations; feeding a high-starch diet may be useful to reduce methane production and reduce the environmental impact of dairying, but it could result in poorer cow health (and welfare) or increased production costs – which is the more important?

## Strategic use of dietary oil supplements

Lipid inclusion in the diet causes a marked decrease in methane production, with the effect being at least partly governed by the fat source used (Dong et al., 1997; Machmuller et al., 1998). This effect is partially but not fully mediated by the depression of protozoal numbers in the rumen (Machmuller et al., 2001, 2003). Ruminal protozoa have been shown to harbour approximately 25% of the methanogens present in the rumen (Newbold et al., 1995), and lipid inclusion appear to represent one of the few practical methods of controlling protozoa in vivo (Newbold and Chamberlain, 1998). However, the effects of fat on methane production are not limited to those mediated via ruminal protozoa, and lipids have been shown to inhibit methanogenesis even in the absence of these protozoa (Broudiscou et al., 1990; Dohme et al., 1999). This may be due to the toxicity of long-chain fatty acids to methanogenic bacteria (Prins et al., 1972; Hendersen, 1973). However, the effect of fat supplementation cannot be viewed in isolation. Fat inclusion in the diet (particularly at levels >5 g/kg DM) can adversely affect ruminal health by significantly inhibiting fibre breakdown in the rumen (Kowalcyk et al., 1977; Machmuller and Kreuzer, 1997). Again, the severity of the effect varies with the type of fat fed (Machmuller et al., 1998).

Another example of a conflict of interests, in this instance a human–economic–environmental dilemma, is the use of palm oils in dairy cow diets. Milk price in some purchasing contracts depends on the percentage of butterfat in milk, and it can be cost effective to boost butterfat in milk by using palm oils (C16 fatty acids). The production of palm oil is generally considered to be severely detrimental to the environment, although it can also provide an income for some of the world's poorest societies. There are clear ethical difficulties in making decisions in which conflicts exist between environmental, animal, economic and human requirements.

## Use of naturally occurring supplements

Feed additives for dairy cattle may represent a future possibility to influence the impact of dairy cows on the environment. There are potential methane-reducing effects from feeding ionophores such as monensin, although this practice is currently banned in the EU. Some unsaturated oils such as linseed, and some essential oils such as extracts from horseradish and garlic, may reduce methane production; more research in this area is needed. Given the forthcoming EU-wide ban on the use of subtherapeutic levels of antibiotics and ionophores as growth promoters in livestock, there has been an explosion of interest in other compounds that might modify microbial activity in the gut. With regard to methane production, attention has focused on plant secondary metabolites, probiotics and propionate precursors. While major EU-funded projects on plant materials to decrease methane production are under way (Wallace, 2004), no details on potential candidate compounds are in the public domain at present. Similarly, the use of probiotics to decrease ruminal methane production has been investigated and, while the development of this approach continues, potential problems with regulation and registration of such substances make it unlikely that commercial products will be released in the near future. Possibly the most promising approach in the short term is the use of propionate precursors – both fumarate and malate have been associated with decreases in methanogenesis in vitro and in vivo (Martin, 1998; Asanuma et al., 1999; López et al., 1999; Bayaru et al., 2001; Newbold et al., 2005; Wallace et al., 2006).

## Genetics

In the future, it is likely that genetics and breeding will play some role in mitigating the environmental impact of dairy farming. A study by Bell et al. (2010) investigated (i) the effect of long-term breeding for kilograms of milk fat plus protein production; and (ii) the influence of parity, genetic line and diet on predicted enteric methane emissions of Holstein-Friesian dairy cows, using 17 years' experimental data from the Langhill herd in Scotland. The Langhill herd comprises genetic lines selected for kilograms of milk fat plus protein (Select) or selected to remain close to the average genetic merit for milk fat plus protein production for all animals evaluated in the UK (Control); it was housed at Langhill, University of Edinburgh (farm 1) between 1990 and 2002 and at the Dairy Research Centre, Scottish Agricultural College (SAC; farm 2) between 2002 and 2007. The study reported that 'Select' cows had a higher weekly DMI and milk yield but a lower predicted enteric methane output per kilogram milk by approximately 12% when compared with 'Control' animals. In terms of diet, the low-forage cows had a higher daily DMI and milk yield, but a lower predicted enteric methane output per kilogram milk, than the high-forage cows at the respective farms.

## Conclusion: Dairy Farming and the Environment

Traditional perspectives of dairy farming have partitioned the issues of food production and environmental impacts as separate components. However, it has become clear that such a narrow view is unhelpful. Food security and the impacts of dairy farming on the environment are also inextricably linked to global energy security and the socio-economic aspects of agriculture for communities worldwide. The dairy industry is expected to reduce the contribution that it makes to global warming, yet the significance of improved cow health and reproductive performance in mitigation of environmental impacts is often underestimated. Above all, herd health advisors have a central role in balancing the interrelated factors involved while ensuring the health and welfare of the animals under their care.

## References and Further Reading

Asanuma, N., Iwamoto, M. and Hino, T. (1999) Effect of the addition of fumarate on methane production by ruminal microorganisms in vitro. *Journal of Dairy Science* 82, 780–787.

Baker, S.K. (1995) Method for improving utilization of nutrients by ruminant or ruminant-like animals. *International Patent No WO9511041.*

Bauman, D.E., McCutcheon, S.N., Steinhour, W.D., Eppard, P.J. and Sechen, S.J. (1985) Sources of variation and prospects for improvement of productive efficiency in the dairy cow: a review. *Journal of Animal Science* 60, 583–592.

Bayaru, E., Kanda, S., Kamada, T., Itabashi, H., Andoh, S., Nishida, T. *et al.* (2001) Effect of fumaric acid on methane production, rumen fermentation and digestibility of cattle fed roughage alone. *Animal Science Journal* 72, 139–146.

Beddington, J. (2011) *The Future of Food and Farming: Challenges and Choices for Global Sustainability.* Government Office for Science, London.

Bell, M.J., Wall, E., Russell, G., Morgan, C. and Simm, G. (2010) Effect of breeding for milk yield, diet and management on enteric methane emissions from dairy cows. *Animal Production Science* 50, 817–826.

Bonnet, P., Lancelot, R., Seegers, H. and Martinez, D. (2011) Contribution of veterinary activities to global food security for food derived from terrestrial and aquatic animals. *Proceedings of the 79th General Session of the World Organisation of Animal Health,* Paris, 22–27 May.

Broudiscou L., van Nevel, C.J. and Demeyer, D.I. (1990) Incorporation of soya oil hydrolysate in the diet of defaunated or refaunated sheep: effect on rumen fermentation in vitro. *Archives Tierernahr* 40, 329–337.

Cabinet Office Report (2008) *Food Matters. Towards a Strategy for the 21st Century.* Cabinet Office, London.

Capper, J.L., Cady, R.A. and Bauman, D.E. (2009) The environmental impact of dairy production: 1944 compared with 2007. *Journal of Animal Science* 87, 2160–2167.

Chadwick, D.R., del Prado, A., Mills, J.A.N., Crompton, L.A., Dragosits, U., Scholefield, D. *et al.* (2007) The implications of farm-scale methane mitigation measures for long-term national methane emissions. Final report to DEFRA on project CC0270, DEFRA, London.

Chagunda, M.G.G., Römer, D.A.M. and Roberts, D.J. (2009) Effect of genotype and feeding regime on enteric methane, non-milk nitrogen and performance of dairy cows during the winter feeding period. *Livestock Science* 122, 323–332.

Convention on Biological Diversity (2011) www.cbd.int (accessed 3 August 2011).

DairyCo Factsheets (2010) *Efficient Milk Production: Climate Change*. Available at http://www.dairyco.org.uk/library/research–development/climate-change.aspx

DairyCo Roadmap (2010) www.dairyco.org.uk/library/research-development/environment/dairy-roadmap.aspx

DeJarnette, J.M., Marshall, C.E., Lenz, R.W., Monke, D.R., Ayars, W.H. and Sattler, C.G. (2004) Sustaining the fertility of artificially inseminated cattle: The role of the artificial insemination industry. *Journal of Dairy Science* 87 (e-Suppl.), E93–E104.

DEFRA (2009) *Protecting our Water, Soil and Air. A Code of Good Agricultural Practice for Farmers, Growers and Land Managers*. DEFRA, London.

Dereck, K., Graham, D., Balkwill, T., Garner, P., Hodgman, C., Flint, A. *et al.* (2010) Occurrence of a quadruplex motif in a unique insert within exon C of the bovine estrogen receptor α gene (ESR1). *Biochemistry* 49, 7625–7633.

Dohme, F., Machmüller, A., Estermann, B.L., Pfister, P., Wasserfallen, A. and Kreuzer, M. (1999) The role of the rumen ciliate protozoa for methane suppression caused by coconut oil. *Letters in Applied Microbiology* 29, 187–192.

Dong, Y., Bae, H.D., McAllister, T.A., Mathison, G.W. and Cheng, K.J. (1997) Lipid-induced depression of methane production and digestibility in the artificial rumen system (RUSITEC). *Canadian Journal of Animal Science* 77, 269–278.

Eastridge, M.L. (2006) Major advances in applied dairy cattle nutrition. *Journal of Dairy Science* 89, 1311–1323.

Esselmont, R.J. (2003) The costs of poor fertility and what to do about reducing them. *Cattle Practice* 11, 237–250.

European Biodiesel Board (2009) *The EU Biodiesel Industry*, available at http://www.ebb-eu.org/stats.php.

European Commission (2000) *Green Paper: Towards a European Strategy for the Security of Energy Supply*, available at http://ec.europa.eu/energy/green-paper-energy-supply/doc/green_paper_energy_supply_en.pdf, p4.

Farm Animal Welfare Council (2009) *Farm Animal Welfare in Great Britain: Past, Present and Future*. Report, FAWC, London.

FAO (2008) *How to Feed the World in 2050*. FAO, Rome.

FAO (2010) *Greenhouse Gas Emissions from the Dairy Sector. A Life Cycle Assessment*. FAO, Rome.

Garnsworthy, P.C. (2004) The environmental impact of fertility in dairy cows: a modelling approach to predict methane and ammonia emissions. *Animal Feed Science and Technology* 112, 211–223.

Green, M.J., Husband, J.A., Huxley, J.N. and Statham, J.M. (2011) Role of the veterinary surgeon in managing the impact of dairy farming on the environment. *In Practice* 33, 366–373.

Hegarty, R.S. (2004) Genotype differences and their impact on digestive tract function of ruminants: a review. *Australian Journal of Experimental Agriculture* 44, 459–467.

Henderson, C. (1973) The effects of fatty acids on pure cultures of rumen bacteria. *Journal of Agricultural Science, Cambridge* 81, 107–112.

HM Government (2010) The 2007/08 *Agricultural Price Spikes: Causes and Policy Implications*, available at http://www.defra.gov.uk/foodfarm/food/pdf/ag-price100105.pdf, pp. 114.

Holter, J.B. and Young, A.J. (1992) Methane prediction in dry and lactating Holstein cows. *Journal of Dairy Science* 75, 2165–2175.

Intergovernmental Panel on Climate Change (2007) *Climate Change 2007: Synthesis Report*. IPCC, Geneva, Switzerland.

International Energy Agency (2007) Renewables in global energy supply: an IEA factsheet, available at http://www.iea.org/papers/2006/renewable_factsheet.pdf, p. 15.

Johnson, K.A. and Johnson, D.E. (1995) Methane emissions from cattle. *Journal of Animal Science* 73, 2483–2492.

Kebreab, E., France, J., McBride, B.W., Odongo, N., Bannink, A., Mills, J.A.N. *et al.* (2006) Evaluation of models to predict methane emissions from enteric fermentation in North American dairy cattle. In: Kebreab, E., Dijkstra, D., Gerrits, W., Bannick, A. and France, J. (eds) *Nutrient Digestion and Utilization in Farm Animals: Modelling Approaches*. CAB International, Wallingford, UK, pp. 299–313.

Kowalcyk, J., Ørskov, E.R., Robinson, J.J. and Stewart, C.S. (1977) Effect of fat supplementation on voluntary food intake and rumen metabolism in sheep. *British Journal of Nutrition* 37, 251–257.

Kyoto Protocol to the United Nations Framework Convention on Climate Change (1998), art 3.1. UNFCCC, Bonn, Germany.

Lana, R.P., Russell, J.B. and Van Amburgh, M.E. (1998) The role of pH in regulating methane and ammonia production. *Journal of Animal Science* 76, 2190–2196.

López, S., Valdes, C., Newbold, C.J. and Wallace, R.J. (1999) Influence of sodium fumarate addition on rumen fermentation in vitro. *British Journal of Nutrition* 81, 59–64.

Lovett, D.K., Shalloo, L., Dillon, P. and O'Mara, F.P. (2006) A systems approach to quantify greenhouse gas fluxes from pastoral dairy production as affected by management regime. *Agricultural Systems* 88, 156–179.

Machmuller, A. and Kreuzer, M. (1997) Methane suppression by coconut oil and associated effects on nutrient and energy balance in sheep, *Proceedings of the Society of Nutrition and Physiology* 6, 65–72.

Machmuller, A., Ossowski, D.A., Wanner, M. and Kreuzer, M. (1998) Potential of various fatty feeds to reduce methane release from rumen fermentation in vitro (Rusitec). *Animal Feed Science and Technology* 77, 117–130.

Machmüller, A., Dohme, F., Soliva, C.R., Wanner, M. and Kreuzer, M. (2001) Diet composition affects the level of ruminal methane suppression by medium-chain fatty acids. *Australian Journal of Agricultural Research* 52, 713–722.

Machmüller, A., Soliva, C.R. and Kreuzer, M. (2003) Effect of coconut oil and defaunation treatment on methanogenesis in sheep. *Reproduction Nutrition Development* 43, 41–55.

Maplecroft (2011) *Maplecroft Food Security Index and Interactive Global Map*. Maplecroft, Bath, UK (http://maps.maplecroft.com, accessed December 2010).

Martin, S.A. (1998) Manipulation of ruminal fermentation with organic acids: a review. *Journal of Animal Science* 76, 3123–3132.

Moss, A.R., Jouany, J.-P. and Newbold, J. (2000) Methane production by ruminants: its contribution to global warming. *Annales de Zootechnie* 49, 231–253.

Newbold, C.J. and Chamberlain, D.G. (1998) Lipids as rumen defaunating agents. *Proceedings of the Nutrition Society* 47, 154A.

Newbold, C.J., Lassalas, B. and Jouany, J.-P. (1995) The importance of methanogenesis associated with ciliate protozoa in ruminal methane production *in vitro*. *Letters in Applied Microbiology* 21, 230–234.

Newbold, C.J., Lopez, S., Nelson, N., Ouda, J.O., Wallace, R.J. and Moss A.R. (2005) Proprionate precursors and other metabolic intermediates as possible alternative electron acceptors to methanogenesis in ruminal fermentation in vitro. *British Journal of Nutrition* 94, 27–35.

Nuffield Council Report (2011) *Biofuels: Ethical Issues*. Nuffield Council on Bioethics, London.

Pinares-Patiño, C.S., Baumont, R. and Martin, D.R. (2004) Methane emissions by Charolais cows grazing a monospecific pasture of timothy at four stages of maturity. *Canadian Journal of Animal Science* 78, 769–777.

Prins, R.A., Van Nevel, C.J. and Demeyer, D.I. (1972) Pure culture studies of inhibitors for methanogenic bacteria. *Ant Van Leeuwen* 38, 281–287.

Renewable Fuels Agency (2008) *The Gallagher Review of the Indirect Effects of Biofuels Production*, available at http://www.renewablefuelsagency.gov.uk/sites/renewablefuelsagency.gov.uk/files/_documents/Report.

Renewable Fuels Association (2010) *Climate of Opportunity: 2010 Ethanol Industry Outlook*, available at http://ethanolrfa.org/page/-/objects/pdf/outlook/RFAoutlook2010_fin.pdf?nocdn=1, p6.

Shu, Q., Gill, H.S., Hennessy, D.W., Leng, R.A., Bird, S.H. and Rowe, J.B. (1999) Immunisation against lactic acidosis in cattle. *Research into Veterinary Science* 67, 65–71.

Steinfeld, H., Gerber, P., Wassenaar, T., Castel, V., Rosales, M. and de Haan, C. (2006) Livestock's long shadow; environmental issues and options. A report prepared by FAO, Animal Production and Health Division, Rome.

Tamminga, S., Bannink, A., Dijkstra, J. and Zom, R. (2007) Feeding strategies to reduce methane loss in cattle. Animal Science Group report, Wageningen, The Netherlands.

UK Biodiversity Partnership (2007) *Conserving Biodiversity – The UK Approach*. DEFRA, London.

Ulyatt, M.J. and Lassey, K.R. (2001) Methane emissions from pastoral systems: the situation in New Zealand. *Archivos Latinoamericanos de Produccion Animal* 9, 118–126.

United Nations (1992) *Convention on Biological Diversity*. UN, Rome.

US Energy Information Administration (2010) International energy outlook 2010 highlights, available at http://www.eia.doe.gov/oiaf/ieo/highlights.html.

Van Soest, P.J. (1982) *Nutritional Ecology of the Ruminant*. O and B Books, Oregon, pp. 40–41.

Wallace, R.J. (2004) Antimicrobial properties of plant secondary metabolites. *Proceedings of the Nutrition Society* 63, 621–629.

Wallace, R.J., Wood, T.A., Rowe, A., Price, J., Yanez, D.R., Williams, S.P. *et al.* (2006) Encapsulated fumaric acid as a means of decreasing ruminal methane emissions. *International Congress Series* 1293, 148–151.

Wright, A.D., Kennedy, P., O'Neill, C.J., Toovey, A.F., Popovski, S., Rea, S.M. *et al.* (2004) Reducing methane emissions in sheep by immunization against rumen methanogens. *Vaccine* 22, 3976–3985.

Yan, T. and Mayne, C.S. (2007) Mitigation strategies to reduce methane emission from dairy cows. In: Hopkins, J.J., Duncan, A.J., McCracken, D.I., Peel, S. and Tallowin, J.R.B. (eds) *High-value Grassland: Providing Biodiversity, a Clean Environment and Premium Products*. University of Keele, UK, pp. 345–348.

# Appendix 1  Sample Sizes and Disease Prevalence Estimates

**Martin Green[1] and Laura Green[2]**
[1]*School of Veterinary Medicine and Science, University of Nottingham, Sutton Bonington Campus, Leicestershire LE12 5RD, UK;* [2]*School of Life Sciences, The University of Warwick, Coventry, CV4 7AL, UK*

---

## Sample Size Estimates

In many situations it is important to make an accurate estimate of the level of a disease, condition or metabolic state within a population of dairy cows. The population of interest may be the whole herd but may also be a smaller subset, such as the cows within the first 30 days after calving. Whilst it is possible to test all cows within a population of interest, financial constraints often mean that a smaller sample is preferred to make an estimate of the population status.

This raises the question, 'How many do I need to test to get an accurate estimate of the population prevalence?' This is an important question and has to be answered in a variety of situations. However, the answer to the question depends on specific circumstances, because the size of the sample needed varies according to the following factors:

**1.** The number of cows in the population of interest (target population). For example, this may be the whole herd (in the case of an infectious disease such as Johne's disease) or a smaller group (in the case of the metabolic status of cows within 30 days of calving).
**2.** The prevalence of the condition of interest in the target population. This is the level of the condition in the target population that you want to detect to indicate that

a herd is positive or has a problem. For example, in the case of bovine viral diarrhoea (BVD) virus it may be important to detect whether infection is present at all (prevalence >0) or, in the case of raised non-esterified fatty acids just prior to calving, it may be that a threshold of 15% is set before further investigations are considered worthwhile.
**3.** The certainty you require of detecting a given prevalence. When testing a sample of cows you cannot be 100% positive that you have made an absolutely accurate estimate of the prevalence in the target population, and statistical sampling theory allows us to calculate how certain we are in our prevalence estimate. This raises the necessary question of how certain we need to be in order to make a decision based on the results of our sample? For some conditions, where the consequences are severe, it may be necessary to be very certain before making decisions and thus a certainty of over 95% might be chosen. For other situations – for example, when the results will lead to further investigations rather than large financial decisions – a lower certainty is often sufficient, for example 70–80%.

Here, we use a statistical method based on the hypergeometric distribution to estimate the appropriate probabilities. This is a discrete probability distribution because the number of cows has to be a whole number – we cannot have 9.5 affected cows in a population. The distribution is used to estimate the probability of selecting a certain number of disease-positive cows in a specific sample size, given that the disease level in the overall population of interest is at a specified level. A key feature of this distribution is that it describes the number of positive animals in a sample from a larger population, given that once cows have been selected they are no longer available to be chosen again.

A simple sample size calculator is provided online to accompany this book and can be found at www.cabi.org/resources/dhhmg. A calculator that extends sample size estimates to include imperfect sensitivity and specificity can be found at www.ausvet.com.au/content.php?page=software#freecalc.

The following examples can be followed by using the calculator, and are provided to give an illustration of how to estimate the number of animals to sample in different disease situations.

### Example 1: Testing a group of maiden heifers for BVD antigen (virus) status

Target population = 40 (= number of heifers in the whole group). Prevalence of interest: 1 or more affected animals in 40 (i.e. we want to detect a prevalence of ≥2.5%; sensitivity and specificity of the test are assumed to be 100%).

| Sample size taken | Certainty of identifying one diseased animal in your sample given a prevalence in the target population of 2.5% (only 1 diseased animal is actually present) | Certainty of identifying ≥1 positive animal in your sample given a prevalence in the target population of 5.0% (2 positive animals present) |
|---|---|---|
| 6 | 0.15 | 0.28 |
| 12 | 0.30 | 0.52 |
| 15 | 0.38 | 0.62 |
| 20 | 0.50 | 0.76 |
| 30 | 0.75 | 0.94 |
| 35 | 0.88 | 0.99 |

### Example 2: Testing a group of maiden heifers for BVD antibody status

Target population = 40 (= number of heifers in the whole group). Prevalence of interest: 4 or more affected animals in 40 (i.e. we want to detect a prevalence of ≥10%; sensitivity and specificity of the test are assumed to be 100%).

| Sample size taken | Certainty of identifying ≥1 positive animal in your sample given a prevalence in the target population ≥10% |
|---|---|
| 6 | 0.49 |
| 12 | 0.78 |
| 15 | 0.86 |
| 20 | 0.95 |

### Example 3: Testing a group of cows after calving for betahydroxybutyrate levels

Target population = 20 (= number of cows within 30 days of calving in a 240 cow dairy herd). Prevalence of interest: 3 or more animals positive (i.e. we want to detect a prevalence of ≥15%; sensitivity and specificity of the test are assumed to be 100%).

| Sample size taken | Certainty of identifying ≥1 positive animal in your sample given a prevalence in the target population ≥15% |
|---|---|
| 6 | 0.68 |
| 7 | 0.75 |
| 8 | 0.81 |
| 9 | 0.86 |
| 12 | 0.95 |

## Estimating Disease Prevalence from Test Results

Having chosen the relevant sample size using the method above and having obtained test results, we can now estimate the probability that the true disease prevalence in the population is above a given level. This will depend upon the actual number of test-positive animals that we identify in our sample and the degree of certainty that we require. Again, the online calculator provided (www.cabi.org/resources/dhhmg.) can be used to make these estimates and we provide examples below to illustrate how this can be done.

### Example 1: Testing a group of maiden heifers for BVD antibody status

Target population = 40 (= number of heifers in the whole group). Prevalence of interest: 4 or more affected animals in 40 (i.e. we want to detect a prevalence of $\geq 10\%$). Sample size used = 12 (i.e. number of heifers tested; sensitivity and specificity of the test are assumed to be 100%).

| Number positive in sample | Probability that population prevalence is $\geq 10\%$ |
|---|---|
| 0 | 0.22 |
| 1 | 0.65 |
| 2 | 0.93 |
| 3 | 1.00 |
| 4 | 1.00 |

### Example 2: Testing a group of cows after calving for betahydroxybutyrate levels

Target population = 20 (= number of cows within 30 days of calving in a 240 cow dairy herd). Prevalence of interest: 3 or more animals positive (i.e. we want to detect a prevalence of $\geq 15\%$). Sample size used = 6 (i.e. number of heifers tested; sensitivity and specificity of the test are assumed to be ~100%).

| Number positive in sample | Probability that population prevalence is $\geq 15\%$ |
|---|---|
| 0 | 0.32 |
| 1 | 0.80 |
| 2 | 0.98 |
| 3 | 0.99 |

# Appendix 2 Genetics and Herd Health

## Jonathan Statham[1] and Martin Green[2]

[1]*Bishopton Veterinary Group, Mill Farm, Studley Road, Ripon, North Yorkshire HG4 2QR, UK;* [2]*School of Veterinary Medicine and Science, University of Nottingham, Sutton Bonington Campus, Leicestershire LE12 5RD, UK*

## Introduction

Genetics plays an important role in dairy cow health and production, and while this book focuses on herd health in relation to farm management, we provide here an outline of the principles of genetic evaluations to enable the reader to gain a basic understanding. To fully incorporate genetic selection into a herd health programme, we recommend working collaboratively with independent specialists in this field.

Average milk production in the Holstein breed has increased from around 5000 kg/year in the 1980s to over 8000 kg/year today, and it has been estimated that genetics is responsible for more than half of this increase. The breeding priorities of commercial dairy farmers are ultimately driven by profitability, whatever the farming system (intensive, extensive, etc.) and fundamental to this is milk volume, fat and protein production. Consequently, total milk solids often drive long-term breeding policy in many herds. However, lifespan and fertility are increasingly recognized as driving profitability on a lifetime basis and so are becoming significant in breeding decisions.

We outline below the terms and concepts commonly used in genetic evaluations and note the increasing importance of traits relating to health and longevity (Dairy Co, 2011).

## Genetic Indices

A genetic index 'GI' (often known as a 'proof') provides a measure of an animal's ability to pass its genes on to the next generation. Genetic indices are calculated from data from a variety of sources to produce estimate of an animal's genetic worth. For a bull, the most important component of his proof is his daughters' performance, while for a cow the most important component is her own performance. When either a bull or cow is too young to have any performance information of its own, its proof will be calculated from family information.

Statistical models are used to calculate genetic indices using milk recording and animal data, and the models account to some extent for offspring being present in a variety of farm environments. In the UK and in a variety of dairy nations, genetic indices are expressed as predicted transmitting abilities (PTA). These predict the extent a given trait will be passed on to an animal's offspring. That is, the amount of a trait the offspring will receive from its parents. Genetic progress over long periods of time necessitates recalibration of the indices. Thus, every five years (UK), the national average for every trait is recalculated and reset to zero. For example, in 2010 the genetic base was re-calculated for all breeds and the PTA should precisely be referred to as PTA 2010.

## UK indices

### Production traits

Production traits were the first to be introduced into genetic indices. All male and female dairy cattle are assigned a PTA for milk (kg), fat (kg), fat (%), protein (kg) and protein (%). In a baseline year, the daughters of a bull with a PTA of 650 kg milk are on average predicted to produce 650 kg more milk in a lactation than the daughters of an 'average' bull, whose PTA is zero. *Persistency* of milk production is derived from yield at 280 days as a percentage of yield at 60 days.

### *Health, welfare and fitness traits*

Increased significance is being attached to health, welfare and fitness traits to address lifetime profitability and consumer concerns.

1. Somatic cell count (SCC). PTAs are expressed as a percentage and generally fall within the range +30 to −30. For every 1% increase in a bull's SCC PTA, an increase of 1% in his daughters' SCC is predicted. Negative PTA for SCC are desirable.
2. Fertility. Fertility Index (FI) provides a prediction of female fertility expressed as a financial figure (£) (generally −15 to +15) and is based largely on a combination of calving interval and non-return rates. On average, every £1 increase in a bull's FI is predicted to deliver just under half a day's reduction in his daughters' calving interval and 0.5% improvement in non-return rate at 56 days.

3. Lifespan. PTAs are expressed in terms of lactations (i.e. the extra number of lactations predicted for survival), and are calculated from actual daughter survival information if available; otherwise, information on type (feet, legs and udder), cell count and family is used. Range is typically −0.5 to + 0.5.
4. Locomotion. The PTA is expressed on a scale of around −3 to +3. The best locomotion scores of +3 or higher predict the transmission of an excellent gait.

### *Management traits*

Management traits refer to those traits facilitating a streamlined and undisrupted milking routine and include:

1. Temperament (−3 to +3, as increasingly placid).
2. Ease of milking (−3 to +3, from hard-milkers to very fast with risk of running milk).
3. Calving ease (−3 to +3, from more difficult to easier calvings) in regard to two aspects:

- Direct calving ease (dCE %) gives a prediction of the ease with which a calf by that sire will be born.
- Maternal calving ease (mCE %) predicts the ease with which a daughter of that sire will give birth.

### *Type traits*

Seventeen 'type' traits (e.g. stature, angularity, teat length) are used to assess cow conformation. Data are usually collected from first-lactation cows, often by breed societies, each of which determines its own breed standards. A score of zero represents the breed average, and such traits are commonly expressed on a bar chart (linear score).

## Genetic indices for selection
### (£PIN and PLI)

Selection indices such as profit index (£PIN) and profitable lifetime index (PLI) bring together a variety of traits into one figure:

- £PIN: profit index predicts the additional margin over food and quota costs per lactation that a bull or cow is expected to pass on to its progeny compared with an average baseline £PIN of zero, and is based purely on production traits (milk, fat and protein).
- PLI: this has been designed as a primary selection tool to identify animals predicted to transmit the greatest financial improvement in their lifetime. PLI improves on PIN by adding health, welfare, fitness and lifespan components to the same production formula. Each trait is weighted by its relative economic value and the resulting single figure represents the financial improvement an animal is, on average, predicted to pass on to its offspring expressed on a lifetime basis. The PLI's revised formula for 2007 increased its emphasis on health, welfare and fitness traits and reduced the emphasis on production traits to 45%.

### Genetic indices outside the UK

Most dairying countries publish selection indices similar to UK £PIN and PLI, although a detailed description of these is beyond the scope of this book. Since genetic indices in different countries are based on different economic and management conditions and breeding priorities, they should not be used to select bulls outside the national farming conditions. However, methods have been developed to provide foreign-proven bulls with UK-equivalent figures. Originally, a simple conversion formula was applied to each component of the proof, but today the process is more complex and uses a technique

called multiple-trait across-country evaluation (MACE), undertaken by an organization called Interbull. The UK and Interbull coordinate their work so that all the genetic indices are published simultaneously three times per year.

### Reliability of genetic indices

The reliability of GI varies widely depending on the amount and source of information available. For example, a GI for production traits based on a parent average typically has a reliability of around 30–40% but a proof for a bull based on the performance of his daughters in several hundred herds could have a reliability of up to 99%. The lower the reliability of the proof, the more likely it is to change as more daughters are added, so it is important to use young bulls with caution. However, using a variety of young sire semen has a place in most herd breeding programmes and may offer large rewards if proved successful. Care should be taken not to overuse a particular young unproven sire of low reliability.

### Heritability

Some traits are more heritable than others and the more heritable a trait, the easier it is to improve through breeding. Highly heritable traits include fat (0.68) or protein (0.68) percentage of milk. Heritability estimates for major health and production characteristics of dairy cows are shown below in Table A2.1.

### Genetic defects

A number of recessive genetic defects cause problems in dairy breeding: (i) bovine leukocyte adhesion deficiency (BLAD), causing a fatal deficiency of the immune system; (ii) complex vertebral malformation (CVM), causing stillbirths or, more commonly, abortion or fetal death before 260 days of gestation; and (iii) mule foot (MF), causing the two claws of the hoof to become fused. All artificial insemination (AI) sires are tested and any carrying the defective gene will be identified by the suffixes *BL, *CV and *MF, respectively. Matings should be avoided between carrier parents, to prevent any risk of expressing a genetic defect.

**Table A2.1.** Heritability estimates for major health and production characteristics of dairy cows (based on www.dairyco.org.uk/library/farming-info-centre/breeding/breeding-briefs.aspx).

| Trait | Heritability |
|---|---|
| *Production* | |
| Milk yield | 0.55 |
| Protein yield | 0.51 |
| Protein percentage | 0.68 |
| Fat yield | 0.47 |
| Fat percentage | 0.68 |
| *Linear type* | |
| Stature (ST) | 0.41 |
| Body depth (BD) | 0.33 |
| Rump angle (RA) | 0.30 |
| Rear leg side (RLS) | 0.20 |
| Fore udder attachment | 0.22 |
| Udder support (US) | 0.19 |
| Teat placement rear (TPR) | 0.29 |
| Teat length (TL) | 0.29 |
| Chest width (CW) | 0.25 |
| Angularity (ANG) | 0.34 |
| Rump width (RW) | 0.26 |
| Foot angle (FA) | 0.10 |
| Rear udder height (RUH) | 0.23 |
| Udder depth (UD) | 0.35 |
| Teat placement rear (TPS) | 0.29 |
| *Composite type* | |
| Mammary | 0.27 |
| Legs and feet | 0.16 |
| Type merit/type score | 0.32 |
| *Management* | |
| Lifespan | 0.06 |
| Somatic cell count | 0.11 |
| Temperament | 0.11 |
| Body condition score | 0.27 |
| Maternal calving ease | 0.04 |
| Locomotion | 0.10 |
| Fertility | 0.03 |
| Ease of milking | 0.21 |
| Direct calving ease | 0.07 |

# Reference

DairyCo (2011) *Breeding Briefs: A Quick Guide to Genetic Indexes in Dairy Cattle*. DairyCo Breeding + AHDB, Kenilworth, UK.

# Index

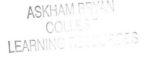